Design for Mental and Behavioral Health

Studies confirm that the physical environment influences health outcomes, emotional state, preference, satisfaction, and orientation, but very little research has focused on mental and behavioral health settings. This book summarizes design principles and design research for individuals who are intending to design new mental and behavioral health facilities and those wishing to evaluate the quality of their existing facilities. The authors discuss mental and behavioral health systems, design guidelines, design research, and existing standards, and provide examples of best practice. As behavioral and mental health populations vary in their needs, the primary focus is limited to environments that support acute care, outpatient and emergency care, residential care, veterans, pediatric patients, and the treatment of chemical dependency.

Mardelle McCuskey Shepley, M.Arch., M.A., D.Arch., EDAC, FAIA, FACHA, LEED BD+C, is a professor in the Department of Design & Environmental Analysis and associate director of the Healthy Futures Institute at Cornell University. Dr. Shepley has authored/co-authored five books, most recently *Design for Critical Care* (2009), *Health Facility Evaluation for Design Practitioners (2010)*, and *Design for Pediatric and Neonatal Critical Care* (2014). To enhance the link between research and practice, Dr. Shepley has worked in professional practice, full-time and part-time, for 25 years. She is founder of ART+Science, design research consultants.

Samira Pasha, M.Arch., Ph.D., AIA, LSSGB, EDAC, LEED BD+C, is an architect and researcher at CallisonRTKL, Washington, DC. As part of the healthcare studio team, her work includes programming, planning, and evaluation of healthcare environments ranging from small unit renovations to health campus master plans, including domestic and international projects. Since 2012 Samira has been involved with NCARB intern think tank, AIAS, and District Architecture Center (DAC) as an advocate for integrating research into practice of architecture.

Design for Mental and Behavioral Health

Mardelle McCuskey Shepley and
Samira Pasha

Routledge
Taylor & Francis Group
LONDON AND NEW YORK

First published 2017
by Routledge
2 Park Square, Milton Park, Abingdon, Oxon OX14 4RN

and by Routledge
711 Third Avenue, New York, NY 10017

Routledge is an imprint of the Taylor & Francis Group, an Informa business

British Library Cataloguing-in-Publication Data
A catalogue record for this book is available from the British Library

Library of Congress Cataloging-in-Publication Data
Names: Shepley, Mardelle McCuskey, author. | Pasha, Samira, author.
Title: Design for mental and behavioral health / Mardelle McCuskey Shepley and Samira Pasha.
Description: Milton Park, Abingdon, Oxon ; New York : Routledge, 2017. | Includes bibliographical references and index.
Identifiers: LCCN 2016050179 | ISBN 9781138126350 (hb : alk. paper) | ISBN 9781138126367 (pb : alk. paper) | ISBN 9781315646916 (ebook)
Subjects: | MESH: Facility Design and Construction—methods | Community Mental Health Centers | Interior Design and Furnishings—methods | Psychiatric Department, Hospital
Classification: LCC RA790.5 | NLM WM 27.1 | DDC 362.2/2—dc23
LC record available at https://lccn.loc.gov/2016050179

ISBN: 978-1-138-12635-0 (hbk)
ISBN: 978-1-138-12636-7 (pbk)
ISBN: 978-1-315-64691-6 (ebk)

Typeset in Syntax LT Std
by Apex CoVantage, LLC

Contents

List of figures

Acknowledgements

We would like to thank Kimia Erfani, Andrea Fronsman, Adisa Soren, and Janhawi Kelkar, who supported the gathering of data during the production of this book, and Chery Manniello for her editorial assistance. We also appreciate the support of the Center for Health Design (CHD) that allowed us to base portions of the content of Chapters 2, 9, and 10 on a white paper authored by Shepley and Pasha and published on the CHD website in 2013. We are grateful for the contributions of the white paper co-authors: Pamela Ferguson, Jamie C. Huffcut, Guy Kiyokawa, Joe Martere, Terri Meyerhoeffer, Brenda McDermott, Gabriel Oproescu, Jean Young, Rana Sagha Zadeh, Terri Zborowsky, and Craig Zimring.

Introduction

Wire, briar, limber, lock.
Three geese in a flock.
One flew east.
One flew west.
And one flew over the cuckoo's nest.

This nursery rhyme was the inspiration for the title of Kesey's well-known work of fiction, *One Flew Over the Cuckoo's Nest* (1962). The novel and the subsequent film (1975) have served to characterize our perception of mental health environments. Filmed at the Oregon State Mental Hospital, Kesey drew our attention to a critical social issue – the need to provide better environments for persons coping with mental health challenges. While contemporary behavioral and mental health facilities are not typically as dismal as those portrayed in the novel, the quality and availability of these physical settings are profoundly lacking.

News stories regarding mental health issues pepper the press. In the United States approximately 55% of individuals with behavioral health disorders and 88% of those with addiction disorders lack access to appropriate care (SAMHSA, 2015). Global shortcomings have been identified in both developed regions, such as Canada, Australia, Western Europe, and the United Kingdom, and the developing world. We are in desperate need of facilities for children and adults in inpatient, outpatient, and emergency settings. Many existing behavioral and mental health facilities are substandard; these environments inhibit the treatment process and undermine the activities of staff and patients. Unfortunately, patients in behavioral and mental health inpatient and outpatient settings are often treated in spaces that would be demoralizing for healthy individuals.

The public recognizes that most of us will spend time in hospitals at some point during the course of our lives. Recognizing this, socially responsible design practitioners have been using research-based design interventions to enhance general hospital settings for the last 30 years. However, behavioral and mental health facilities have received little attention. Our 2013 review of more than 300 publications concluded that research focusing on behavioral health environments was very limited and insufficient to support the design process (Shepley & Pasha, 2013).

We don't have to look far to find reasons for the lack of attention to these settings. Among the most prominent are limited funds for the construction of appropriate inpatient and outpatient facilities, limited support for research that demonstrates the impact of psychiatric facilities, and the pervasive stigma regarding mental and behavioral illness relative to "physical" illness. People with diagnoses such as cancer or cardiac disease are embraced by society more readily than individuals diagnosed with schizophrenia or bipolar disorders. Poor mental health is still closeted; mental health patients may be perceived as culpable for their health status and therefore less deserving than individuals with other illnesses.

Awareness of the importance of design research is critical to public welfare. Multiple studies confirm that the physical environment can influence health outcomes, emotional state, preference, satisfaction, orientation, and other physical and mental health-related factors. In some cases, appropriate environments may even save lives. Examples of life-supportive design features of hospitals are materials and mechanical systems that limit the communication of infection and lighting that reduces medical errors.

Regarding life-saving features of behavioral health facilities per se, the physical environment can mitigate suicide attempts by excluding fixtures and furnishings that support ligature. Some aspects of the environment may help reduce stress, pathological behaviors, and aggression. Environmental features that might positively impact outcomes include the private rooms, visual and physical access to the outdoors, heterogeneous lighting schemes, access to diversions such as music and entertainment, movable furniture, better acoustics, representational art, higher daylight exposure, homelike design, and proximity and visibility of common spaces from staff stations.

The means of enhancing awareness of the poor quality of many psychiatric facilities and increasing knowledge regarding the positive impact of good design are clear. First, the public must express its desire for these services and facilities via interaction with governmental representatives. Second, funding agencies must acknowledge the critical nature of behavioral health evidence-based design by allocating monies in support of design research. Third, architects, landscape architects, and interior designers must link arms with clinical staff and facility managers to gather data to increase our understanding of good mental health facility design.

Admittedly, resources are rare and service and facility requirements are complex and extensive. However, in light of the 2015 finding that 18.1% of adults experienced some form of mental illness in the previous year (CBHSQ, 2015), and considering the personal devastation that takes place when suicidal or violent individuals go untreated, we cannot ignore the need to develop appropriate behavioral and mental health facilities.

This book responds to this situation by providing a history of mental health and mental health design, design guidelines, information regarding various mental and behavioral health settings, design research, case studies, and a summary of standards and regulations. As mental and behavioral health are global issues, we attempted to integrate information outside North America when the resources were available.

The purpose of *Design for Mental and Behavioral Health* is to provide a foundation that will serve as a reference for designers, researchers, and organizations that are evaluating their current behavioral health environments or planning new facilities. More broadly, we hope to contribute to the provision of humane and healing environments for mental and behavioral health patients.

References

Center for Behavioral Health Statistics and Quality (CBHSQ). (2015). *Behavioral health trends in the United States: Results from the 2014 national survey on drug use and health* (HHS Publication No. SMA 15–4927, NSDUH Series H-50).

Kesey, K. (1962). *One flew over the cuckoo's nest*. Madison, WI: Turtleback Books.
Shepley, M., & Pasha, S. (2013). *Design research and behavioral health facilities*. Concord, CA: Center for Health Design.
Substance Abuse and Mental Health Services Administration (SAMHSA). (2015). *More Americans continue to receive mental health services, but substance use treatment levels remain low*. Retrieved from www.samhsa.gov/newsroom/press-announcements/201509170900

Part One: Mental and behavioral health context

Mental and behavioral health history and context

1

1.1 Historical perspective

1.1.1 History of psychiatric care

Individuals have attempted to define mental illness as long as we have endeavored to find cures. As a result of a variety of viewpoints, attitudes toward those inflicted with mental illness have ranged from punishing the ill to treating them with compassion. During the Middle Ages in Europe, hospices, workhouses, jails, and asylums housed mentally ill patients. Reports of Germany's asylums around 1800 describe "mad-cages" where patients were locked up "like criminals." The French government erected facilities as part of general hospitals, in which the psychiatric patients represented a portion of the residents. Around the same time in England, some psychiatric patients were hospitalized in public or private asylums, with a larger portion hospitalized in the private "nervous clinics" (Shorter, 1997).

Mental illness was originally perceived to be a function of the mind rather than organic in nature and, as a result, patients were treated harshly. By the end of the nineteenth century, developments in medicine and an enhanced understanding of mental illnesses led to more individualized care and better-trained attendants, which reduced reliance on mechanical restraints (Caplan, 1969). With the evolution of treatment methods, the focus of treatment also changed. Later in the twentieth century, custody and security were not the chief concerns of the facilities. Rather, the emphasis was on providing efficient treatment and successful discharge of patients (Blain, 1956). A summary of scientific/social stances from 4 BC to the present is provided in Figure 1.1.

1.1.2 History of psychiatric facilities

In 1796 the York Retreat, an asylum that pioneered moral treatment, was established by an English businessman, William Tuke. Samuel Tuke, grandson of William, authored the book *Practical Hints*, in which he discussed design features that can support concepts of moral treatment. Tuke questioned the design of the asylums of the period, which, up to that time, focused on the secure incarceration of patients. Security, he recommended, was to be achieved through direct observation of patients rather than use of physical restraints (Tuke, 1815). He recommended design that allows flexible and liberal access of patients to daylit spaces with fresh air. To reduce anxiety and restlessness and to enhance a sense of autonomy, he recommended employing a variety of scenery and spaces such as galleries for indoor exercise, courts for outdoor exercise, and dayrooms for activity and social interaction. Tuke's ideal asylum was one in the form of a double-cross or H-shape and included a chapel, baths, and accommodations for patients who also worked at the asylum or became ill (Tuke, 1815).

Figure 1.1: *History of significant events and design implications regarding psychiatric care – pre-twentieth-century events*

Pre-twentieth-century events

Timeline	*Major influences*	*Scientific/social stance*	*Architectural response*
4 BC	Hippocrates	Symptoms of mental disorder are due to disease originating in brain.	
	Plato	Imbalance of mind, body, and spirit could cause distress and thus mental illness.	
3 BC	Patanjali	Emphasis on self-realization.	15-bed hospital and school located in Chingleput District
8th–11th century	Avicenna	Connection between the body and soul.	Specialized mental health hospitals in Baghdad, Fès, and Cairo
13th century	Bishop-elect of Bethlehem	Focus on punishment and confinement rather than treatment.	Bethlehem Hospital in England
1656	Louis XIV, Robert Burton	No greater cause to melancholy than idleness. Knowledge of the human mind is humankind's greatest need.	Public Hospital System in France for those suffering from mental illnesses
18th century	Romantic Era Jean Jacques Rousseau	Compassion toward people with mental illness. Trauma in childhood could have negative implications in adulthood.	
1758	Enlightenment period William Battie	Mental illness requires compassionate treatment. Mental disorder is result of dysfunction of material brain and body rather than internal working of the mind – criticism of Bethlehem's treatment.	
1761	George III's remission after recovering from mental treatment	Mental illness known as something that can be cured.	
1790s to early 1800	Philippe Pinel, William Tuke, Jean-Baptiste Pussin, Jean Esquirol	Introduction of moral treatment. Banned physical punishment and confinement of patients.	Creation of York Retreat for 30 patients living as part of a community in a small country house who would rest, talk, and do manual work; establishment of 10 new mental hospitals in France replacing dark, dungeon-like asylums with sunny, well-ventilated rooms

Pre-twentieth-century events

Timeline	*Major influences*	*Scientific/social stance*	*Architectural response*
19th century	Georg Wilhelm Friedrich Hegel, Sigmund Freud	Origins of talk therapy, psychotherapy based on ideas of human experiences and natural human effort to make sense of the world.	
1838–1839	Édouard Séguin	Systematic approach to train "lunatics."	The first school for the severely retarded in France
1842	Dorothea Lynde Dix	U.S. law initiated erection of state asylums.	Erection of state hospitals based on Kirkbride model that was believed to have therapeutic effects
1845	Anthony Ashley-Cooper	Lunacy act in England, changing status of lunatics to patients who need treatment. Commissioner in "lunacy" empowered.	Evaluation of private asylums

In 1751 the Pennsylvania Hospital in Philadelphia became the first U.S. hospital that accepted psychiatric patients. Shortly thereafter, psychiatric facilities were incorporated into New York Hospital as well as Massachusetts General Hospital. Later hospitals separated psychiatric patient wards from other patients and moved on to create a new form of management (Kirkbride, 1854). Although these mid-eighteenth- to early-nineteenth-century facilities were originally intended to cure patients, they were eventually used for custodial purposes and run by lay administrators who would seek physician consultations. Physical restraints and extreme temperatures were used, since the common belief at the time was that the mentally ill were insensitive to pain and that extreme conditions could shock them back to sanity (Talbott, 1978).

"For most of the nineteenth-century, doctors believed that between 70 and 90 percent of insanity cases were curable, but only if patients were treated in specially designed buildings" (Yanni, 2007, p. 1). U.S. asylums of the period followed a building style introduced by Dr. Thomas Kirkbride, who early in his career at the Institute of Pennsylvania Hospital wrote a book titled *On the Construction, Organization and General Arrangements of Hospitals for the Insane*. The proposed model included a series of designated patient wards that were staggered to form canted wings that were attached to a central section of the building housing common functions.

Kirkbride's prototype provided separate wards dedicated to different groups of patients based on their mental state and gender. In his book, he recommends that each ward include chambers for patients and attendants as well as a dayroom, dining room, bathrooms, housekeeping and storage rooms, and dumbwaiters and staircases to access the common sections of the building. Areas of the building housing more violent or noisy patients were only one story and utilized the single-loaded corridor model. A ward for patients who needed quiet and seclusion was also located at grade. These wards had access to dedicated gymnasiums, yards, and activity areas. The building's common areas included a lecture room (also used as a lab for experimental purposes),

Figure 1.2: *Number of beds per facility and cost, 1887 (Data source: Wilbur, 1887, cited by Yanni, 2007)*

Facility location	*Number of beds*	*Cost*	*Cost/bed*
Massachusetts	450	$1,250,000	$2,778
Massachusetts	450	$1,600,000	$3,556
Connecticut	450	$600,000	$1,333
New York	600	$2,000,000	$3,333
New York	500	$1,800,000	$3,600
New York	300	$900,000	$3,000
New Jersey	800	$2,500,000	$3,125
Pennsylvania	500	$1,000,000	$2,000
Maryland	300	$803,000	$2,677
Kentucky	375	$162,000	$432
Ohio	900	$1,800,000	$2,000
Ohio	600	$950,000	$1,583
Michigan	580	$653,000	$1,126
Illinois	450	$534,000	$1,187
Wisconsin	500	$552,000	$1,104
Iowa	300	$600,000	$2,000
Minnesota	500	$480,000	$960
Missouri	250	$209,000	$836
Nebraska	80	$113,000	$1,413
California	900	$1,000,000	$1,111
Average	**489**		**$1,958**

reception, private and common visitation rooms, and the medical and administrative offices. The superintending physician's residential suite was on the third floor. The basement included building service spaces (kitchens, baker's room, and laundry) and female workers' rooms. Patient workrooms, museum, and reading rooms were located in another area (Kirkbride, 1854). Mental hospitals, as reported by Wilbur in 1877, were large and expensive, typically costing more to construct than the equivalent of $2,000 per bed – considerably more than a luxury hotel at the time (see Figure 1.2) (Yanni, 2007).

The concept of moral treatment was challenged at the end of the nineteenth century when the facilities faced the issue of overcrowding and discharge rates could not keep up with admission rates, which were often determined by court rulings. This problem was exacerbated as immigrant populations increased and state legislatures were reluctant to financially support these facilities. The inevitable imbalance led facilities to use more physical restraints to control patients, limit activities, and employ custodial care in place of moral treatment once again (Talbott, 1978).

The ever-growing patient rate necessitated implementing programs for early discharge of treated patients and preparing them for living in the community. A review of the available design literature at this point (e.g., the design process for the rehabilitation program in the state of Missouri) suggests that the major concern for discharge was that existing hospitals were overcrowded and lacked modern fireproof construction (Bowen, 1939).

As a result of the analysis of data from World War I troops, new principles of care for mental illnesses were established: "proximity, immediacy, and expectancy." These terms suggest that treatment should take place near where the patient lives, should be provided immediately after the crisis, and that recovery should be expected (Salmon, 1917). The discovery of effective psychopharmacological agents in the 1950s fomented significant developments in the care of serious psychiatric conditions. With these developments, the need for constant observation, seclusion, or physical restraints in hospitals was reduced. More importantly, more patients could function at a level that would allow them to be discharged, which was a promising solution for the issue of overcrowding (Talbott, 1978).

Arguments against overcrowding and quality of residential services discouraged expansion of existing mental health hospitals in the 1950s (Caplan, 1969). Empowered by new methods of treatment and principles of care, discussions began concerning the provision of mental healthcare in different settings and contexts including outpatient clinics, home visiting, community mental health centers as well as the psychiatric units of the mental health hospitals (Caplan, 1969). Many new ideas emerged at this time regarding new forms of care settings such as branch hospitals for the aged as well as geriatric hospitals, day and night hospitals, halfway homes, psychiatric shelter workshops and rehabilitation centers, colonies for the mentally deficient, and therapeutic farms (Blain, 1956).

A series of articles dedicated to the design of mental hospitals appeared in *Architectural Record* in 1953. The articles were written by psychiatrists and hospital architects and covered new models of care and prototypes of new hospitals and outpatient buildings. Blain, medical director of the American Psychiatric Association at the time, discussed the need for a therapeutic regimen by "combining and focusing on a patient or a group of patients all the influences a hospital could muster to push the patient to recover" (Blain, 1953). Until this time, and based on the work of Salmon, the ideal model of care was to diagnose and treat patients with the goal of returning them to outpatient status as quickly as possible, and hence architects were called on to create environments that would help patients to heal (Guttersen, 1953a). The articles appearing in this issue of *Architectural Record* described a return to principles of design for moral care as mentioned by Tuke in 1815 (Guttersen, 1953a; 1953b).

However, as early as 1970, concerns were raised regarding the effectiveness of the new models of care that focused on increasing patient discharge rates and outpatient care (Talbott, 1978). Following research on the status of discharged psychiatric patients, a 1977 report sponsored by the National Institute of Mental Health (NIMH) was submitted to Congress addressing chronically mentally ill patients living within the community (Barchrach, 1976). The phenomenon of readmission became problematic at this time, with rates rising from 43% in 1963 to 70% in 1974 in some states (U.S. Comptroller General, 1977).

1.1.3 Post-nineteenth-century history of legislation

The development of laws protecting psychiatric patients was a sign of growing public awareness, and included a twofold shift: the shift from a focus limited to public safety to the provision of care with dignity for the mentally ill, and the shift in responsibility of care from the public sector to the state. By 1890 in the United States, every state had built at least one mental hospital that was publicly supported. Admission and discharge rates in these hospitals were regulated by court referrals rather than professional diagnosis, which resulted in overcrowding (Caplan, 1969).

In 1946, President Harry Truman signed the National Mental Health Act. This act provided funds for the creation of the National Institute of Mental Health (NIMH) (Public Law 79–487). The purpose was to improve:

> the mental health of the people of the United States through the conducting of researches, investigations, experiments, and demonstrations relating to the cause, diagnosis, and treatment of psychiatric disorders; assisting and fostering such research activities by public and private agencies, and promoting the coordination of all such researches and activities and the useful application of their results; training personnel in matters relating to mental health; and developing, and assisting States in the use of, the most effective methods of prevention, diagnosis, and treatment of psychiatric disorders.
>
> (Public Law 79–487)

The research conducted by the NIMH concerning the issues of overcrowding in state hospitals, combined with developments in medicine, resulted in a shift toward the creation of community mental health centers (CMHC). The Enactment of Public Law 88–164 (October 1963) made funds available to create CMHCs, which were to be tailored for the immediate community and patient population they served. The law required a single state agency for each state that would develop a master plan taking into consideration existing resources and estimates of need and evaluating priorities. Once the state plan was approved, private and nonprofit organizations could submit proposals for federal construction assistance (Dorsett & Brown, 1965).

A U.S. court ruling in 1971 (*Wyatt v. Stickney*, 1971) acknowledged psychiatric patients' rights to quality physical environments that supported their treatment goals (Sommer & Kroll, 1979). Improvements were slow in coming. In 1985 at the Joint Hearings before the Subcommittee on the Handicapped, staff presented findings from 31 facilities and 600 interviews indicating that hospital patients and staff were subject to injury and that living conditions were unacceptable (U.S. Senate, Senate Committee on Appropriations, 1985). Subsequently, the United Nations General Assembly adopted a resolution of "Principles for the Protection of Persons with Mental Illness and Improvement of Mental Health Care" (United Nations, 1991).

Recent legislation has supported the provision of mental health services. The Paul Wellstone and Pete Domenici Mental Health Parity and Addiction Equity Act of 2008 (MHPAEA) required group health plans and health insurance issuers that provide mental health or substance use disorder benefits to provide such services at parity with medical/surgical benefits. The Patient Protection and Affordable Care Act (PPACA) was signed into law in 2010. By 2014, it was required that all new small group and individual market plans cover mental health and substance use disorder services, and at parity with medical and surgical benefits. The significance of the act was in providing more Americans with access to quality healthcare, as well as mental health and substance use disorder services (Beronio, Po, Skopec, Glied, 2013).

A summary of post-nineteenth-century significant events and design implications regarding psychiatric care is provided in Figure 1.3.

Figure 1.3: *History of significant events and design implications regarding psychiatric care – post-nineteenth-century events in the United States*

Twentieth- and Twenty-First-Century Developments in the United States

Timeline	*Major influences*	*Scientific/social stance*	*Architectural response*
1908	Clifford Beers	National Committee for Mental Hygiene: Early detection of mental illnesses as a preventive practice institutionalized in the network of child guidance clinics.	
1917	Thomas Salmon	Analysis of data from World War I troops led to findings that formed principles of proximity, immediacy, and expectancy.	First local decentralized outpatient clinics.
1946	H. Truman	National Mental Health Act: National Institute of Mental Health to conduct research into reducing mental illness.	
1963	J. F. Kennedy	Public Law 88–164: a single state agency for each state to develop a master plan considering existing resources and estimates of need and evaluating priorities.	Creation of community-based mental health centers in the United States.
1965	NIMH, U.S. Public Health Service, the Western Institute for Research in Mental Health	Research on programming, planning, and design of mental health facilities.	Generation of design considerations for four patient groups: children, adults, geriatric patients, and alcoholics.
1993	American Institute of Architects	Supportive evidence that design can contribute to better treatment and patient safety.	Publication of "Design Consideration for Mental Health Facilities."
2010	Department of Veterans Affairs	In response to needs of veterans of war seeking treatment in VHA (America's largest integrated healthcare system, serving 8.76 million veterans each year).	Publication of "Design Guidelines – Department of Veterans Affairs (DVA) Office of Construction and Facilities Management."
2014	Hunt & Sine		Published *Design Guide for the Built Environment of Behavioral Health Facilities*.
2014	Facility Guidelines Institute (FGI)	The national organization could establish consensus standards for health and residential care facilities.	*Design Guide for the Built Environment of Behavioral Health Facilities* was moved into the FGI website, which started in 1974 to develop guidelines for the planning, design, and construction of healthcare facilities.

Twentieth- and Twenty-First-Century Developments in the United States

Timeline	*Major influences*	*Scientific/social stance*	*Architectural response*
2015	Department of Veterans Affairs		Checklist was developed to ensure compliance of all Veterans Health Administration (VHA) hospitals with safety measures.
2015	Department of Defense		Guidelines to provide objective criteria for developing space requirements for different clinical and support areas.

1.2 Challenges to mental and behavioral health research and design

Fueled by the trend toward evidence-based design (EBD), research on healthcare facilities has increased over the last 25 years. A variety of topics have been covered in this effort. However, studies addressing the design of mental and behavioral health (MBH) environments are few. The absence of research in this area of specialization is surprising, as legal precedents have spoken to the need for quality environments for many years. Challenges to providing mental and behavioral health environments include a variety of settings and a variety of diagnoses.

1.2.1 Variety of settings

One of the complications associated with conducting MBH research and generating guidelines is the variety of potential settings. Psychiatric facilities include psychiatric hospitals, psychiatric and neuro-psychiatric nursing units of general hospitals, facilities for the psychiatric medically infirm, gero-psychiatric units, alcohol and drug addiction treatment facilities (both inpatient and out-patient), mental health clinics, day hospitals, day treatment centers, and others (Carr, 2011). (A summary of patient categories and settings is provided in Figure 1.4.)

The settings in which patients find themselves vary dramatically. Apart from inpatient and outpatient environments, there are multiple residential hybrids, such as halfway houses. Some settings are not designed to deal with the care needs of individuals with MBH diagnoses. For example, Rabins et al. (1996) point out the high prevalence of psychiatric disorders in senior residents of public housing facilities that lack services to support these individuals.

1.2.2 Variety of diagnoses

Models introduced by Tuke (1815) and Kirkbride (1854) suggested segregation of patients based on their diagnosis. Recent studies recommend that patient and staff satisfaction could be improved by separation of cognitively impaired (e.g., dementia) from functionally challenged (e.g., depressed) patients (Craig, Patel, Lee-Jones, & Hatton, 2000). However, available research does not provide enough evidence to draw conclusions regarding specific design guidelines for each patient group or groups of patients that need a separate environment of care.

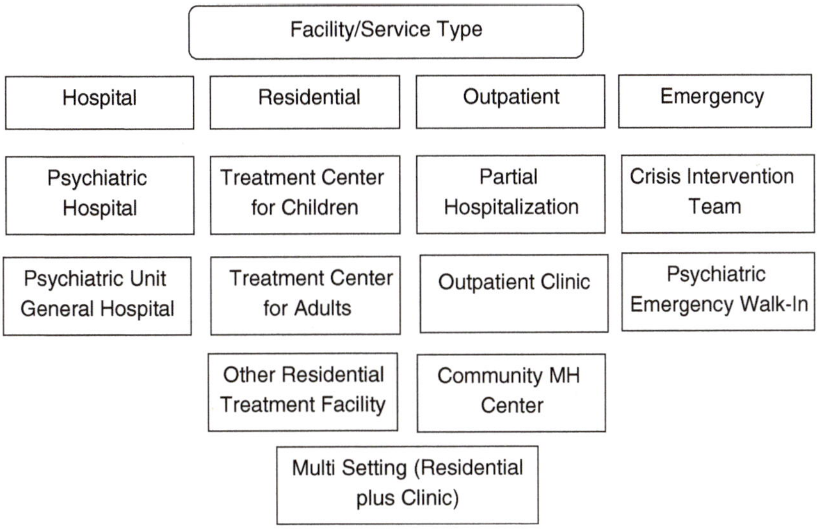

Figure 1.4: *Populations and categories of behavioral health facilities (Derived from Substance Abuse and Mental Health Services Administration, U.S. Department of Health and Human Services "Behavioral Health Treatment Services Locator" [SAMHSA, 2016])*

A discussion of the variety of diagnoses leads to an understanding of the definition of mental illness. Halpern defines mental illness as "a range of chronic subjectively unpleasant psychological conditions," ranging from a group of symptoms such as mild listlessness, depression, and anxiety, to extreme pathology (Halpern, 1995). The National Institute of Mental Health identifies 11 primary topics in the discussion of mental health in relation to diagnosis:

- Anxiety disorders
- Attention deficit hyperactivity disorder
- Autism spectrum disorders
- Bipolar disorder
- Borderline personality disorder
- Depression
- Eating disorders
- Prevention
- Research on HIV and AIDS
- Schizophrenia
- Suicide prevention

Within the discussion of anxiety disorders are generalized anxiety disorder, obsessive-compulsive disorder, panic disorder, post-traumatic stress disorder, and social phobia (NIMH, 2013).

Designers and providers find it difficult to simultaneously support the needs of such a wide variety of individuals, many with multiple diagnoses, sensory processing deficits, and cognitive disorders. In addition, categorizing patients becomes more complicated since the severity of mental disorders is not simply defined by diagnosis but rather as a byproduct of distress, dysfunction, and consequently the disabilities it causes for the individual (Sanderson & Andrews, 2002; Sartorius, 2009). In addition, certain characteristics of the population may influence their evaluation of the environment. A study conducted by Klett, Berger, Sewall, and Rice (1963) suggests that, while education and length of hospitalization did not influence patient evaluations of the ward environment, variables such as age, gender, and patients' predicted date of discharge significantly correlated with their responses. Among these variables, predicted date of discharge merits attention because it reflects patients' mental readiness to cope with a permanent versus short-term situation. Consequently, research on MBH patients is challenging due to each patient's unique needs, preferences, symptoms, and behaviors, ranging from suicide risk (Appleby, 1992) to short-term memory deficiencies (Tek et al., 2002), or absconding (running away from the facility) (Nijman et al., 2011).

1.3 Global issues

In order to more thoroughly understand these challenges, we must address the national and international context. The remainder of this chapter provides documentation of recent findings regarding international status of services and suicide rates.

1.3.1 North American context

The following provides a brief overview of developments and data in Canada, the United States, and Mexico. Although there are significant geographic and fiscal distinctions among these countries, there are similar issues regarding mental and behavioral services.

The Mental Health Commission of Canada (MHCC) released a national-level set of indicators for mental health care in Canada that covers the following topics: access and treatment, adults, caregiving, children and youth, diversity, economic prosperity, housing and homelessness, population well-being, recovery, seniors, stigma, and suicide. The tool has been introduced as the first step toward identifying important areas that need further research and data to enable evidence-based policies and decisions (MHCC, 2015). According to the Canadian Mental Health Association (CMHA) (2016), 20% of Canadians experience a mental illness at some point in their lifetime. Suicide is prevalent, with rates as high as 24% of deaths among 15–24 year olds, and 16% among 25–44 year olds. The CMHA estimates that 3.2 million children between 12 and 19 years old in Canada are at risk of developing depression. According to the WHO Mental Health Atlas 2011, the suicide rate for males is 16.8 per 100,000 population and for females is 5.5 per 100,000 population.

In the United States, suicide was the tenth leading cause of death in 2011 (38,285 individuals) (Hoyert & Xu, 2012). The suicide rate for males in the United States is 17.7 per 100,000 population and for females is 4.5 per 100,000 population (WHO, 2011). Between 2009 and 2012 about 3% of people over 12 years old in the United States had severe depressive symptoms, and approximately 22% had other depression symptoms. Only 35% of people with severe depressive symptoms had sought professional care (Pratt & Brody, 2014). The rates show a 20% increase in the number of individuals seeking mental health treatment since 2011, greater than all other

Figure 1.5: *U.S. trends in mental health and substance abuse relative to other medical needs, 2011–2014 (HRSA, 2015)*

Services (# of patients)	*2011*	*2012*	*2013*	*2014*	*2011–2014 trend change*
Medical	17,354,833	18,034,338	18,592,375	19,495,235	12.33%
Dental	4,037,384	4,332,314	4,442,177	4,776,465	18.31%
Mental Health	932,950	1,035,537	1,119,706	1,251,498	34.14%
Substance Abuse	105,084	114,037	105,605	100,238	–4.61%
Enabling	1,873,745	1,970,511	2,077,351	2,205,003	17.68%

modalities other than vision (Figure 1.5). Interestingly, access to substance abuse treatment has remained relatively constant.

Mexico, which is considered in the upper middle income group based on 2010 World Bank criteria, struggles with public health problems and maladaptive behaviors such as aggressiveness, alcoholism, delinquency, substance abuse, and prostitution that negatively impact families (Latigue & Vives, 2015). In Mexico, the suicide rate for males is 6.8 per 100,000 population and for females is 1.3 per 100,000 population (WHO, 2011).

1.3.2 European context

Several European countries have developed their mental healthcare systems to eliminate the need for traditional psychiatric hospitals. These countries, including Iceland, Italy, and Sweden, are exclusively reliant on community-based systems of care (WHO, 2011). However, a large difference exists among the European countries in terms of mental health services. For example, the number of nurses that work in mental healthcare range from 163 per 100,000 persons in Finland to 4 per 100,000 persons in Bosnia and Herzegovina and 3 per 100,000 population in Greece. In 2014, six European countries were among the top twenty countries with the highest estimated suicide rates globally. These countries included Lithuania (28.2 per 100,000), Kazakhstan (23.8 per 100,000), and Turkmenistan (19.6 per 100,000) (WHO, 2014).

1.3.3 Middle Eastern context

Perhaps the most vulnerable population in the Middle East includes displaced people who have endured military conflicts and wars. This population struggles with post-traumatic stress disorder (PTSD) and lives in unacceptable conditions or lacks access to care. Another large at-risk population in the region is composed of expatriates who hold jobs as blue-collar and domestic workers (Yahia, 2012).

Natural disasters, mainly earthquakes, are responsible for several traumatic events, reinforced by the region's water scarcity. Climate variability and a fast-growing urban population settled in insecure structures and unplanned urban areas are other challenges to mental health in this region (The World Bank, 2014). Studies on the aftermath of an earthquake in Bam (Parvaresh & Bahramnezhad, 2009) and Marmara (Basoglu, Kilic, Salcioglu, & Livanou, 2004) show that a high level of PTSD was detected among the survivors.

Suicide rates for the majority of Arab countries are not available. Syria had a reported suicide rate of 0.4 per 100,000 persons before the recent conflicts. Iran and Turkey were reported in 2011 to have suicide rates of 5.2 and 4.0 per 100,000 persons. Breaking down by gender, Israel reported suicide rates of 8.7 for males and 3.3 for females per 100,000 population (WHO, 2011).

1.3.4 Asian context

The Asian context can be divided into the Southeast Asian and Western Pacific regions. The countries in the region have highly varied political systems that translate into a wide range of healthcare systems and education. In most countries psychiatrist to population rates (1:80,000 in China, 1:330,000 in India, 1:460,000 in Indonesia) are very low. Moreover, the specialists are not distributed evenly and are mostly concentrated in large urban areas and megacities (Meshvara, 2002). Among the 79 countries that provide data about psychiatric inpatient admissions, the Southeast Asian and Western Pacific regions have the highest rate of involuntary admission rates to psychiatric hospitals (60% versus 17% global average) (WHO, 2014).

Suicide statistics in Asian countries are significant, with rates as high as 35.8 for males and 13.7 for females per 100,000 persons in Japan. High rates are also reported in China (13.8 male and 12.2 female per 100,000 persons), Korea (29.6 male and 14.1 female per 100,000 persons), India (12 male and 9.1 female per 100,000 persons), and Sri Lanka (44.6 male and 16.8 female per 100,000 persons) (WHO, 2011).

1.3.5 Central and South American context

Migration, domestic violence, sociopolitical unrest, and natural disasters are ever-present sources of trauma in most Latin American and Caribbean countries, which, despite the need, devote less than 2% of their total health budget to mental health (Alarcon, 2003). These limited resources are concentrated in metropolitan areas, leaving 45% of the population unattended (Cruz, 2015). The role of mental health in primary care is limited in most parts of Central and South America. According to the 2013 WHO AIMS report, mental health systems are not adequate to respond to the needs of the population in Latin America. Integration of mental health into primary care lacks financial support, as most resources are absorbed by psychiatric hospitals (PAHO, 2013).

Among the Central and South American countries that reported suicide rates to WHO, a wide range of rates was observed between various countries and between male and female genders. Rates were as high as 19.6 male and 4.9 female per 100,000 population in Cuba. Brazil had an average suicide rate of 7.3 per 100,000 population. Costa Rica (31.2 male and 2.5 female) and Belize (13.4 male and 1.6 female) were among the countries that displayed a large difference between suicide rates of male and female citizens (WHO, 2011).

1.3.6 African context

The 48 sub-Saharan African countries have consistently dominated the list of least developed countries since 1971 according to the United Nations (Essoungou, 2011). One in seven children and adolescents in sub-Saharan Africa suffers from psychiatric difficulties, including depression and anxiety disorders as well as conduct, disruptive, and reactive behavior disorders (Cortina, Sodha,

Fazel, & Ramchamdani, 2012). Liu et al. (2016) systematically reviewed literature on interventions concerning mental health worker training in Africa and found that the training outcomes were focused on changes in knowledge and attitude. However, few studies evaluated health workers' skills and assessed the clinical outcomes. Suicide rates for the majority of African countries are not available. Among the very few that reported their data to WHO, Zimbabwe had suicide rates of 10.6 for male and 5.2 for female per 100,000 population.

1.3.7 General international challenges

1.3.7.1 Impact of natural disasters and emergency situations on care providers

Humanitarian healthcare providers in emergency settings face mental health issues exacerbated by three main conditions: preexisting social or psychological issues, emergency-induced issues (the aftermath of the traumatic event), and humanitarian aid-induced problems (overcrowding, lack of privacy, community structure fragmentation, anxiety about continuation of aid) (Inter-Agency Standing Committee, 2010). Neria (2015) suggests that a proactive response to the outbreak of Ebola in West Africa should have incorporated an assessment of psychological stressors associated with the outbreak for both civilians and healthcare providers.

1.3.7.2 Scarcity of resources and economic instability

A nationally representative survey of Afghans reported lack of food and water were the most common sources of trauma (Cardozo et al., 2004). Economic instability can also be a source of stress and cause mental health issues in countries with better resources. An analysis of multi-decade and nationwide data on suicide in Greece revealed a positive correlation between occurrences of austerity-related events and rates of suicide (Branas et al., 2015).

1.3.7.3 War, conflicts, and human rights violations

PTSD, anxiety, and depression have been reported among survivors of war, conflict, or human rights violations in Yugoslavia (Basoglu et al., 2005), Eastern Afghanistan (Scholte et al., 2004), the Central African Republic (Vinck & Pham, 2010), Liberia (Johnson et al., 2008), Nepal (Kohrt et al., 2008), and Congo (Johnson et al., 2010), among many others. According to UNHCR (2015), in 2014, an average of 42,500 individuals per day had to seek protection from conflict and persecution at home.

1.3.7.4 Forced displacement and migration

Global forced displacement had an unprecedented increase in 2014, reaching 59.5 million individuals worldwide, 8.3 million persons more than 2013 (UNHCR, 2015). Forced displacement can be a traumatic experience in itself and is usually accompanied by underlying social and economic deficits. As an example, research shows that among residents of the Jaffna District in Sri Lanka, the prevalence of symptoms of PTSD, anxiety, and depression was high and significantly associated with displacement status and previous trauma exposure (Husain et al., 2011). Twenty years after the Guatemalan civil conflict, psychiatric morbidity was prevalent among refugees to Mexico (Sabin, Cardazo, Nackerud, Kaisar, & Varese, 2003).

Immigration and the stress resulting from relocation can also lead to psychosis. Research shows that psychosis is more significantly prevalent among immigrants (Morgan & Hutchinson, 2009). It is noteworthy that this population brings a new set of standards of normality or patterns of disorder. Applying the assumptions, knowledge, and practices customary in the destination country without considering the cultural background can interfere with the treatment and may produce treatment-induced problems (Marsella, 2011).

1.4 Mental and behavioral health context summary

Mental and behavioral disorders are the leading cause of disability worldwide. An estimated 22.2% of all years lived with disability are due to mental and behavioral disorders (Murray, Vos, Lozano, Naghavi, Flaxman, 2013). Moreover, this group of disorders can co-occur with other diseases, leading to increases in morbidity and mortality risk for chronic diseases such as angina, arthritis, asthma, diabetes, cancer, and coronary artery disease (CAD). When an individual is facing other physical health conditions, mental illness can cause interruption in treatment seeking and adherence, resulting in poorer health outcomes (Pike, Susser, Galea, Pincus, 2013).

The study of mental health goes beyond individual attributes such as thoughts, emotions, behaviors, and interactions with others. Social, cultural, economic, political, and environmental factors can determine mental health for individuals or groups of people. Each year, individuals or groups of individuals around the world become vulnerable by being exposed to traumatic situations and environments (WHO, 2013). To improve access to care, the WHO (2013) recommends that countries develop comprehensive community-based mental health and social care services, and integrate mental healthcare into general hospitals and primary care settings. However, despite the need, very limited resources are dedicated to mental health research and in-service provision (Kakuma, Minas, van Ginneken, Dal Poz, & Desiraju, 2011). Stigma and accessibility barriers make the limited existing services even harder to reach (Pike, Susser, Galea, & Pincus 2013).

References

Alarcon, R. D. (2003). Mental health and mental healthcare in Latin America. *World Psychiatry*, *2*(1), 54–56.

Appleby, L. (1992). Suicide in psychiatric patients: Risk and prevention. *British Journal of Psychiatry*, *161*, 749–758.

Barchrach, L. L. (1976). *Deinstitutionalization: An analytical review and sociological perspective*. Rockville, MD: Department of Health, Education and Welfare.

Basoglu, M., Kilic, C., Salcioglu, E., & Livanou, M. (2004). Prevalence of posttraumatic stress disorder and comorbid depression in earthquake survivors in Turkey: An epidemiological study. *Journal of Traumatic Stress*, *17*, 133–141.

Basoglu, M., Livanou, M., Crnobaric, C., Franciskovic, T., Suljic, E., Duric, D., & Vranesic, M. (2005). Psychiatric and cognitive effects of war in former Yugoslavia: Association of lack of redress for trauma and posttraumatic stress reactions. *Journal of American Medical Association*, *249*(5), 581–590.

Beronio, K., Po, R., Skopec, L., & Glied, S. (2013). *Affordable care act expands mental health and substance use disorder benefits and federal parity protections for 62 million Americans.* Office of the Assistant Secretary for Planning and Evaluation. U.S. Department of Health and Human Services. Retrieved from https://aspe.hhs.gov/report/affordable-care-act-expands-mental-health-and-substance-use-disorder-benefits-and-federal-parity-protections-62-million-americans

Blain, D. (1953, November). Mental patients can be cured. *Architectural Records*, 181–182.
Blain, D. (1956, November). Psychiatric facilities of the future. *Architectural Record*, 205.
Bowen, L. R. (1939, February). Planning for state hospitals. *The Modern Hospital*, *52*(2), 61–65.
Branas, C., Kastanaki, A., Michalodimitrakis, M., Tzougas, J., Kranioti, E., Theodorakis, P., & Wiebe, D. (2015). The impact of economic austerity and prosperity events on suicide in Greece: A 30 year interrupted time series analysis. *BMJ Open*, *5*, e005619.
Canadian Mental Health Association. (2016). *Fast facts about mental illness*. Retrieved from www.cmha.ca/media/fast-facts-about-mental-illness/#.V0Ej25ErLIW
Caplan, R. B. (1969). *Psychiatry and the community in nineteenth century America*. New York: Basic Books.
Cardozo, B. L., Bilukha, O. O., Crawford, C., Shaikh, I., Wolfe, M., Gerber, M., & Anderson, M. (2004). Mental health, social functioning, and disability in post war Afghanistan. *Journal of American Medical Association*, *292*(5), 575–584.
Carr, R. (2011). Psychiatric facility. *Whole Building Design Guide*. Retrieved from www.wbdg.org/design/psychiatric.php
Cortina, M. A., Sodha, A., Fazel, M., & Ramchamdani, P. G. (2012). Prevalence of child mental health problems in sub-Saharan Africa, a systematic review. *Archives of Pediatrics and Adolescent Medicine*, *166*(3), 276–281.
Craig, J. S., Patel, J., Lee-Jones, C., & Hatton, C. (2000). Psychiatric assessment wards for older adults: A qualitative evaluation of two ward models. *International Journal of Geriatric Psychiatry*, *15*(8), 721–728.
Cruz, A., (2015). Poor mental health, an obstacle to development in Latin America. *The World Bank*. Retrieved from www.worldbank.org/en/news/feature/2015/07/13/bad-mental-health-obstacle-development-latin-america
Dorsett, C., & Brown, B. (1965). *Planning, programming, and design for the community mental health center*. Pittsburgh, PA: National Institute for Mental Health.
Essoungou, A. (2011). Africa's least developed: Lands of opportunity. *Africa Renewal*. Retrieved from www.un.org/africarenewal/magazine/august-2011/africas-least-developed-lands-opportunity
Guttersen, A. G. (1953a). Design of intensive treatment building. *Architectural Record*, *204*, 189–203.
Guttersen, A. G. (1953b). Psychiatric service in the general hospital. *Architectural Record*, *204*, 204–212.
Halpern, D. (1995). *Mental health and the built environment: More than bricks and mortar?* London, UK: Taylor & Francis.
Hoyert, D. L., & Xu, J. (2012). Deaths: preliminary data for 2011. *National Vital Statistics*, *61*(6). Retrieved from www.cdc.gov/ nchs/data/nvsr/nvsr61/nvsr61_06.pdf
HRSA. (2015). *Program grantee comparison data*. HRSA Health Center Program, U.S. Department of Health and Human Services. Retrieved from http://bphc.hrsa.gov/uds/datacenter.aspx?year=2014&state=&compare=Nat
Husain, F., Anderson, M., Cardozo, B. L., Becknell, K., Blanton, C., Araki, D., & Vithana, E. K. (2011). Prevalence of war-related mental health conditions, association with displacement status in post-war Jaffna district, Sri Lanka. *Journal of American Medical Association*, *306*(5), 522–531.
Inter-Agency Standing Committee. (2010). *Mental health and psychological support in humanitarian emergencies: What should humanitarian health actors know?* Geneva, Switzerland: WHO.
Johnson, K., Asher, J., Rosenberg, S., Raja, A., Panjabi, R., Beadling, C., & Lawry, L. (2008). Association of combatant status and sexual violence with health and mental health outcomes in post conflict Liberia. *Journal of American Medical Association*, *300*(6), 676–690.

Johnson, K., Scott, J., Rughita, B., Kisielewski, M., Asher, J., Ong, R., & Lawry, L. (2010). Association of sexual violence and human rights violations with physical and mental health in territories of Eastern Democratic Republic of the Congo. *Journal of American Medical Association, 304*(5), 553–562.

Kakuma, R., Minas, H., van Ginneken, N., Dal Poz, M. R., & Desiraju, K. (2011). Human resources for mental health care: Current situation and strategies for action. *Lancet, 378*, 5–11.

Kirkbride, T. (1854). *On the construction, organization, and general arrangement of the hospitals for the insane*. New York: Arno Press.

Klett, S., Berger, D., Sewall, L., & Rice, C. (1963). Patient evaluation of the psychiatric ward. *Journal of Clinical Psychology, 19*, 347–351.

Kohrt, B., Jordans, M., Tol, W., Speckman, R., Maharjan, S., Worthman, C., & Komproe, I. (2008). Comparison of mental health between former child soldiers and children never conscripted by armed groups in Nepal. *Journal of American Medical Association, 300*(6), 691–702.

Lartigue and Vives, J. (1991). Mental Health Services in Mexico. *The Journal of Sociology & Social Welfare: 18*(2). Retrieved on January 27, 2017, from http://scholarworks.wmich.edu/jssw/vol18/iss2/5

Liu, G., Jack, H., Piette, A., Mangezi, W., Machando, D., Rwafa, . . . Abas, M. (2016). Mental health training for health workers in Africa: A systematic review. *The Lancet Psychiatry, 3*(1), 65–76.

Marsella, A. (2011, October). *Twelve critical issues for mental health professionals working with ethno-culturally diverse populations*. American Psychological Association. Retrieved from www.apa.org/international/pi/2011/10/critical-issues.aspx

Mental Health Commission of Canada. (2015). *Informing the future: Mental health indicators for Canada, Ottawa, Ontario*. Mental Health Commission. Retrieved from www.mentalhealthcommission.ca/English/system/files/private/document/Informing%20the%20Future%20-%20Mental%20Health%20Indicators%20for%20Canada.pdf

Meshvara, D. (2002). Mental health and mental healthcare in Asia. *World Psychiatry, 1*(2), 118–120.

Morgan, C., & Hutchinson, G. (2009). The social determinants of psychosis in migrant and ethnic minority population: A public health tragedy. *Psychological Medicine, 1*, 1–5.

Murray, C. J., Vos, T., Lozano, R., Naghavi, M., & Flaxman, A. D. (2013). Disability adjusted life years (DALYs) for 291 diseases and injuries in 21 regions, 1990–2010: A systematic analysis for the Global Burden of Disease Study 2010. *Lancet, 380*, 2197–2223.

National Institute of Mental Health (NIMH). (2013). *National Institute of Mental Health*. Retrieved February 8, 2013, from www.nimh.nih.gov/index.shtml

Neria, Y. (2015). The 2014 Ebola outbreak and mental health. *Journal of American Medical Association, 313*(6), 567–568.

Nijman, H., Bower, L., Haglund, K., Muir, E., Simpson, A., & Vender Merwe, M. (2011). Door locking and exit security measures on acute psychiatric admission wards. *Journal of Psychiatric and Mental Health Nursing, 18*, 614–621.

Pan American Health Organization. (2013). *WHO AIMS: Report on mental health systems in Latin America and the Caribbean*. World Health Organization. Retrieved from www.paho.org/hq/index.php?option=com_docman&task=doc_view&gid=21325&Itemid

Parvaresh, N., & Bahramnezhad, A. (2009). Post-traumatic stress disorder in Bam-survived students who immigrated to Kerman, four months after the earthquake. *Archives of Iranian Medicine, 12*, 244–249.

Pike, K., Susser, E., Galea, S., & Pincus, H. (2013). Towards a healthier 2020: Advancing mental health as a global health priority. *Public Health Reviews*, *35*(1). Retrieved June 26, 2016, from www.publichealthreviews.eu/upload/pdf_files/13/00_Pike.pdf

Pratt, L. A., & Brody, D. (2014). *Depression in the U.S. household population, 2009–2012*. National CERNER for Health Statistics, Centers for Disease Control and Prevention. Retrieved June 2, 2016, from www.cdc.gov/nchs/data/databriefs/db172.htm

Public Law 79–487. (1946). *National Mental Health Act*. Retrieved June 26, 2016, from https://history.nih.gov/research/downloads/PL79–487.pdf

Public Law 88–164. (1963). *Mental Retardation Facilities and Community Health Centers Construction Act of 1963*. National Archives Catalog. Retrieved June 26, 2016, from https://research.archives.gov/id/299883

Rabins, P., Black, B., German, P., Roca, R., McGuire, M., Brant, L., & Cook, J. (1996). The prevalence of psychiatric disorders in elderly residents of public housing. *Journal of Gerontology*, *51A*(6), M319–M324.

Sabin, M., Cardazo, B. L., Nackerud, L., Kaisar, R., & Varese, L. (2003). Factors associated with poor mental health among Guatemalan refugees living in Mexico 20 years after civil conflict. *Journal of American Medical Association*, *290*(5), 635–642.

Salmon, T. W. (1917). War neuroses: Shell Shock. *Military Surgeon*, *41*, 674–693.

SAMHSA. (2016). *SAMHSA service locator*. Retrieved June 26, 2016, from https://findtreatment.samhsa.gov/locator?sAddr=&submit=Go

Sanderson, K., & Andrews, G. (2002). Prevalence and severity of mental health-related disability and relationship to diagnosis. *Psychiatric Services*, *53*, 80–86. doi:10.1176/appi.ps.53.1.80

Sartorius, N. (2009). Disability and mental illness are different entities and should be assessed separately. *World Psychiatry*, *8*, 86. doi:10.1002/j.2051–5545.2009.tb00220.x

Scholte, W., Olff, M., Ventevogel, P., de Vries, G.-J., Jansveld, E., Cardozo, B. L., & Crawford, C. (2004). Mental health symptoms following war and repression in Eastern Afghanistan. *Journal of American Medical Association*, *292*(5), 585–593.

Shorter, E. (1997). *A history of psychiatry: From the era of the asylum to the age of Prozac*. New York: John Wiley & Sons.

Sommer, R., & Kroll, B. (1979). Mental patients and nurses rate habitability. In D. Canter & S. Canter (Eds.), *Designing for therapeutic environments* (pp. 199–212). Sussex, UK: John Wiley & Sons.

Talbott, J. A. (1978). *The death of the asylum*. New York: Grune & Stratton.

Tek, C., Gold, J., Blaxton, T., Wilk, C., McMahon, R. P., & Buchanan, R. W. (2002). Visual perceptual and working memory impairments in schizophrenia. *Archives of general psychiatry*, *59*(2), 146.

Tuke, S. (1815). *Practical hints on the construction and economy of Pauper Lunatic Asylums*. York: Alexander.

United Nations. (1991). *Principles for the protection of persons with mental illness*. Retrieved June 16, 2016, from United Nations website: www.un.org/documents/ga/res/46/a46r119.htm

United Nations High Commissioner for Refugees. (2015). A world at war. UNHCR Global Trends 2014. Retrieved from www.unhcr.org/556725e69.pdf

U.S. Comptroller General. (1977). *Returning the mentally disabled to the community: Government needs to do more*. Washington, DC: U.S. Government Accountability Office.

U.S. Congress. (1985). Care of Institutionalized Mentally Disabled Persons. Joint Hearings before the Subcommittee on the Handicapped. *United States Senate*, Ninety-Ninth Congress, First Session. Retrieved June 26, 2016, from http://files.eric.ed.gov/fulltext/ED263712.pdf

Vinck, P., & Pham, P. (2010). Association of exposure to violence and potential traumatic events with self-reported physical and mental health status in the Central African Republic. *Journal of American Medical Association*, *304*(5), 544–552.

Wilbur, H. B. (1877). *Buildings for the Insane: A report*. Boston, MA: Albert J. Wright.

The World Bank. (2014). *Natural disasters in the Middle East and North Africa: A regional Overview*. The International Bank for Reconstruction and Development. Retrieved from www.wds.worldbank.org/external/default/WDSContentServer/WDSP/IB/2014/03/06/000442464_20140306122711/Rendered/PDF/816580WP0REPLA0140same0box00PUBLIC0.pdf

World Health Organization. (2011). *World mental health Atlas*. World Health Organization. Retrieved from www.who.int/mental_health/publications/mental_health_atlas_2011/en/

World Health Organization. (2013). *Mental health action plan, 2013–2020*. World Health Organization. Retrieved from http://apps.who.int/iris/bitstream/10665/89966/1/9789241506021_eng.pdf

World Health Organization. (2014). *World mental health Atlas*. World Health Organization. Retrieved from http://apps.who.int/iris/bitstream/10665/178879/1/9789241565011_eng.pdf?ua=1&ua=1

World Health Organization, Regional Office for Europe. (2014). *Data and statistics*. Retrieved from www.euro.who.int/en/health-topics/noncommunicable-diseases/mental-health/data-and-statistics

Wyatt v. Stickney, (1971).

Yahia, M. (2012). Dealing with the mental illness in the Middle East. *Nature Middle East*. Retrieved from www.natureasia.com/en/nmiddleeast/article/10.1038/nmiddleeast.2012.103

Yanni, C. (2007). *Architecture of madness: Insane asylums in the United States*. Minneapolis: University of Minnesota Press.

General design considerations

2

> Patients were exquisitely sensitive to the physical environment. Their senses open to a barrage of stimuli, they seemed unable to sort out the signal from the noise. Subtle "messages," non-verbal and graphic, which lay buried in the design of settings were abundantly clear to patients. Patients reacted to the information, coded into the environment by designers and by the culture, as if it had been "written" only for them. Misinformation and accidental malformations in the settings created illusions which were very close to, and sometimes seemed to trigger, hallucinations.
>
> (Spivak, 1984, p. 12)

This observation by Spivak in the 1980s underlines the impact of the environment on healing in behavioral and mental health facilities and provides the context for this chapter. Designers of the period knew that the need for care was not being met in the United States and that the life cycle of existing state institutions was ending; a mandate to deliver care was evident and facilities of the future required change.

Rivlin and Wolfe (1979) point out that operational protocols supersede the impact of the physical environment, but acknowledge that the environment can serve to support therapy objectives. While there are naysayers who challenge the potential impact of the physical environment, we support the theory of affordances developed by J. J. Gibson (1979), who posits that the environment serves to support or undermine human activity.

> The possibilities of the environment and the way of life of the animal go together inseparably. The environment constrains what the animal can do, and the concept of a niche in ecology reflects this fact. Within limits, the human animal can alter the affordances of the environment but is still the creature of his or her situation.
>
> (Gibson, 1979, p. 143)

While we also acknowledge the role of the science of medicine and the art of human relationships to the healing process, we emphasize the role the environment plays in supporting or undermining these contributors. By acknowledging the importance of the physical environment, we must recognize the need for reliable guidelines. These guidelines are critical to the creation of environments that support the psychological needs and functional requirements of a well-designed facility and are the topic of this chapter.

Apart from addressing specific design objectives, we find it useful to create a context by summarizing design theories that impact the design of psychiatric facilities. This discussion will be followed by summarizing design recommendations provided by a series of academics and practitioners, some of which are substantiated by research and some of which are founded on personal experience and perspective. While this chapter describes the theories and concepts associated with the design of behavioral and mental health facilities, Chapter 9 addresses the research more specifically and Chapter 10 describes formally developed standards documents intended to guide the design process.

2.1 Theories behind psychiatric facility design

Each designer embraces his or her own hybrid theory of design regarding psychiatric facilities, but there are several approaches around which individuals have coalesced. They are anthroposophy, evidence-based design, generative design, Planetree, salutogenic design, and specialist versus generalist theories.

2.1.1 *Anthroposophy*

The Anthroposophical Society was founded by Rudolf Steiner in 1924 and supports a philosophy of using conscious understanding to be open to the "various spiritual realms" linked to human life (Allgemeine Anthroposophische Gesellshaft, 1999). The objective of anthroposophical design is to provide a "sense of living order" (Logsdon, 1995). One of the philosophical principles is the evolution of the patient from high control and containment to exploration. Anthroposophic treatment for psychiatric conditions such as depression differs from traditional treatment in its use of physical therapies, nonverbal artistic therapies, and anthroposophic medications (Hamre et al., 2006). Hospitals with anthroposophic behavioral health units include:

- Filderklinik, Filderstadt, Germany (pediatric psychiatry, psychosomatic medicine),
- Ita Wegman Klinik, Arlesheim, Switzerland (psychiatry),
- Friedrich-Husemann-Klinik, Buchenbach, Germany (psychiatry), and
- Lievegoed Kliniek, Bilhoven, Netherlands (psychiatry) (Evans & Rodger, 1992).

Anthroposophic design features soft forms that are intended to be playful and human-friendly. Anton Alberts, a Dutch architect (1927–1999), once said that form is "spirit made visible." While rectilinear shapes reflect development of a concrete mind and quantitative intelligence, softer forms are believed by anthroposophists to be a reflection of advanced intuition (Visionesse, 2008).

2.1.2 *Evidence-based design and research-informed design*

Sackett, Rosenber, and Muir (1996) described evidence-based medicine as "the conscientious, explicit and judicious use of current best evidence in making decisions about the care of individual patients" (p. 71). In response, Hamilton and Watkins define EBD as: "a process for the conscientious, explicit and judicious use of current best evidence from research and practice in making critical decisions, together with an informed client, about the design of each individual and unique project" (Hamilton & Watkins, 2009, p. 9). One of the early misinterpretations of the term was that EBD was a product rather than a process. The objective for evidence-based design in healthcare is to inform design decisions with the objective of enhancing the patient and family care experience and the work environment for staff (Stichler & Hamilton, 2008).

The actual contribution of EBD has been a source of great debate in two main areas. First, misunderstanding about the scope – those who challenge it assume that EBD claims to provide proof of outcomes for building approaches. In reality current EBD is only intended to add information to the decision-making process. Research never provides "proof," but rather deals in probabilities. Second, many are concerned that the emphasis on science will undermine the art of the design process. However, we argue that design strategies are so numerous that information provided by researchers will likely never exceed more than 5%–10% of the design decisions. The intent of EBD healthcare architecture should be "improving the organization's clinical, economic, productivity, satisfaction, and cultural measures" (Hamilton, 2003).

Research-informed design is an alternative expression for describing the intent of EBD, and may be an option to the implied rigidity of the term "evidence." However, those interested in EBD or research-informed design are both advocating for the use of science to help resolve design questions that otherwise lack sufficient information to allow for confident decision-making.

2.1.3 *Generative design*

Generative environments are described as the third type of space in addition to physical and social environment (Ruga, 2008, 2010). Generative space "is social space that is informed, conditioned and reinforced by the physical environment. Generative space is generative in that it encourages, supports, and reinforces improvements to health and well-being; it is intended to be progressively 'life-enhancing' " (Ruga, 2008, 2010). As an example, the Arlington Free Clinic in Virginia employed a generative approach by emphasizing social interaction (The Caritas Project, 2014). Due to the multiple settings for social interaction in psychiatric facilities, generative space is an approach that is particularly relevant.

2.1.4 *Planetree and the Institute for Patient-Centered Design*

Both Planetree and the Institute for Patient-Centered Design are discussed in this section due to their focus on the patient. While Planetree addresses healthcare patient overall needs, the Institute for Patient-Centered Design focuses specifically on the physical environment.

The mission of Planetree is "the development and implementation of innovative models of healthcare that focus on healing and nurturing body, mind and spirit" (Planetree, 2014) and was founded by Angela Thieriot in response to personal negative hospital experiences. Planetree embraces physical environments that support patient-centered care and are of particular interest to designers. In terms of physical plant, Planetree recommends the inclusion of a patient/family resource center to provide health information. Planetree environments are intended to be accessible and homelike. Spaces are available for patient privacy as well as social opportunities. Break areas are provided for staff to allow them to reenergize. The first Planetree unit was at the San Francisco General Hospital (Frampton & Charmel, 2009; Orr, 1995).

To achieve Planetree goals Stamford Hospital added several physical environmental features in their psychiatric unit, including a water system in lieu of water bottles, a remodeled activity room, a chalkboard in the community room with a soft green and white color scheme, a refurnished waiting area with wall art, opaque window film that allows light in while preserving patient privacy rather than a vertical blind window treatment located between the waiting area and activity room, and inspirational quotes added to walls (Planetree, 2014). The modifications were associated with increased satisfaction, as reflected in the data shown in Figure 2.1.

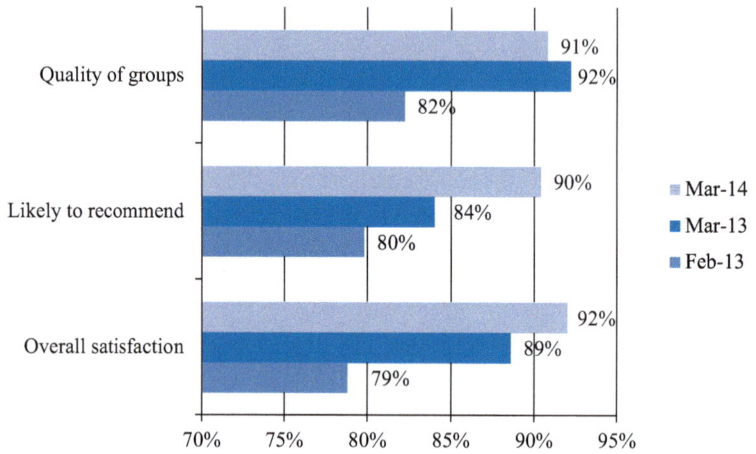

Figure 2.1: *Satisfaction rates (%) at the Stamford Planetree inpatient mental health facility, February 2013, March 2013, March 2014 (Planetree, 2014)*

Griffin Hospital also has a Planetree psychiatric unit. Among the principles employed there were increased natural daylight, reduction of number of beds from 16 to 14, a more open floor plan to enable communication and visibility between patients and staff, and more open nurse stations (Turlington, 2004). Turlington (2004) proposes that these enhanced links reduce the loss of control felt by patients and encourage social interaction. Other interventions included private and semiprivate rooms, an entertainment lounge, a residential kitchen, and a dining area. Individual and group therapy rooms that also support patient education, aromatherapy and arts, natural woodwork, and indirect lighting were also introduced (Turlington, 2004). Similar to Stamford, positive outcomes were found. Evaluations rose to 97% and were maintained at least until 2004, the date of the publication of "Creating a Planetree Inpatient Psychiatric Unit." Inpatient revenues were found to rise by 4% due to an increased number of patients.

In 2011, New York Presbyterian was the first psychiatric hospital to earn the Planetree designation (New York Presbyterian, 2012). Other Planetree behavioral health facilities (both units and hospitals) include:

- Centra voor Psychisch Herstel (the Netherlands) (since 2015),
- Fatima Zorg (the Netherlands) (since 2014),
- GGzE (the Netherlands),
- Griffin Hospital (USA) (since 2008), and
- Stamford Hospital (USA) (since 2012) (Planetree, "Designated Sites," 2014).

The recently formed Institute for Patient-Centered Design, Inc., has a related mission and focuses on encouraging the contributions of patients in the development of the healing environment (Institute for Patient-Centered Design, Inc., n.d.). Since 2010, the institute has advocated for family and patient collaboration with healthcare providers and design teams as a key component of developing a successful project (Institute for Patient-Centered Design, Inc., n.d.). In 2015 the institute took on the mission of raising awareness regarding behavioral health facilities, sponsored a design competition on the topic, and produced a patient room prototype in 2016 for the Veterans Administration.

Under the Affordable Care Act patient-centered care has evolved into a primary objective of the U.S. healthcare system (Cliff, 2012). By addressing the needs of patients, improvements in clinical outcomes, satisfaction, and return on investment can occur (Cliff, 2012). Cliff argues that the reform in healthcare pushes hospitals to improve patient outcomes with fewer resources, which may result in shortened length of stay, fewer visits to the emergency department and readmissions, and improved patient adherence to plans of care (Cliff, 2012).

2.1.5 Salutogenic design

Antonovsky's salutogenic theory suggests that improved health results from a mental state that is fortified by coherence (Golembiewski, 2010); the theory proposes that coherence is supported by an individual's ability to comprehend the environment, to be efficacious in his or her actions, and to find meaningfulness (Golembiewski, 2010). The salutogenic approach intends to eliminate features that generate high stress and to enhance the environment by adding elements that foment access to nature and daylight, personal control, areas dedicated to private and public relaxation, and aesthetic spaces (Heerwagen, Heubach, Montgomery, & Weimer 1995).

Dilani (2008) asserts that salutogenic design is the foundation for psychosocially supportive design, resulting in improved health and well-being. The framework for salutogenic design emphasizes an ecological and holistic approach by embracing interconnections between people, events, procedures, and places (Heerwagen et al., 1995). This framework includes the following components: (1) social cohesion and opportunities for formal and casual interactions, (2) personal control of daylight, electric light, temperature, and noise as well as access to private rooms, and (3) opportunities for relaxation and rejuvenation via quiet rooms, outdoor spaces, and diffuse lighting (Heerwagen et al., 1995). Psychosocially supportive design is only effective when salutogenic management by the entire organization is achieved (Dilani, 2008). The salutogenic model must be implemented through empirical studies associated with well-being factors in the context of psychosocially supportive design (Dilani, 2008).

In his 2010 paper, "Applying a Salutogenic Model to Architectural Design for Psychiatric Care," Golembiewski describes the critical relationship between perceptual dysfunction and psychiatric illness, and notes that mental health imbalances may be the result of distortions in perceptual systems resulting in hallucinations, unpredictability, and delusions. To achieve a salutogenic environment, the design must be (1) comprehensible and easy to read, (2) manageable and able to allow the patient to feel like he or she can make a difference, and (3) meaningful; the latter is the most critical and can be achieved through environmental richness (Golembiewski, 2010).

2.1.6 Specialist versus generalist

Chrysikou (2014) writes that there are two competing theories regarding the planning of mental and behavioral health facilities – one focusing on a specialist approach and the other focusing on a generalist approach. The former suggests that environments should be specialized to meet the needs of specific populations; the latter recommends a more normalized environment for all populations (Chrysikou, 2014). The latter is associated with homelikeness, which is advocated by many designers. However, according to Chrysikou, normalization theory constitutes a useful tool but is not a panacea and cannot be evenly applied to all facilities.

2.2 Planning and programming considerations

Strategic planning and program considerations have been raised in the literature. Some of the broader considerations relate to physical, fiscal, and social sustainability (energy conservation, cost-effectiveness, and contextual relationship with the community). As a core principle of programming, Davis, Glick, and Rosow (1979) argue that it is possible to address the requirements of a psychotherapeutic milieu within the confines of code and budgetary restrictions through creative and flexible design. However, the programmatic elements, which fully address treatment, training, and research goals, must be clearly defined in advance, and all those involved should be participating in the programming and design process.

Porter and Easter (1980) make the following thoughtful recommendations for programming a behavioral health facility:

1. Residential facilities should use environmental quality rather than medication as a guiding philosophy.
2. The patient is the center of the treatment plan.
3. Programming should allow for flexibility and growth.
4. Support should be provided to patients, staff, and family.
5. Requirements should be discussed with all levels of building occupants (Porter & Easter, 1980).

Regarding the last point, Von Sommaruga Howard (2004) suggests group involvement in programming for mental and behavioral health facilities, but notes that participants may bring their own fears into the discussion; they may seek control and project this onto the patient group. As such, appropriate moderating must be provided. Service users, in particular, should be involved (Fitzgerald, Kirk, & Bristow, 2011). Multiple perspectives are essential and will address the issue that "many apparent amenities are not simply frills, but significant resources in milieu therapy and psychotherapy, and can be trimmed only at some risk to patients and their treatment" (Davis et al., 1979, p. 460).

2.3 Transdisciplinary collaboration

In a series of interviews with eight specialists in health facility design and construction on the topic of future leaders, Shepley (2016) noted that the interviewees all believed that the most successful individuals will be those who embrace change and a transdisciplinary approach, which aims to blend various disciplines, to problem solving. The nature of change in MBH facilities may be limited to new knowledge regarding pharmacology and genetics.

An effective relationship between mental health clinicians and designers is critical to the process of design:

> Effective collaboration between psychiatrists and architects is essential to avoid repetition of past errors. Care must be taken to create a facility to survive the test of usage, as well as building to survive the test of time.
>
> (Foley & Lacy, 1967, pp. 1017–1018)

However, the interactions between disciplines are not without peril. Foley and Lacy (1967) note that collaborations between psychiatry and architecture face the following challenges:

- Semantic differences: Words such as "program" and "design" are thought of differently. For an architect, a program connotes spatial relationships, while a psychiatrist is likely thinking of a group of services; the term "design" to an architect usually involves the broad process associated with problem solving, while the psychiatrist may think of design as a floor plan.
- Dichotomous role of the psychologist: The psychologist is seeking the expertise of a designer while at the same time is the expert in his or her field.
- Communication of expertise: Both psychiatrists and architects are accustomed to being authorities in their fields, yet each has trouble providing the appropriate information to support the process as each lacks experience in the others' field (Foley & Lacy, 1967).

Shepley and Watson (2012) note the lack of collaboration between healthcare practitioners and health facilities designers as extending beyond the design process to creating barriers to design research. The lack of collaboration was demonstrated in a meta-review of literature that explored the frequency of collaboration between the two disciplines. They found that of the 269 articles reviewed only 2% represented collaborations between disciplines and conclude with the following appeal:

> As architects, we make this entreaty to those who believe that the physical environment plays an important role in staff and patient outcomes – we need medical practitioners to help champion this cause. Together we have the capability of creating safer, more efficient and more curative healthcare environments.
>
> (Shepley & Watson, 2012)

2.4 Design considerations

In our literature review of 2013 (Shepley & Pasha, 2013), we encountered multiple articles advocating for particular design approaches to mental and behavioral health facilities. Some of these recommendations were by designers who were building on their experience with psychiatric facilities, and others were offered by design researchers but not necessarily supported by evidence from the studies they were describing. Experience and inference cannot be ruled out as being essential in the design process. This is particularly true in light of the limited amount of science available to inform the multiple decisions that must be made. Common understandings of behavior and experience from existing practice suggest that these are viable concepts. Many competent design decisions have been made based on the knowledge brought to the table by designers and MBH clinicians.

The following design considerations are an amalgamation of the design recommendations of multiple authors. Some guidelines were drawn from governmental entities, such as the Department of Veterans Affairs (2010) and other large organizations (Facilities Guidelines Institute, 2014) and the National Association of Psychiatric Health Systems (Hunt & Sine, 2012), and are discussed in Chapter 10.

Some of these recommendations predate the year 2000, and the characteristics of the residential populations served over this period have changed. Most notably, the number of patients in residential care has decreased significantly. Only the most acute patients have been retained in traditional psychiatric settings, a circumstance that impacts the design goals of that environment. However, we noted that the distinctions between the recommendations made by older studies and newer studies, which are primary proffered by organizations, are minimal, perhaps due to the lack of research.

Unfortunately, the majority of the studies conducted on psychiatric facilities do not elaborate on the type of mental disorders that characterize their population, likely due to the circumstance that psychiatric facilities serve a wide range of patients. Therefore, we provide generic design guidelines and considerations that apply to design of behavioral and mental health facilities in general.

As mentioned, some of the guidelines addressed in the subsequent sections are not based on specific research. However, they are included here due to the credentials of the authors and experts who were consulted in the absence of a broad research database. The content for Sections 2.5 and 2.6 is based on information from Shepley et al. (2013) and other publications. The recommendations have been divided into two categories, one summarizing issues associated with environmental psychology (Section 2.5) and the other summarizing recommendations for specific environmental settings (Section 2.6).

2.5 Environmental psychology issues

Environmental psychology issues focus on eleven topics: (1) personal space and density, (2) stress choice and control, (3) sensory considerations, (4) spatial clarity and organization, (5) comfortable and homelike surroundings, (6) high-quality, well-maintained environment, (7) positive distraction, (8) social interaction, (9) access to nature and daylight, (10) safety, and (11) supervision.

2.5.1 Personal space and density

Personal space is defined by Robert Sommer (2008) as "an area with invisible boundaries surrounding a person's body into which intruders may not come." Personal space has been described as the conceptual spatial envelope around an individual that defines that person's relationships with others (Shepley, 2017). Privacy is a related concept and a common objective in psychiatric facility design (e.g., Dvoskin et al., 2002). According to Altman (1975), privacy is the ability to control social interaction. Izumi (1968) suggests that the provision of privacy and density control, coupled with unambiguous, cohesive, and reassuring design, can support treatment goals in psychiatric units. Patients benefit from the opportunity for emotional attachment to and ownership of space. For example, a bedroom that has features supporting embellishment with personal objects that help patients express their identity is recommended (Bailey, 2002).

Density in the context of this book refers to the number of people per room or per unit. Several authors advocate for lower density patient rooms (e.g., Chou, Lu, & Mao, 2002; Forster, Cavness, &

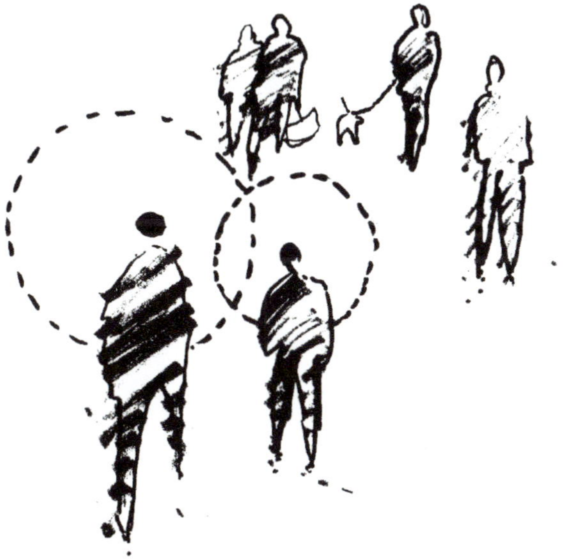

Personal space

Phelps, 1999; Izumi, 1968; Lynch, Plant, & Ryan, 2005; Martin, 1995; Salerno, Forcella, Di Fabio, Figa Talamance, & Boscolo, 2012; Turlington, 2004; Ulrich, Bogren, & Lundin, 2012; Wilson, Soth, & Robak, 1992; Wolfe, 1975), but research is lacking regarding room density and safety.

Design teams should be aware of the impact of culture, ethnicity, and race on spatial density and personal space needs. Evans et al. (2003) found that some ethnicities/races, such as African, may be more sensitive to increased densities.

2.5.2 Choice and control

Offering choices increases an individual's sense of control and thereby reduces stress. The provision of a sense of control is one of Ulrich's four primary health facility design guidelines (see Ulrich, 1999, 2000, 2001; Ulrich et al., 2008; Ulrich, Berry, Quan, & Parish, 2010) and a factor in achieving patient-centered care (Devlin & Arneill, 2003). The principle of locus of control has its foundation in personality theory and is associated with the perceived center of social control (Shepley, 2016). Mental health environments have been described as being "overshadowed" by issues of control (Johansson, Skärsäter, & Danielson, 2006).

Related to choice and control, several authors suggest that the ward environment should support patient autonomy and spontaneity. These variables are two of the ten components of the Ward Atmosphere Scale tool that evaluates facility social environment. In studies that incorporated this tool, patients subjected to coercive measures perceived less autonomy (Middelboe, Schjodt, Byrsting, & Gjerris, 2001). Von Sommaruga Howard (2004) emphasizes the need for patients to be able to modify their spaces in some way and notes that gaining new experience in the treatment facility may suggest the possibility of personal change.

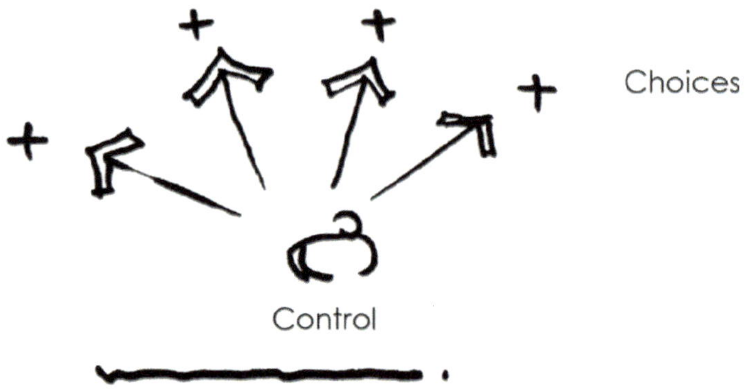

Choice and control

Staff also need options, the most significant of which is the ability to seek respite when necessary. Staff are most effective and caring for patients when their own personal needs are addressed. Therefore, consultation and therapy spaces for staff mental health consultation and therapy should be considered in a facility. One of the stressors on a unit is the potential for patient aggression against staff. Perceived negative health-related quality of life was found to be related to increased workplace violence against nurses by mental health patients (Chen, Huang, Hwang, & Chen, 2010).

2.5.3 Sensory considerations

Psychologists describe the continuum of an individual's information-processing relationship with the outside world as ranging from sensation to perception to cognition. Sensation is our spontaneous, unprocessed absorption of experience, such as the response to heat. Perception involves interpretation of experience, such as the ability to process the location of elements in space. Cognition is most commonly associated with problem solving and interpretation of experience. Sensory experience in a mental and behavioral health setting might involve any of the five senses: sight, hearing, touch, smell, and taste. Inappropriate odor, for example, can undermine the quality of the space.

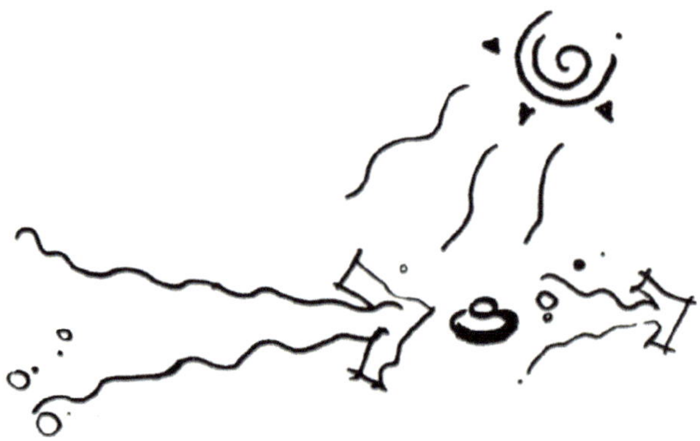

Sensory considerations

2.5.4 Spatial clarity and organization

Making sense of the world is a primary objective of functioning comfortably in the physical environment. Making sense is related to clear expressions of public versus private space, intuitively supportive wayfinding, or storage or placement of materials that meets expectations.

Confusion and conflict may take place if public versus private space is not effectively distinguished. This conflict can occur between patients or between patients and staff. The importance of effective wayfinding that distinguishes public and private space has been clearly articulated (e.g., Carpman & Grant, 2016). While wayfinding within a residential facility might not be as critical due to the scale of the environment and a resident's extended familiarity, wayfinding issues may arise when trying to locate a unit within a bigger complex or when visiting a large clinic. Regarding placement of materials, order (without boredom) is sought. Environmental psychologists discuss the notion of the importance of an enriched environment in the broader context of prospect and refuge theory (Appleton, 1996). The gist of this theory is that an ideal environment offers a balance between interest, challenge, and comprehensibility.

The physical environment, when chaotic and disorganized, can result in individuals reacting in negative ways; when clear, it can provide direction (Bartlett, 1997). Eklund and Hansson (2001) found order and organization among the most crucial contributors to patient satisfaction.

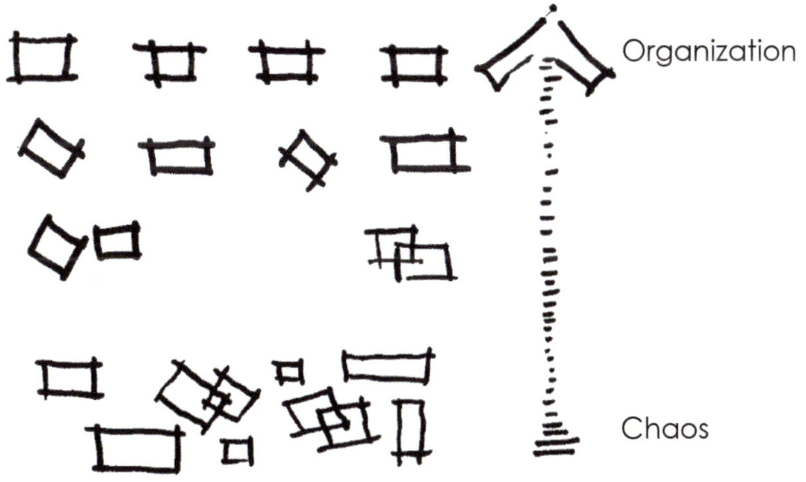

Spatial clarity and organization

2.5.5 Comfortable and homelike surroundings

A deinstitutional environment is often recommended by clinicians and designers (Baltazar, Kapp, Tugny, & Furtado, 2013; Doherty & Sell, 2011). Von Sommaruga Howard (2004) makes the point that in a regular hospital the bedroom is a place of therapy while in a psychiatric facility it is a place to sleep, perhaps with someone we don't know. Shared bedrooms are a hallmark of an institutional setting and may have a negative impact on patients. Residents in Grosenick and Hatmaker's (2000) study said an institutional-looking facility reminded them of treatment and disease.

Defining deinstitutional or homelike environments is challenging for designers and researchers alike. Many consider the notion of home as the setting where we are provided choice and control (Csikszentmihalyi & Rochberg-Halton, 1981) rather than an environment with a specific aesthetic. Spivak identified 13 characteristics that focus on the most fundamental activities of daily living – shelter, sleep, mate, groom, feed, excrete, store, territory, play, route, meet, compete, and work (Spivak, 1984) – and recommends supporting these activities when practical. Another step in deinstitutionalizing a behavioral health environment is reducing the boundaries between staff and patients (Firth, 2004). Homelikeness is one of a variety of gestures conveying meaning in a psychiatric experience about which designers should be aware (Andes & Shattell, 2006; Remen, 1991).

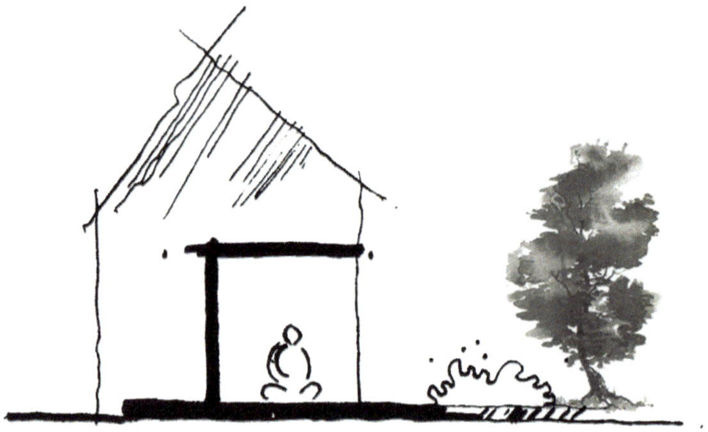

Comfortable and homelike

However, when pressed to address aesthetic qualities, recommendations are that the design should be stylistically familiar to the experience of residents (noninstitutional), safe, have a means of access to nature (windows, courtyards, etc.), and grant privacy through the provision of single-occupant rooms. Carr (2011) also mentions cheerful and noninstitutional materials, reduced noise from building systems, operable lighting, and access to radio and TV. Homelike in the traditional sense might not be appropriate due to the prior experience of patients, who may have negative associations with the traditional aesthetics of homes. Homelike environment extends beyond the building itself to the site. (See Section 2.6.)

2.5.6 High-quality, well-maintained environment

Staff and patients have registered a desire for a higher-quality and well-maintained environment (Davis et al., 1979), and these features are among the guidelines recommended in the *Whole Building Design Guide* produced by the National Institute of Building Sciences (Carr, 2011).

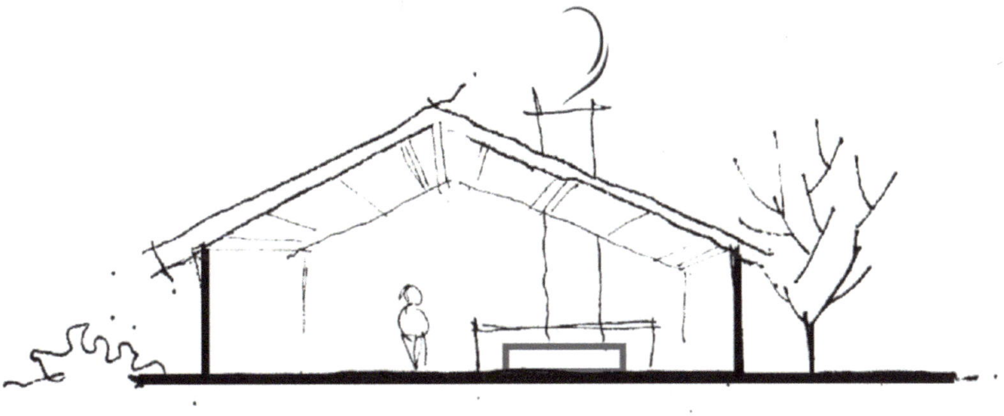

High-quality, well-maintained environment

Grosenick and Hatmaker (2000) surveyed staff in a drug rehabilitation facility and determined that well-maintained, comfortable lounge furniture positively impacted treatment goals. Potthoff (1995) also found that furniture and finishes related to satisfaction in three rehabilitation facilities. Likewise, Holahan and Saegert (1973) found more positive attitudes were associated with a remodeled ward that had new furniture and paint and bedcovers.

Staff are impacted as well. Christenfeld, Wagner, Pastva, and Acrish (1989) conducted a pre- and post-occupancy of two wards that included improvements in finishes and furnishings and found more positive staff mood and lower frequency of unscheduled staff absences.

2.5.7 Positive distraction

In the early 1980s, research on a cluster of potentially supportive environmental dimensions became more widespread. Instead of addressing reduction of the negative aspects of the environment, the focus was redirected at the creation and reinforcement of positive experiences (Shepley, 2006). These experiences are intended to allow a patient to project him or herself into an experience outside the healthcare setting – typically a less threatening and more healing space. The focus of this new research was positive distraction, or "the ability to allow the individual to shift focus from negative foci within the health environment to the more restorative aspects of the non-medical world" (Shepley, 2006, p. S34). Among the factors that contribute to positive distraction are art, music, entertainment (TV, computer-sourced), books/magazines, social interaction, and nature. Art and music find their place in the mental and behavioral health setting in two roles – one in which the patient listens to music or observes art, and one in which the patient uses art and music as tools for therapy.

Researchers found that when art depicting restorative nature was introduced in a psychiatric patient lounge, patients requested less anxiety medication – an indication that art helped lower

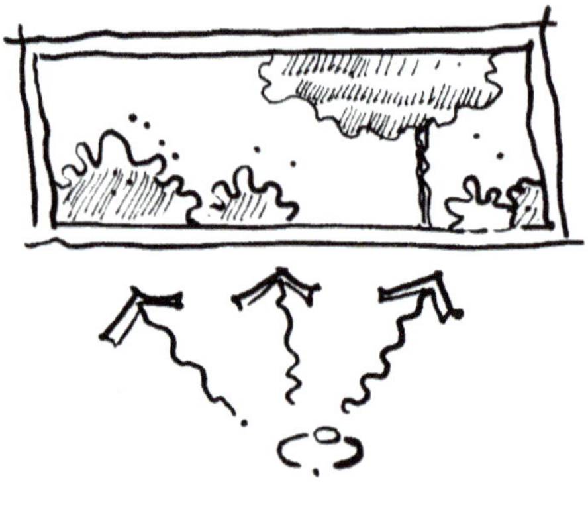

Positive distraction

patient anxiety and agitation (Nanda, Eisen, Zadeh, & Owen, 2011). Nanda, Gaydos, Hathorn, and Watkins (2010) suggest the following for art themes in a behavioral health facility for war veterans:

- Water scenes with nonturbulent water.
- Nature scenes with open foreground, broad-canopy trees, savannah landscapes, and rich vegetation.
- Positive cultural images (e.g., historic neighborhoods).
- Fresh, familiar flowers in gardens with open foregrounds.
- Figurative, emotionally positive people's faces.

Music, sports, and recreational activities may have a healing impact (MacKinnon, 2009). Music has been found to contribute to reduced aggression in psychiatric settings. Cummings, Grandfield, and Coldwell (2010) introduced a space dedicated to relaxation in their unit – a comfort room – that included low light and soft music and found the room reduced patient stress. Overall, the role of music is considered to be an effective tool, although not as effective as other therapies (Choi, 1997).

Social interaction and access to nature are a common means of achieving positive distraction, but because of their significance, they are addressed separately in the following two sections.

2.5.8 Social interaction

Designers and clinicians encourage interaction between patients, staff, and visitors for the purpose of socialization and exposure to real-world environments (Porter & Easter, 1980). Spaces for one-on-one interaction are specifically recommended, as well as dayrooms and common areas to encourage interaction and community (Davis et al., 1979; Devlin, 1992; Gutkowski,

Ginath, & Guttmann, 1992; Sidman & Moos, 1973; Turlington, 2004). Furniture arrangement, both chairs and group tables, is also critical and has been found to impact interaction (Gutkowski et al., 1992; Timko, 1996). While the majority of interactions take place in activity and dining areas, the dayroom, nurse station area, and halls are also commonly used (Fairbanks et al., 1977).

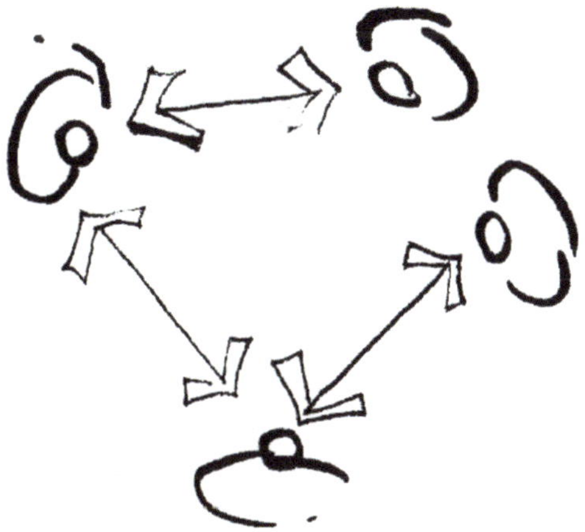

Social interaction

2.5.9 Access to nature and daylight

Of all the guidelines endorsed by designers and researchers regarding healthcare settings, access to nature, both direct and indirect, has received the greatest support, perhaps due to its intuitive reasonableness. Among the many researchers who have found evidence in support of this approach in behavioral and mental health settings are Perkins (2013), Shepley (1995), and Ulrich et al. (2012). Benedetti, Colombo, Barbini, Campori, and Smeraldi (2001) found that sunlight reduced length of stay in hospitalized bipolar patients, and Olver, Love, Daniel, Norman, and Nicholls (2009) found a reduction in seclusion episodes when patients were relocated to a new unit with higher levels of daylight.

Apart from passive interaction, Paget and White (2004) recommend access to nature as a tool in the therapy process and as a means to support social interaction. Additionally, interaction may play a special developmental role with regard to children and adolescents (Bailey, 2002).

Daylight and views are important factors in a healing environment (Arneill, 1959; Davis et al., 1979; Gutkowski & Guttman, 1992; Turlington, 2004; Ulrich et al., 2012). Bakos, Bozic, Chapin, and Neuman (1980) found that the introduction of improved lighting in conjunction with other modifications resulted in improved behavioral changes in a state geriatric facility.

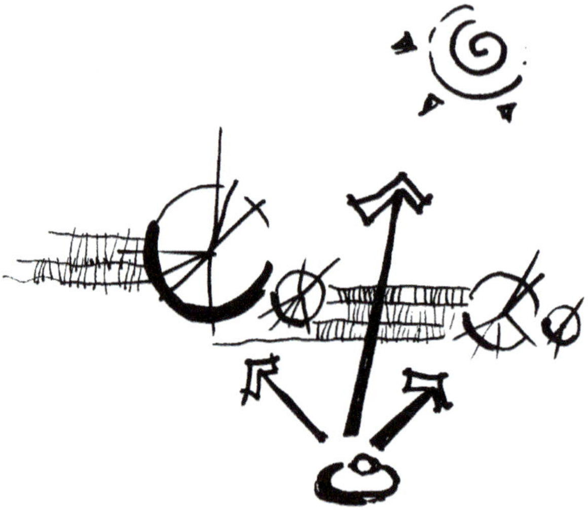

Access to nature and daylight

2.5.10 Safety

The provision of security while avoiding patient intimidation is a goal for designers seeking patient and staff safety (Porter & Easter, 1980). Jeffers (1991) reminds us that supervision protocols are essential to creating a safe environment for patients. Dix (2001) recommends that mental health facility staff consider safety measures against aggression, impulsive behavior, and absconding, while accommodating a range of therapeutic activities.

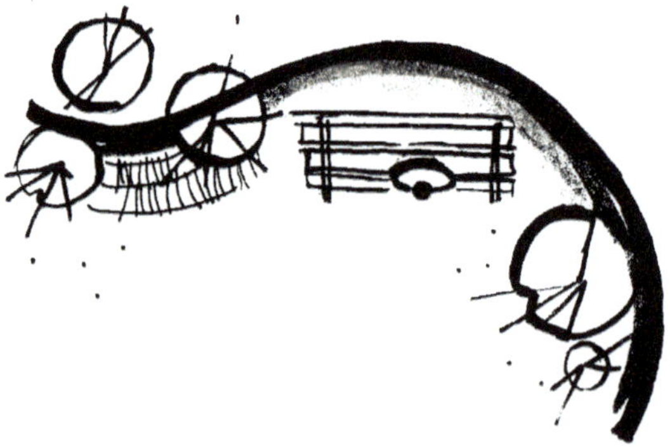

Safety

Staff safety and security are impacted by both operational and physical environmental features. Concern for patient self-harm or aggressive behavior is a primary issue for staff in a psychiatric patient ward (Salerno et al., 2012). Poor environment and locked doors may contribute to these undesirable outcomes. While trying to achieve safety, the appearance of intimidation must be limited. Von Sommaruga Howard (2004) makes a distinction between "being held safe, being restrained or being imprisoned. . . . A locked door does not necessarily provide security, but it does restrict physical access and provide a powerfully restrictive emotional symbol" (p. 74). She also notes that poorly designed surveillance windows create an atmosphere that will not be therapeutic. Security needs vary depending on diagnosis, from those who are very aggressive to those who are very withdrawn (Davis et al., 1979).

2.5.11 *Supervision*

Supervision is critical to the safety of patients. Whitehead, Polsky, Crookshank, and Fik (1984) found that an open nurse station encouraged staff to interact more frequently with patients and that patients feel the configuration increased their sense of wellness. Ulrich et al. (2012) found reductions in the use of restraints when a more open nurse station was part of a bundle of environmental features.

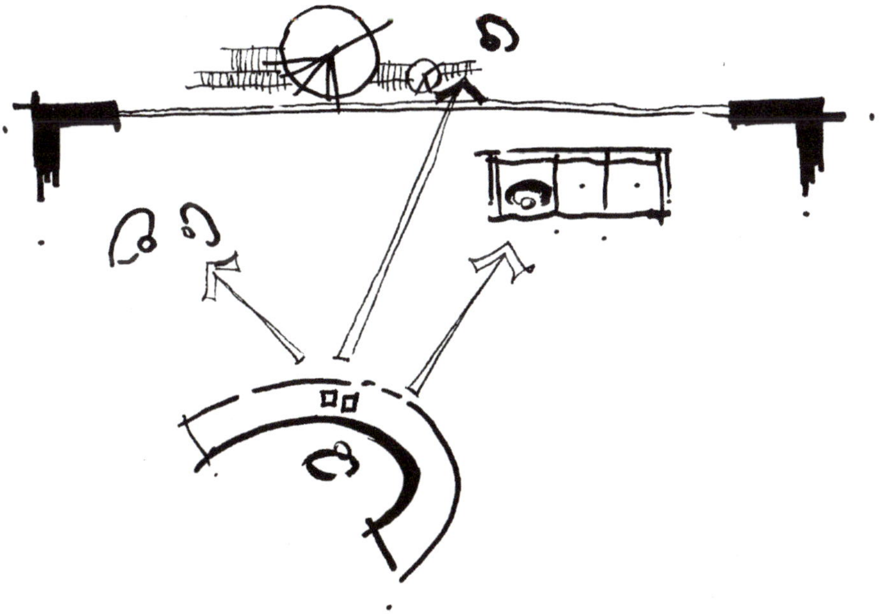

Supervision

Open nurse stations are basic to the Planetree philosophy (Turlington, 2004). Christenfeld et al. (1989) describe the impact of a nurse station that was relocated to increase supervision of the dayroom, entry, and adjoining area, and resulted in improved staff mood, fewer unscheduled absences, enhanced patient self-image, greater satisfaction, and less violence.

2.6 Specific setting issues

2.6.1 *Inpatient common areas, inpatient patient spaces, and overall recommendations*

Common areas include entries, circulation spaces, open spaces near nurse stations, dayrooms, lounges, activity rooms, kitchens, multipurpose rooms, and similar shared items. *Patient spaces* focus on patient private and semiprivate spaces such as bedrooms and bathrooms. Recommendations are summarized in Figure 2.2.

Figure 2.2: *Recommendations for residential/inpatient settings*

	Residential/inpatient overall space	*Residential/inpatient patient space*
Privacy, personal space, density	Avoid overcrowding. Densities can vary depending on the activity and the ethnic/racial background of the patient population per the previous literature review; increase the body-buffer zones for individuals with schizophrenia. Provide acoustical privacy in therapeutic spaces.	Clusters of <11 patients (ideally 8) per pod. Use open layout, with no unnecessary barriers; avoid overcrowding. Use a combination of double and single patient rooms. Provide a minimum of one restroom per two patients attached to patient room. Include a shower, if possible. If not, provide at least one shower per four patients adjacent to patient room.
Stress, choice, control	Provide access to a kitchen and a variety of portions of the facility when possible; group kitchens may provide therapeutic milieu. Provide access to facilities for physical exercise. Design spaces that support a range of treatment activities; provide spaces for autonomy; provide spatial flexibility. Introduce blues in areas where calming is important.	Provide opportunities to personalize the bedroom. In shared room settings provide options external to the room for privacy. Offer options for bedding and artwork. Seclusion rooms should be painted with pale colors, probably blues and greens, not white or gray.
Sensory considerations	Incorporate moderate noise light stimulation via soft, indirect, full-spectrum lighting. Neutralize odors through proper air exchange and the use of cleaning materials with minimal scent. Control for noise; avoid long corridors and reverberant spaces; use color to a adjust corridor proportions.	Provide large windows to enhance the senses and reduce delirium. Consider operable windows with limiters. Allow for individualized control of temperature, within a bracketed range. Provide acoustical control between bedrooms.
Spatial clarity/ organization	Clear separations between functional areas and circulation. Provide visual cues that help building users to understand the function of spaces. Address human scale by providing appropriate transitions between personal, semiprivate, and private space.	Use built-in furniture to delineate bedroom divisions in semiprivate rooms. Create semiprivate vestibules outside rooms to provide an intermediate semiprivate space.

	Residential/inpatient overall space	Residential/inpatient patient space
Comfortable, homelike	Corridors should increase in width, dependent on the population, to accommodate activity level. Provide spaces that parallel functions experienced in the home by focusing on activity type rather than traditional setting. Limit furniture in areas with patients in wheelchairs. Style should be familiar and indigenous, not "decorative" or "trendy."	Offer options for bedding and artwork. Provide wall and shelving space for personal photos or keepsakes. Avoid metal beds or furniture. Provide electric beds for the elderly.
High-quality, well-maintained	Locate service areas accessible to both the unit and service corridor. Locate serviceable parts of patient-room to allow service without entering the room. Select furniture/finishes that minimize frequent need for repair and replacement, while reflecting aesthetic qualities. Provide sufficient housekeeping areas.	Patient rooms should have enough abuse resistance to allow time for an appropriate response team to arrive.
Positive distraction	Provide visual art throughout the unit and in the gardens. Focus on art with restorative image content (primarily nature and positive social content). Provide access to individualized music. Provide opportunities for social interaction and access to nature.	Provide views from the head of the patient bed. Provide comfortable seating with lighting that allows for reading. Provide audio jacks for listening to music.
Social interaction	Gathering areas for patients near the nurse station are encouraged. Include private visiting areas and spaces that support family participation. Maintain links to the local community.	Room configurations that allow for furniture to be located to support a two-person conversation. Cordless check-out phones may be provided to allow the patient to have private conversations when appropriate.
Nature and daylight	Provide windows or access to daylight in all rooms occupied by patients. Provide access to porch areas, outdoor gardens.	Locate windows to serve as focal points in the room and provide views. Provide sunlight and fresh air. Provide multiple windows with views of nature.
Safety	Limit window opening widths in secure facilities; avoid hiding places and blind corners. Adhere to all recommendations in professional guidelines regarding equipment, hardware, and materials. Doors shouldn't swing into areas where people may be moving past.	Patient bedroom doors that can readily be opened by staff in emergencies are essential. Outwardly open doors are preferred but must not swing into the corridor. See guidelines for details regarding specification of furniture, finishes, and equipment.
Supervision	Staff-controlled exits and entrances are necessary. Provide visual access to patients in common spaces except in private, suicide-resistant areas. Make all one-on-one patients with staff visible from a public area to avoid potential abuse or accusations of abuse.	Observation through a door light is recommended.

2.6.2 Outpatient settings

Outpatient settings incorporate all ambulatory care environments including nontraditional (e.g., club/membership) psychiatric care. Recommendations are provided in Figure 2.3.

2.6.3 Staff spaces

Staff are often overlooked in the development of design recommendations. A variety of recommendations are provided in Figure 2.4.

2.6.4 Finishes, furniture, and equipment

Recommendations for finishes, furniture, and equipment are intended to apply to all mental and behavioral health environments, varying depending on the characteristics of the patient population. See Figure 2.5.

Figure 2.3: *Recommendations for outpatient settings*

	Outpatient
Privacy, personal space, density	Provide acoustical privacy at the registration desk and in patient treatment and therapy areas. A minimum of 20 square feet per person has been suggested for standard waiting areas (including space for a receptionist); 30 square feet per person would be a more appropriate standard in a healthcare setting.
Stress, choice, control	Avoid dark, double-loaded therapy room corridors.
Sensory considerations	Provide daylight and acoustical control in patient and staff areas.
Spatial clarity/ organization	The spatial layout of a freestanding clinic should be apparent from the exterior of the building. Whether freestanding or part of a larger structure, landmarks and views outdoors should guide the circulation process.
Comfortable, homelike	Quality chairs, such as what you would find in a traditional healthcare setting, will be appropriate for a clinic facility.
High-quality, well-maintained	Lack of maintenance reflects on patient perception of the quality of care. Furniture and finishes should be selected that are difficult to damage and are easily cleanable.
Positive distraction	Provide views of nature and art in waiting rooms and therapy spaces. When possible, provide books, individualized music, and access to the Internet.
Social interaction	Arrange seating in waiting area to allow for dyads. Provide sufficient space in some therapy rooms to allow for family participation.
Nature and daylight	Provide a courtyard adjacent to therapy areas for outdoor sessions.
Safety	Reception staff should be visible by other staff members. Furniture and finishes should be selected to prevent potential harm to staff and other patients.
Supervision	All patients in the waiting room should be visible from the receptionist station.

Figure 2.4: *Recommendations for staff*

	Staff
Privacy, personal space, density	Nursing station should not serve as a physical barrier that prevents normal interaction between patient and caregiver. Chart rooms and other staff areas should be located so conversations regarding patients and other clinical matters are not overheard by patients or visitors. Staff lounge and outdoor spaces should not be visible by the public.
Stress, choice, control	While open nurse stations are typically preferred, staff in the nursing station should be visible by staff in adjacent locations.
Sensory considerations	Provide daylight and acoustical control in staff areas.
Spatial clarity/ organization	Design an easily identifiable reception area that reflects the treatment goals and expectations.
Comfortable, homelike	Provide staff lockers, group lounge area, and adequate office space for staff.
High-quality, well-maintained	Furniture and finishes should be noninstitutional (e.g., comfortable couch) and easily maintained. Staff lounge should include or be adjacent to locker space with a staff bathroom.
Positive distraction	Include staff lounge and garden.
Social interaction	Furniture arrangements in the staff lounge should support small groups and dyads.
Nature and daylight	Researchers recommend direct access from the lounge to outdoor space. If not possible, a window with a view to nature is recommended. Minimally, "borrowed" daylight from adjacent spaces and nature artwork should be used.
Safety	Locate nursing stations next to seclusion rooms, if possible. Nurse stations should provide the least possible barrier between staff while preventing patients from jumping over the counter.
Supervision	All spaces that are accessible by both patients and staff must be visible by other staff.

Figure 2.5: *Recommendations for furniture, finishes, and equipment*

	Furniture, Finishes, and Equipment
Privacy, personal space, density	Locate furniture to reduce the impression of density by creating seating clusters of various sizes. Varying cluster sizes, from one to four chairs, will also support privacy preferences. Provide open vistas to reduce sense of enclosure.
Stress, choice, control	Use modular furniture so it can be converted and rearranged. Provide soothing artwork and pictures of familiar images. Use framing systems to allow for a changing art program. Select art based on nature images and positive human affect.
Sensory considerations	Avoid artificial materials, complex patterns, color stimulation, monochromic schemes, and reflective surfaces. Provide acoustical control to reduce reverberation.
Spatial clarity/ organization	Create clear divisions between public, semipublic, semiprivate, and private spaces. Provide views to the outdoors that reinforce understanding of interior space relative to the outside. Use finishes to differentiate areas and support activities and space.

	Furniture, Finishes, and Equipment
Comfortable, homelike	Specify upholstered comfortable furniture. Specify noninstitutional furniture. Specify materials for their symbolic meaning rather than for purely functional purposes. Incorporate infrastructure for new technology and access to computers when possible.
High-quality, well-maintained	Use natural wood when possible. Furniture should not be located adjacent to a fence or wall. Use movable furniture, which is heavy to throw; shatterproof glass, tamperproof outlets, and lockable water taps; eliminate sharp corners. Provide durable, cleanable furniture and finishes.
Positive distraction	Artwork can contribute to positive distraction.
Social interaction	Arrange furniture in circular group arrangements as well as dyads.
Nature and daylight	Some seating should be located to allow views to the outdoors or the ability to sit in sun patch areas.
Safety	Furniture must weigh enough so it can't be thrown and sturdy enough so it can't be broken and used to inflict harm. Artwork must be secured to walls.
Supervision	All seating should be visually accessible from the nurse station.

2.7 Site and building envelope and configuration

The external appearance of the clinic or residential building has a significant impact on how clients perceive their care.

- Make the building contextual with the streetscape and easily accessible to vehicles and pedestrians.
- Demonstrate its purpose as a healing environment.
- Use courtyards instead of fenced outdoor areas.
- Avoid placing trees close to the building.
- Provide retreat/private spaces (Shepley et al., 2013).

Chrysikou (2014) presents a matrix of design elements at the site and building envelope/configuration scale focusing on safety and security, competence, and personalization/choice. Chrysikou suggests that layout is the primary element influencing safety, but location, decoration, entrance, capacity, and landscape are also factors. Concerning competence, landscape, layout, decoration, and scale are important. For personalization and choice, landscape, layout, decoration, and scale were pertinent. Interestingly, in Chrysikou's research, façade style was not thought to impact safety, competence, or personalization and choice. This is reasonable, as style preferences tend to vary. Figure 2.6 provides a visual summary of the data from her 2014 publication.

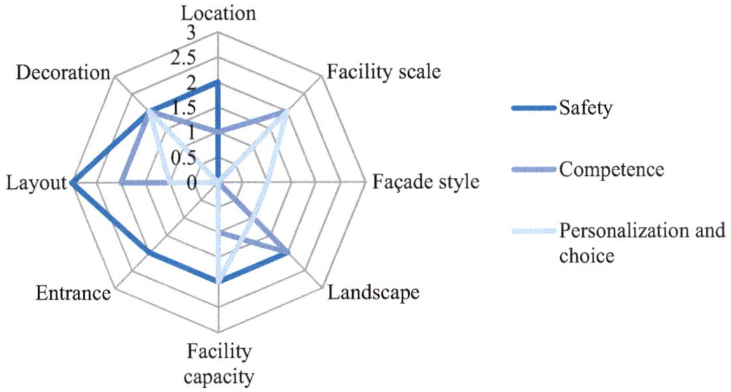

Figure 2.6: *Site scale features and their contribution to safety, competence, and personalization (Data source: Chrysikou, 2014)*

2.8 Case studies

This chapter and the subsequent six chapters conclude with a case study or studies that were selected based on the degree to which the project demonstrated principles addressed in the associated chapter and public acknowledgements of success as demonstrated through recommendations of experts and awards.

2.8.1 Dandenong Hospital

Location:	Melbourne, Australia
Designer/Architect:	Bates Smart in association with the Irwin Alsop Group and LBA Design
Client:	Department of Health/Southern Health
Completion:	Stage 1 – September 2011; Stage 2 – June 2013
Area:	8,200 square meters

Awards: AIA National Award 2014 Public Architecture; AIA Victorian Awards 2014 Public Architecture (New); Australian Timber Design Awards 2014, Overall Award for Timber Design; Australian Timber Design Awards 2014, Excellence in Timber Design, Multi Residential, New Buildings

Client, service users, and services

In 2007, the Australian Department of Human Services appointed Bates Smart in association with the Irwin Alsop Group to design a mental health facility with a 50-bed adult acute unit, a 50-bed secure extended care unit, and a 20-bed aged care assessment unit. Monash Health, the health system operating the facility, is the largest public health service in Melbourne, Australia, and provides services to nearly a quarter of metropolitan Melbourne's population (Monash Health, 2016).

Mission and goals

The goal of the project is to provide an inviting, calm, and safe environment where treatment and healing take place simultaneously. Outdoor and activity areas are intended to promote social interaction. Supervision and observation of patients are facilitated by an open layout floor plan, which increases both accessibility and visibility. Among the objectives of the design are to provide a sense of place and identity for each zone, flexibility of spaces, and blending of indoor and outdoor areas.

Courtyards, while still enclosed and protected by the mass of interior spaces, do not incorporate peripheral standalone walls in an effort to avoid a sense of imprisonment. Patients can freely wander from interior spaces into these courtyards. Flexibility of design, daylit interiors, and timber cladding are intended to reflect a residential environment and thereby avoid an institutional look.

Site

The facility is located in Dandenong, a suburb of Melbourne, approximately 30 kilometers southeast of Melbourne's central business district. The acute mental health facility is nested among suburban residences and incorporates public, semipublic, and private interfaces. The exterior configuration expresses the interior spaces and configuration of surrounding buildings. Diversity in scale, texture, and openness present a variegated streetscape for the adjacent community.

Program

Each of the three units in the facility (Adult Acute, Aged Acute, and SECU) are supported by treatment rooms, staff stations, and consultation and interview rooms, as well as clean and soiled utility rooms. Private patient rooms (with their own separate en suite bathroom) are placed along single-loaded corridors, each wrapped around one of the 16 courtyards in the facility. All bedrooms have external views that enable patients to maintain contact with the outside world. In addition to the courtyards, patients have access to a variety of social spaces on each unit, such as dining areas, activity rooms, and multifunction pavilions. Each unit is also equipped with a laundry room and a patient property storage area. A separate entry is provided for ambulance and police admissions.

A central administrative area contains staff lounge rooms, offices, and a satellite pharmacy. A pneumatic tube system is utilized to deliver medications and prescriptions to key rooms within the unit. The main units are connected to a central Research and Training building.

Configuration and construction

The mass of the facility (composed of four buildings connected through pavilions) incorporates 16 internal glazed courtyards. Common spaces have direct access to these courtyards that provide daylight to the corridors and patient bedrooms. Phase construction was necessary to allow for the maintenance of existing residential mental health units on-site. Blackbutt timber was selected for external cladding and exposed columns. Anti-ligature provisions were employed in all designs, fittings, fixtures, and building systems. Masonry is used in the interior walls to support temperature stability inside the building. In-slab heating and cooling were used in conjunction with fresh air ventilation to enhance the internal thermal environment. All building systems are accessible from the roof space to enable maintenance without disturbing patients or patient activities. The security system is connected to the fire alarm, telephone, and the hospital's duress system. Sustainably designed features such as underground storage of rainwater for irrigation and flushing, recycled and rapidly renewable material, heat recovery in the ventilation system, automatic lighting systems, and bicycle storage are incorporated into the project.

Case study bibliography

Monash Health. (2016). *Monash Health, a world of healthcare: About us*. Retrieved August 10, 2016, from www.monashhealth.org/page/About_Us

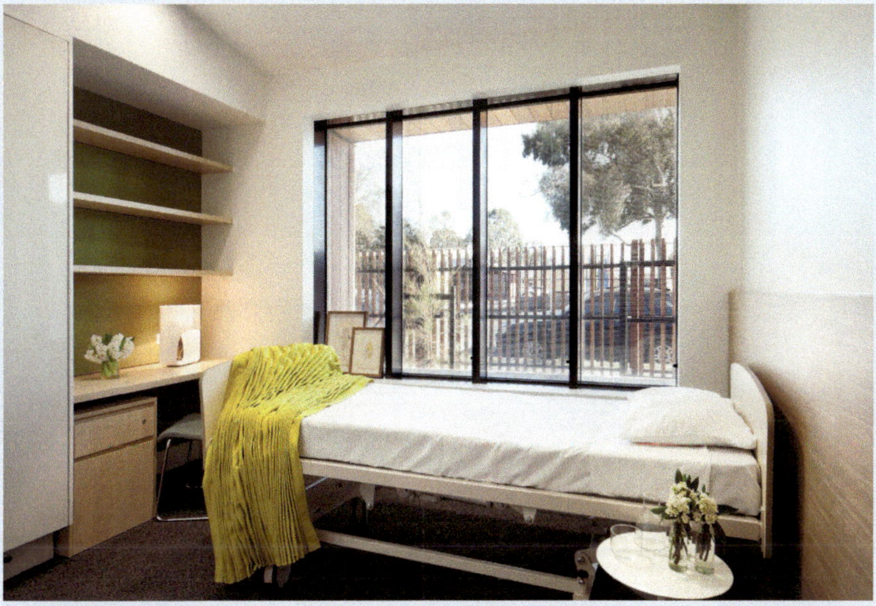

Figure 2.7: *Dandenong – patient bedroom (Architects: Bates Smart in association with Irwin Alsop; Photo credit: John Gollings)*

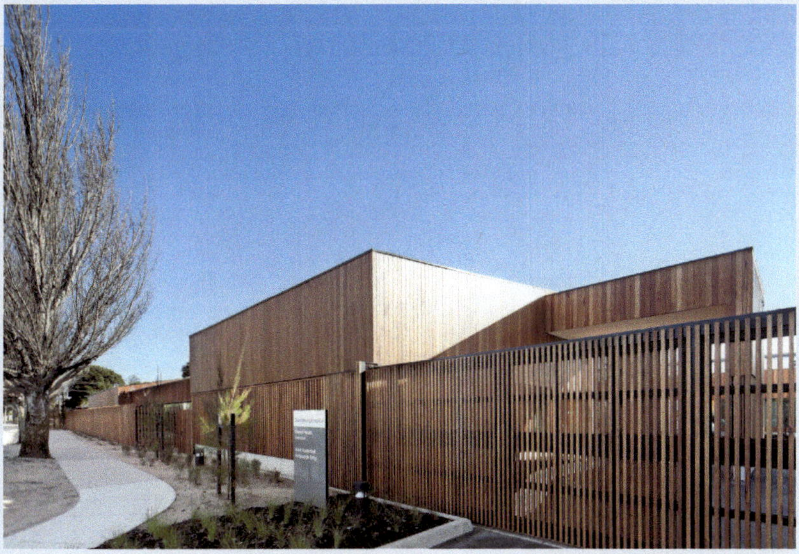

Figure 2.8: *Dandenong – exterior view (Architects: Bates Smart in association with Irwin Alsop; Photo credit: John Gollings)*

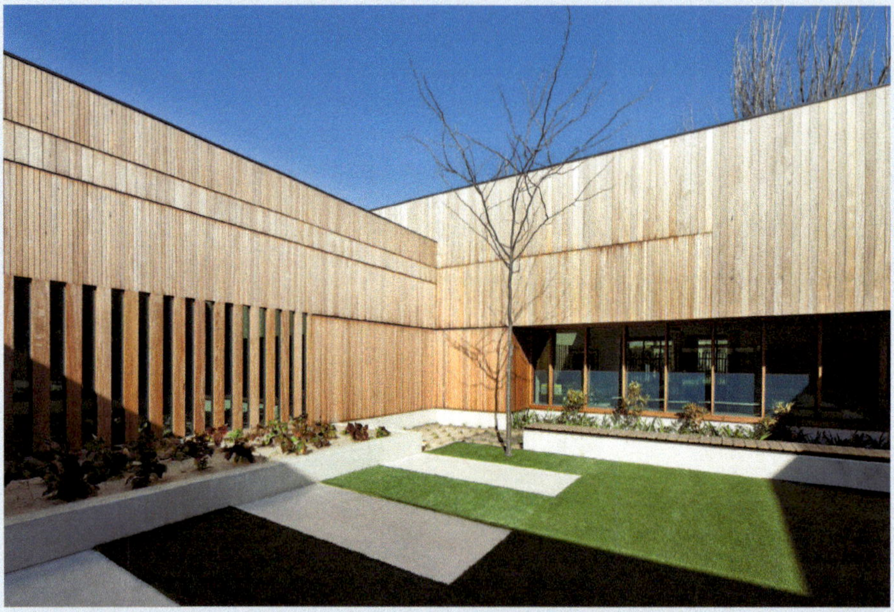

Figure 2.9: *Dandenong – courtyard (Architects: Bates Smart in association with Irwin Alsop; Photo credit: John Gollings)*

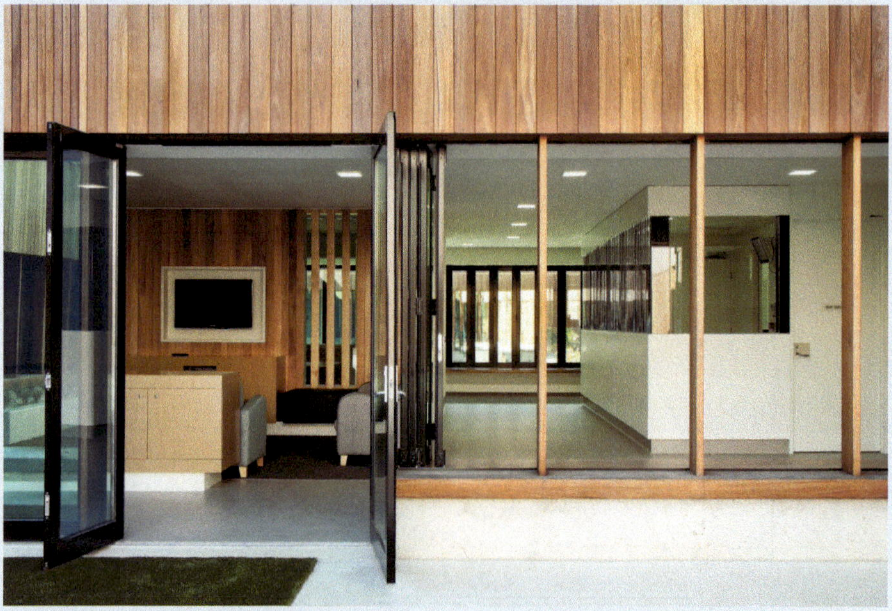

Figure 2.10: *Dandenong – reception, waiting room (Architects: Bates Smart in association with Irwin Alsop; Photo credit: John Gollings)*

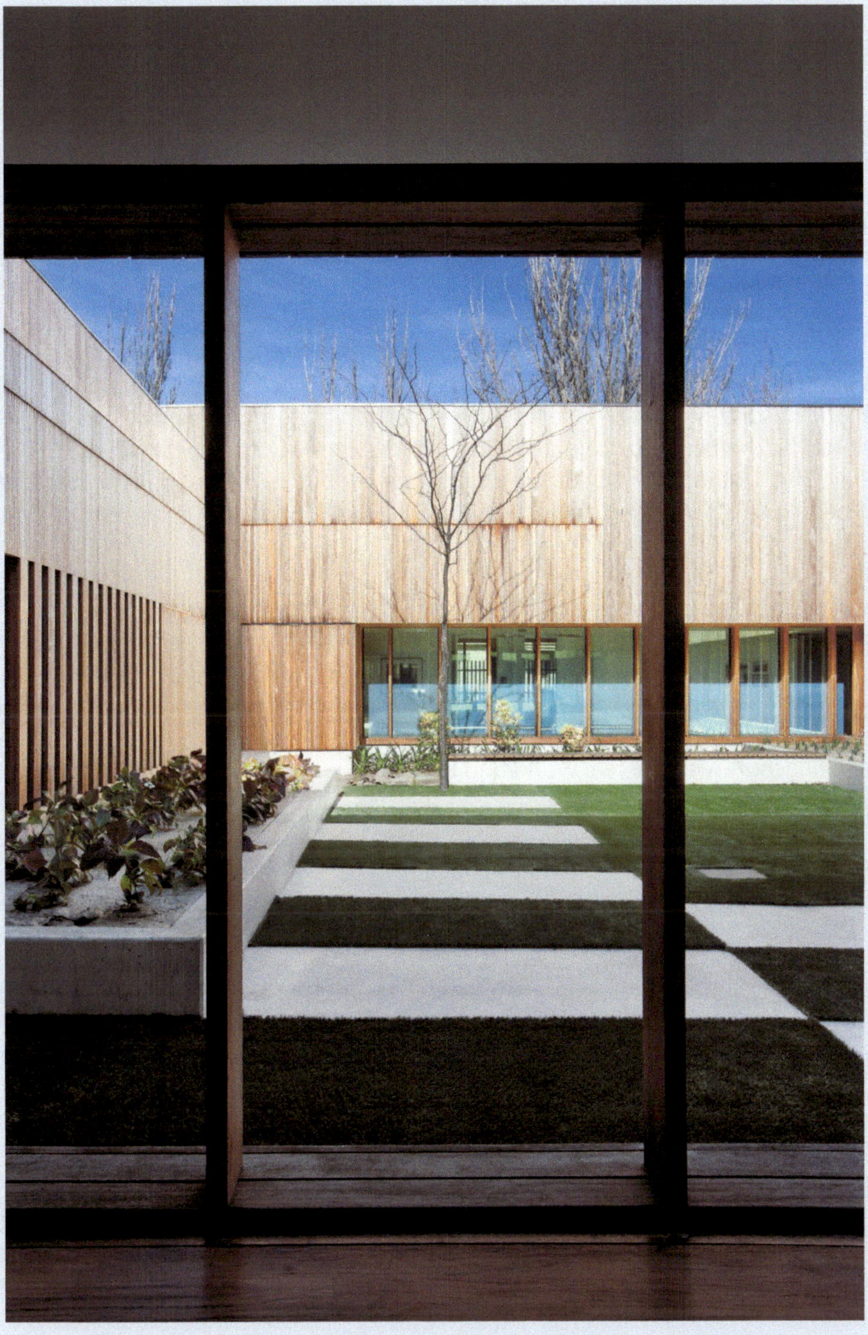

Figure 2.11: *Dandenong – view into courtyard (Architects: Bates Smart in association with Irwin Alsop; Photo credit: John Gollings)*

2.8.2 Psychiatric hospital in Slagelse

Location:	Slagelse, Denmark
Designer/Architect:	Karlsson Arkitekter & Vilhelm Lauritzen Arkitekter
Client:	Region Sjælland (Region Zealand)
Completion:	2015
Area:	44,000 square meters

Awards: The Danish Color Prize 2016; The Construction Client Award 2016; 2016 Healthcare Design Award; Short-listed for WAN Award 2016; Finalist in WAF Award 2016; Finalist in AR Health Awards 2016

Client, service users, and services

The psychiatric hospital supports patients in the Sjælland region and includes 194 inpatient beds and ambulatory and emergency care services with the capacity to support 200 to 300 consultations per day. The 194 inpatient beds are designated as 114 public psychiatric beds, 50 forensic psychiatric beds, and 30 high-security beds dedicated to the Security Department.

Mission and goals

This facility is designated to play a key role in future psychiatric treatment training and research. Another goal of the psychiatric hospital in Slagelse (GAPS) is to support psychiatric patients in developing social competencies and basic skills. Sports and other physical activities are included in the treatment program and subsequently manifested in the built environment. To help patients maintain a connection with the real world and the surrounding community, landscaping and daylighting is used to reflect changing daytime and seasons, and the park surrounding the hospital is accessible to the public. Interior design features include color schemes and poetry created by the artist Malene Landgreen and poet Ursula Andkjær Olsen, respectively.

Site

The site, with an area of 158,463 square meters, is located on the outskirts of a small town 100 kilometers southwest of Copenhagen, Denmark. The woodlands and park surrounding the site are open to the public. The town's tennis club and sports stadium are located adjacent to the health campus. The site is accessible from an expressway connecting Slagelse to Copenhagen.

Program

The psychiatric hospital includes 194 inpatient beds. All the rooms are private with bathrooms and are located on the ground floor. The complex also includes programs for training, recreation, research, and education as well as workspace for 650 employees.

The recreation program consists of two sports halls, a swimming pool, outdoor training areas, and more than 40 courtyards and gardens. The gardens have diverse designs and scales and can host a variety of options for outdoor activities for either patients or staff.

Configuration and construction

The building's exterior has an uncomplicated and simple façade of warm yellow handmade bricks nested in a landscape of wild grass and oak trees. Patient units are all located on the ground floor and are perforated by several courtyards to take advantage of daylight. The wards are connected by a five-story atrium that is enclosed by offices and research and teaching spaces. Specialists work in open activity-based workspaces. Glass has been used along the perimeter of staff working spaces in the wards for better supervision of the ward. The project uses dynamic LED lighting technology that follows the circadian rhythm. Color has been used to enhance identity and wayfinding.

Case study bibliography

Karlsson Arkitekter & Vilhelm Lauritzen Arkitekter. (2015). Project information and other in-house publication materials.

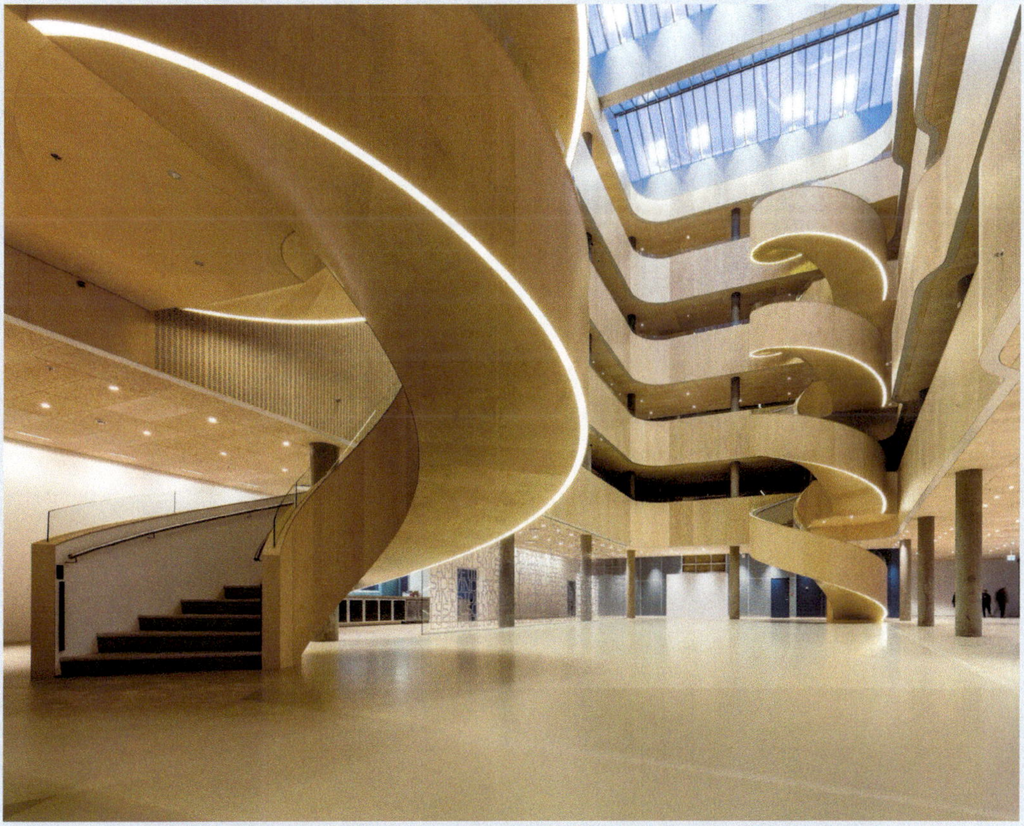

Figure 2.12: *GAPS – outpatient clinic and atrium (Architects: Karlsson Arkitekter/Vilhelm Lauritzen Arkitekter; Photo credit: Jens Lindhe)*

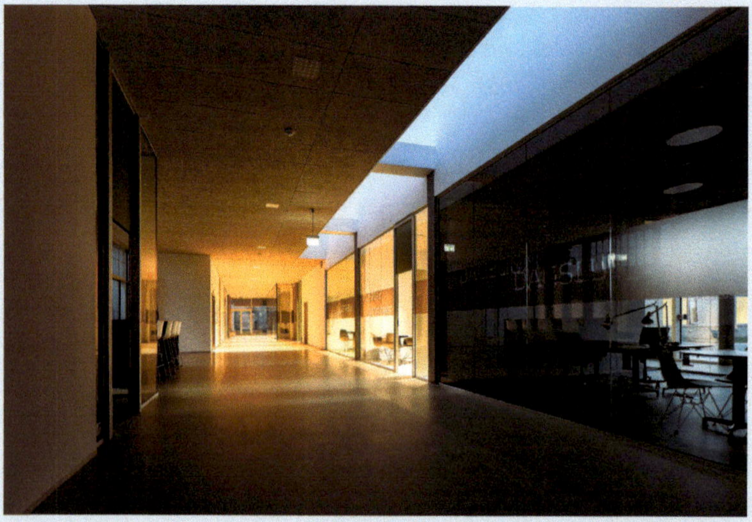

Figure 2.13: *GAPS – common space between wards (Architects: Karlsson Arkitekter/Vilhelm Lauritzen Arkitekter; Photo credit: Jens Lindhe)*

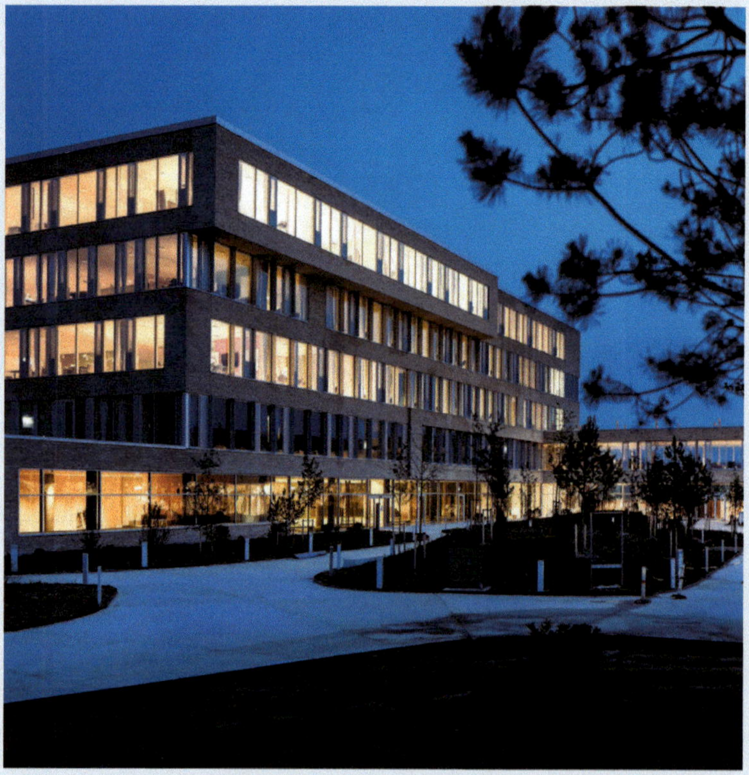

Figure 2.14: *GAPS – exterior night (Architects: Karlsson Arkitekter/Vilhelm Lauritzen Arkitekter; Photo credit: Jens Lindhe)*

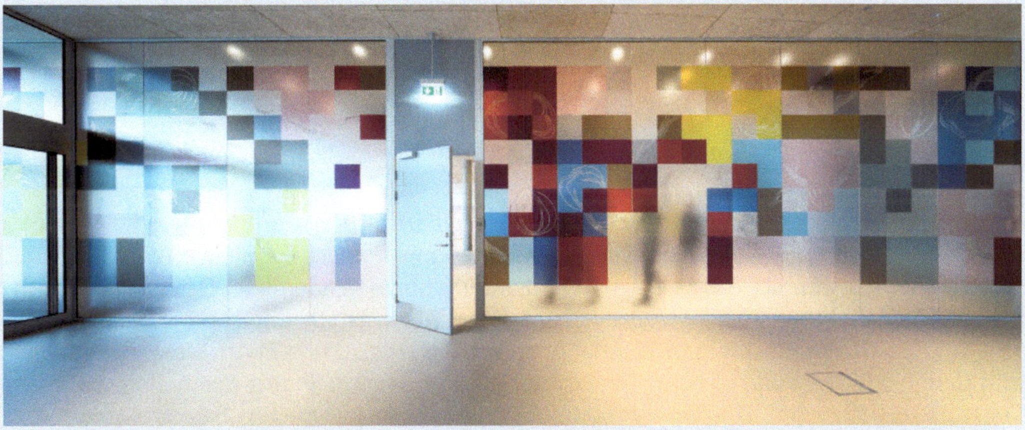

Figure 2.15: *GAPS – glass wall at the main entrance with art by Malene Landgreen (Architects: Karlsson Arkitekter/Vilhelm Lauritzen Arkitekter; Photo credit: Jens Lindhe)*

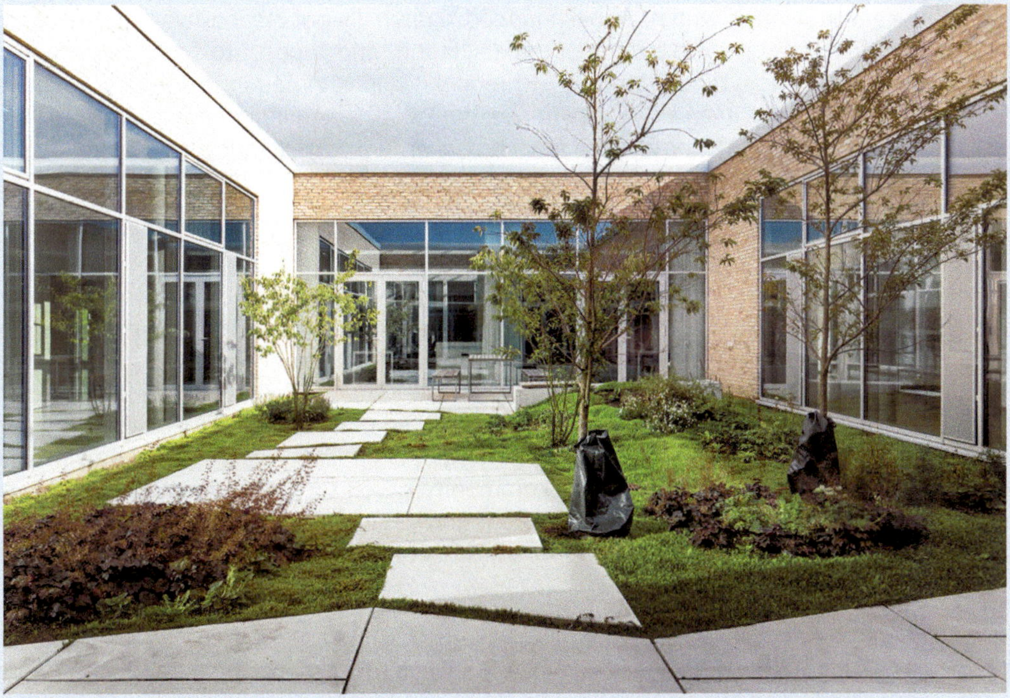

Figure 2.16: *GAPS – courtyard (Architects: Karlsson Arkitekter/Vilhelm Lauritzen Arkitekter; Photo credit: Jens Lindhe)*

2.8.3 *Southwest Centre for Forensic Mental Health Care*

Location:	St. Thomas, Ontario, Canada
Designer/Architect:	Parkin Architects in Joint Venture with Tillmann Ruth Robinson
Client:	St. Joseph's Health Care
Completion:	2013
Area:	235,000 square feet

Awards: 2015 Behavioral Healthcare, Specialty Hospital/Medical Center, Award of Merit (JV aTRR); 2015 London & District Construction Association – Project Excellence Award (JV aTRR); 2014 International Mental Health Design Award, International Academy for Design and Health (JV aTRR); 2013 Institutional Building Achievement Award, Don Smith Commercial Building Awards (JV aTRR); Design and Health International Academy Awards 2014 – Short-listed; Finalist Mental Health Care, Southwest was selected for exhibition and Cameron Shantz made a presentation

Client, service users, and services

The forensic psychiatry program at St. Joseph's Southwest Centre has been established to provide specialized services to individuals with mental illness who have interacted with the criminal justice system. These are individuals who have been judged "criminally not responsible" for their actions and need specialized assessment, treatment, rehabilitation, and support to fulfill their mandated time to heal. A psychosocial rehabilitation (PSR) model is implemented in this facility, which supports patients in recovering in an environment free from stigma and limitations of illness. The PSR model is focused on restoring community functioning of individuals with a psychiatric disability (Dion & Anthony, 1987).

Mission and goals

The center's goal was to create and maintain a "positive, respectful and culturally sensitive environment that respects the unique story of the individual and assists them in their personal journey." To ensure this goal is met, the Ontario Review Board (ORB) annually reviews progress, transition plans, and outpatient management of each patient. The Ontario Review Board has jurisdiction over individuals who, due to mental disorder, are considered unfit to stand trial or assume criminal responsibility. An outreach team works with ORB to assess patients' readiness for thriving in the community as well as connecting them with community-based services in the area. The program also educates healthcare and justice students, staff, and communities in addition to research participation in forensic psychiatry (St. Joseph's Healthcare London, 2015b).

Site

The Forensic Psychiatry Program is located in Central Elgin, a township in southwestern Ontario. The site is located amongst suburban residential areas and farmlands.

Program

The program offers both inpatient and outpatient services. This enables the facility to ensure continuity of care for individuals to increase the safety and security of both the patients and the public.

Inpatient care takes place in units that vary in terms of level of security and care needed and includes a total of 89 single-patient bedrooms. These units include (St. Joseph's Healthcare London, 2015b):

- Forensic Assessment Unit: This unit provides consultation and assessments to evaluate the individual's competency to stand trial or assume criminal responsibility. This unit is a medium secure unit.
- Forensic Treatment Unit: This unit cares for patients who have been deemed qualified to receive longer-term integrated treatment and rehabilitation, and are placed as a result of an Ontario Review Board hearing. Depending on each individual's illness characteristics and security needs, privileges are introduced gradually. This unit is also a medium secure setting.
- Forensic Rehab Readiness Unit: This unit is a minimum secure unit that is managed by keeping it locked. Individuals hosted in this unit have shown improvements in both assessment as well as Ontario Review Board dispositions. These individuals are encouraged to engage in developing their personal goals. They receive initial rehabilitation to prepare for community reintegration.
- Forensic Rehabilitation Unit: This unit is an open minimum secure unit for individuals who have achieved further clinical improvement and rehabilitation development. Rehabilitation is more intensely pursued in this unit to ensure individual competency upon reintegration into the community.

The units, based on level of security, have varying levels of access to two forensic treatment and two rehabilitation courtyards. The centralized services indirectly accessed from the units include:

- food and nutrition,
- patient and family services,
- Ontario Review Board, and
- spiritual care.

Configuration and construction

The inpatient units are arranged in two cross-shaped structures that allow for significant daylight and access to courtyard views for all the patient beds. The two structures are connected at one side through a larger mass that contains supporting programs. The various types of inpatient units represent an individual's journey through recovery. At each unit, security and privileges are determined based on managing risk and balancing autonomy to levels that are appropriate for the individuals residing in that unit (St. Joseph's Healthcare London, 2015b). In addition to the inpatient units, which are intended to represent home to patients, the building utilizes two components consisting of "Neighborhood" and "Downtown." The "Neighborhood" includes functions that are more directly connected to the recovery plan and are adjacent to the units, including team rooms and consult rooms. The "Downtown" component is located farthest from the patient units and includes the functions that are to be used by patients with higher levels of autonomy.

Daylight and views were integral to the design. Large expanses of glass and views to the adjacent heritage landscape give a sense of openness and transparency, deinstitutionalizing and destigmatizing the facility from the occupant and observer's perspectives.

Case study bibliography

Dion, G. L., & Anthony, W. A. (1987). Research in psychiatric rehabilitation: A review of experimental and quasi-experimental studies. *Rehabilitation Counseling, 30,* 177–203.

St. Joseph's Healthcare London. (2015a). *Forensic program: Programs and services.* Retrieved August 20, 2016, from www.sjhc.london.on.ca/mental-health-care/programs-and-services/forensic-program/programs-and-services

St. Joseph's Healthcare London. (2015b). *Southwest Centre for Forensic Mental Health Care.* Retrieved August 20, 2016, from www.sjhc.london.on.ca/sites/default/files/pdf/southwest_centre_brochure_Jan2015.pdf

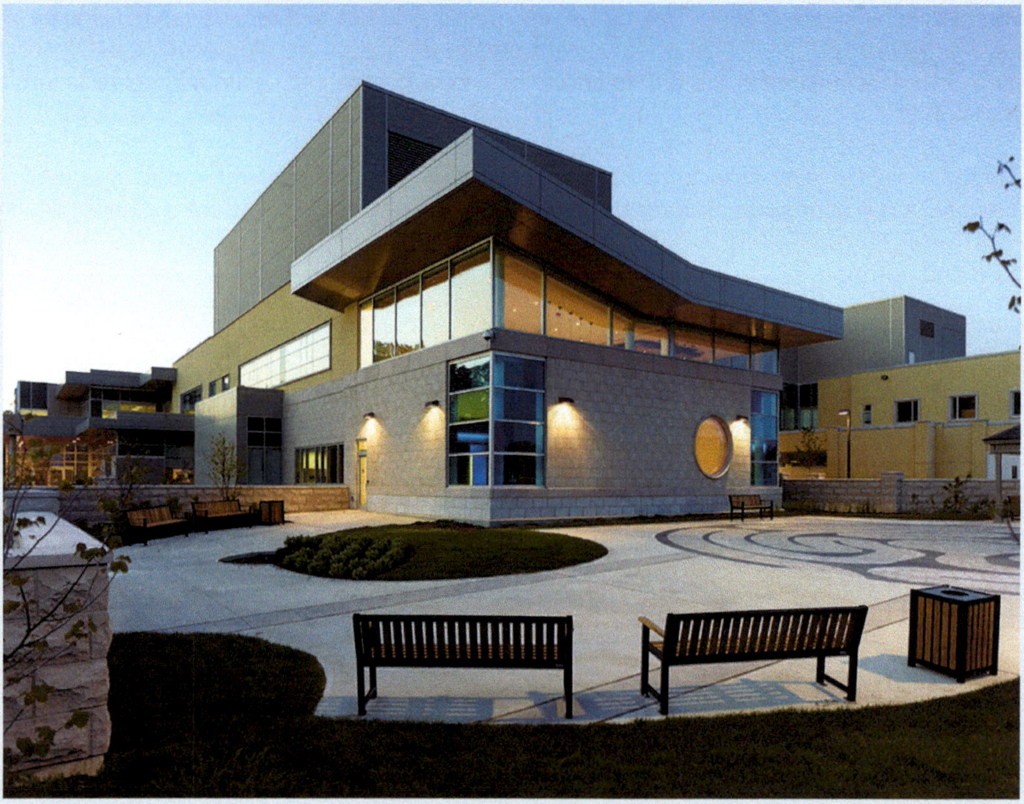

Figure 2.17: *Southwest Centre – chapel exterior (Architects: Parkin Architects/Tillmann Ruth Robinson; Photo credit: Shai Gil Fotography)*

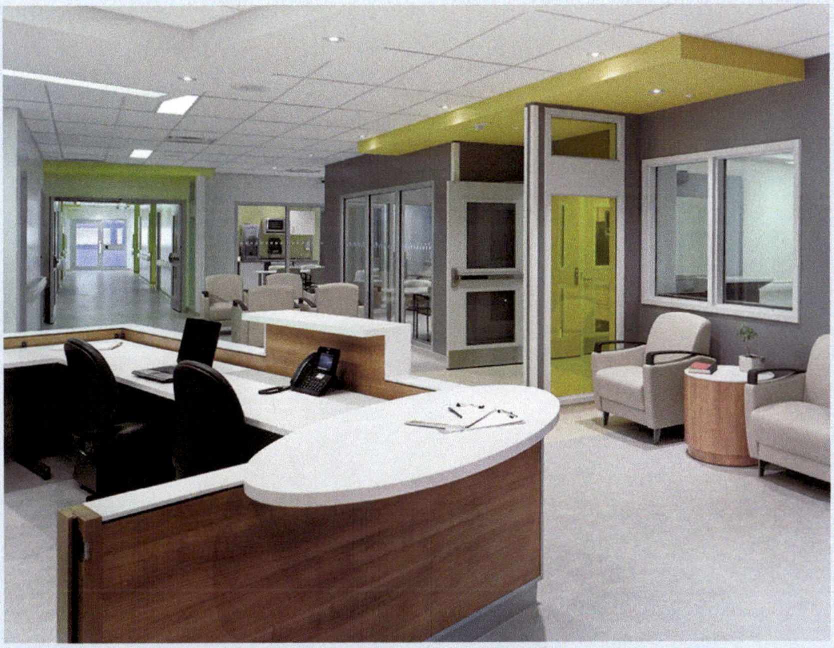

Figure 2.18: *Southwest Centre – inpatient unit (Architects: Parkin Architects/Tillmann Ruth Robinson; Photo credit: Shai Gil Fotography)*

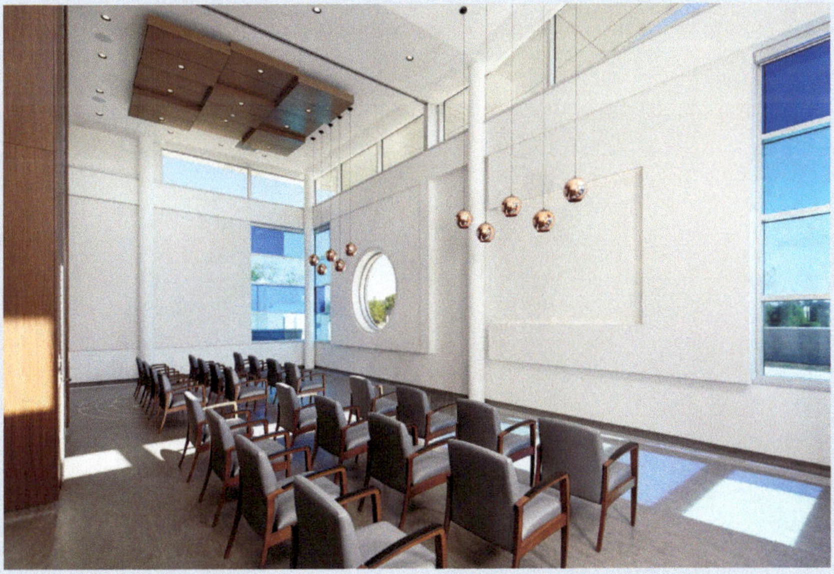

Figure 2.19: *Southwest Centre – chapel (Architects: Parkin Architects/Tillmann Ruth Robinson; Photo credit: Shai Gil Fotography)*

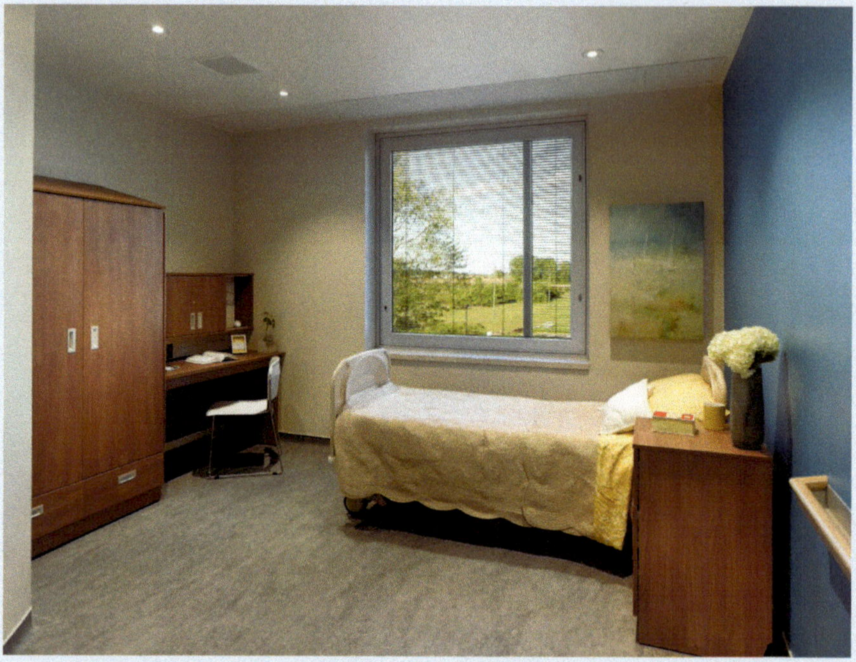

Figure 2.20: *Southwest Centre – patient bedroom (Architects: Parkin Architects/Tillmann Ruth Robinson; Photo credit: Shai Gil Fotography)*

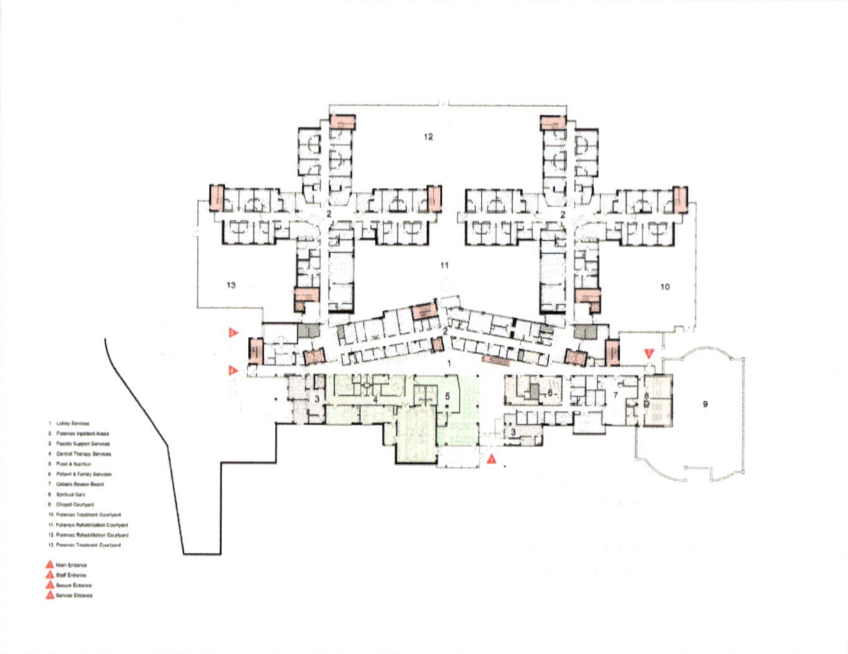

Figure 2.21: *Southwest Centre – floor plan (Architects: Parkin Architects/Tillmann Ruth Robinson; Photo credit: Shai Gil Fotography)*

2.8.4 *Vermont Psychiatric Care Hospital*

Location:	Berlin, VT
Designer/Architect:	architecture+ in collaboration with Black River Design; Landscape architect: Wagner Hodgson
Client:	Vermont Department of Health
Completion:	2014
Area:	53,300 square feet

Awards: Interior Design Project, Overall Winner, Design & Health International Academy Awards, 2015; Mental Health Project, Finalist, Design & Health International Academy Awards, 2015; WAN (World Architecture News) Healthcare Awards Shortlist, 2015; Merit Award, American Institute of Architects, Eastern New York Chapter, 2014

Client, service users, and services

The 25-bed hospital is a replacement to the Vermont State Hospital in Waterbury, which was closed in 2011 after being seriously damaged by Hurricane Irene. Patients admitted to the new psychiatric hospital are individuals above the age of 18 who have been ordered to be hospitalized by a judge as a result of committing a crime. These individuals will be assessed to determine their capacity to stand trial. Other patients may be ordered to undergo hospitalization by a physician who has identified them as having the potential for self-harm or imposing danger to others (Frothingham, 2014). The facility is primarily operated by the Department of Mental Health, which includes staff from various professional backgrounds such as physicians, therapists, administrators, and support personnel (Department of Mental Health, 2016).

Mission and goals

The mission of the Vermont Psychiatric Care Hospital is to provide care and treatment in a "recovery-oriented, safe and respectful environment" that can promote "empowerment, hope and quality of life" for its service users, while acknowledging their rights and their challenges in an involuntary setting. The facility is also committed to education and collaboration with the community, its service users, and its staff (Department of Mental Health, 2016).

Site

Vermont Psychiatric Care Hospital is located on 7.36 acres of land down the road from Central Vermont Medical Center (a 122-bed hospital), in Berlin, Vermont. A few commercial and industrial buildings are scattered in the area surrounding the site, while the majority of residential buildings in the small 2,900-person town are located much farther from the hospital.

Program

The 25 patient beds are distributed between two units, with each unit featuring two separate wings and housing between four to eight patient beds, a kitchenette, and a dining area. Each unit is supported by a secure staff work area, a seclusion room, a treatment planning room, a medications room, exam rooms, a quiet room, a laundry room, and a few staff offices. The two units are connected to more common spaces that include a dining area, library, chapel, art room, activity room, fitness room, and a greenhouse. The chapel can serve as a courtroom or a large family visiting room.

The program also includes a sensory room designed for individual patient-focused therapy. Staff offices and a lounge, classrooms, and administrative functions are also located in this area. Additional exam rooms, consult rooms, and a lab for new admissions are situated near the entrance. The open spaces include a half basketball court, a volleyball court, and a jogging track, as well as a courtyard.

Configuration and construction

Traditional design vernacular of Vermont has been incorporated in the choices of forms and material for the facility. The building has a C-shaped configuration, with patient units at both ends and more common spaces and administrative spaces in the middle. The building wraps around the outdoor activity areas. Each of the inpatient units has a seasonal theme and color and icon palette. The colored linoleum flooring features a creek pattern in the inpatient units, connecting the patient bedrooms and wooden window benches along the way.

Case study bibliography

Department of Mental Health. (2016). *Vermont psychiatric care hospital.* Retrieved August 20, 2016, from http://mentalhealth.vermont.gov/vermont-psychiatric-care-hospital

Frothingham, N. (2014). Vermont Psychiatric Care Hospital: A dramatically different approach. *The Bridge*. Retrieved August 20, 2016, from www.montpelierbridge.com/2014/10/vermont-psychiatric-care-hospital-a-dramatically-different-approach/

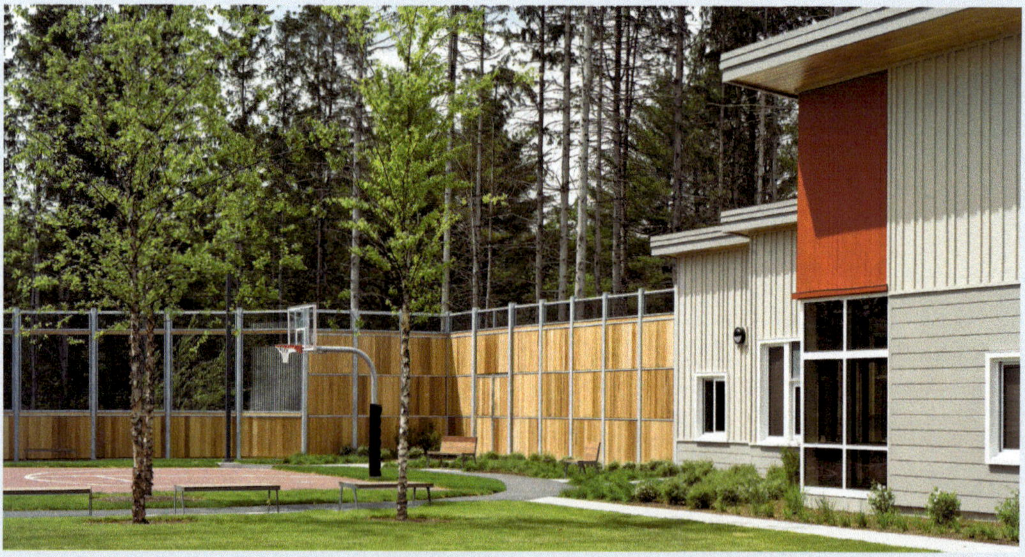

Figure 2.22: *Vermont Psychiatric Care Hospital – exterior view (Architects: architecture+ in collaboration with Black River Design; Photo credit: Jim Westphalen)*

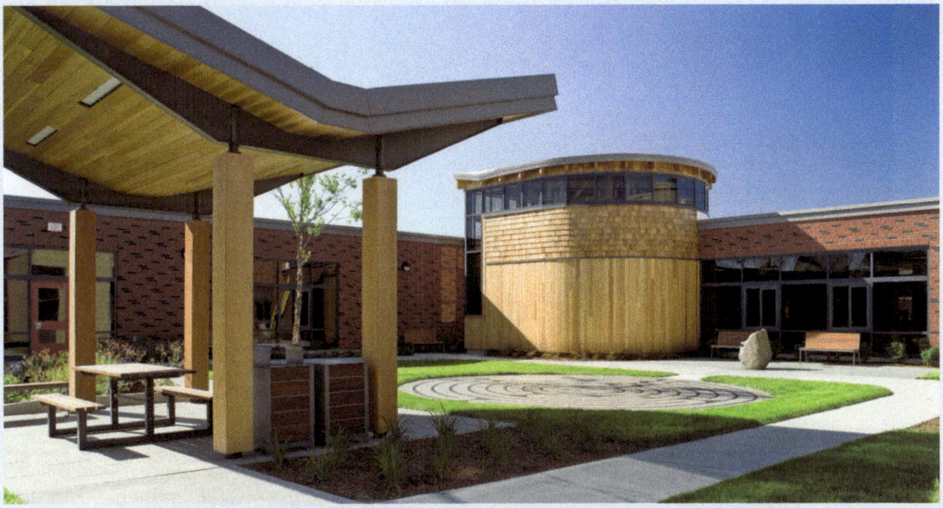

Figure 2.23: *Vermont Psychiatric Care Hospital – courtyard view of pergola and chapel court (Architects: architecture+ in collaboration with Black River Design; Photo credit: Jim Westphalen)*

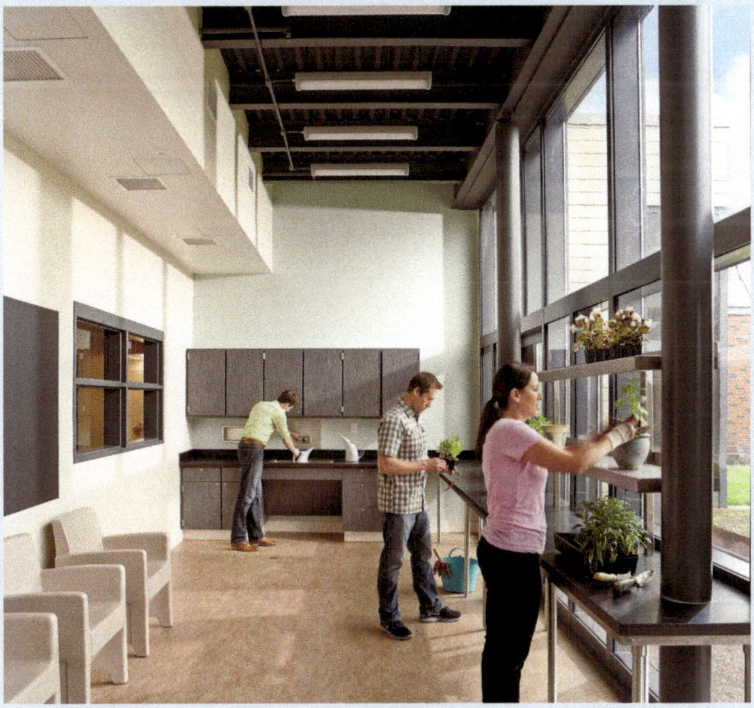

Figure 2.24: *Vermont Psychiatric Care Hospital – horticultural activity room (Architects: architecture+ in collaboration with Black River Design; Photo credit: Jim Westphalen)*

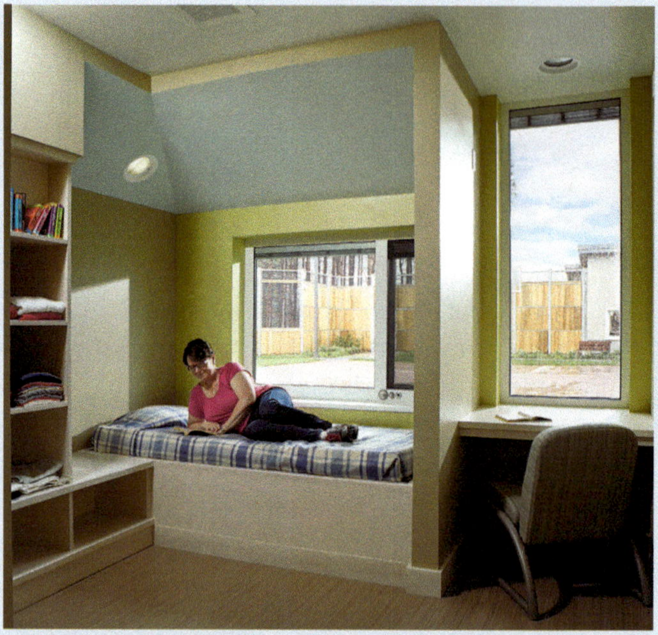

Figure 2.25: *Vermont Psychiatric Care Hospital – patient bedroom (Architects: architecture+ in collaboration with Black River Design; Photo credit: Jim Westphalen)*

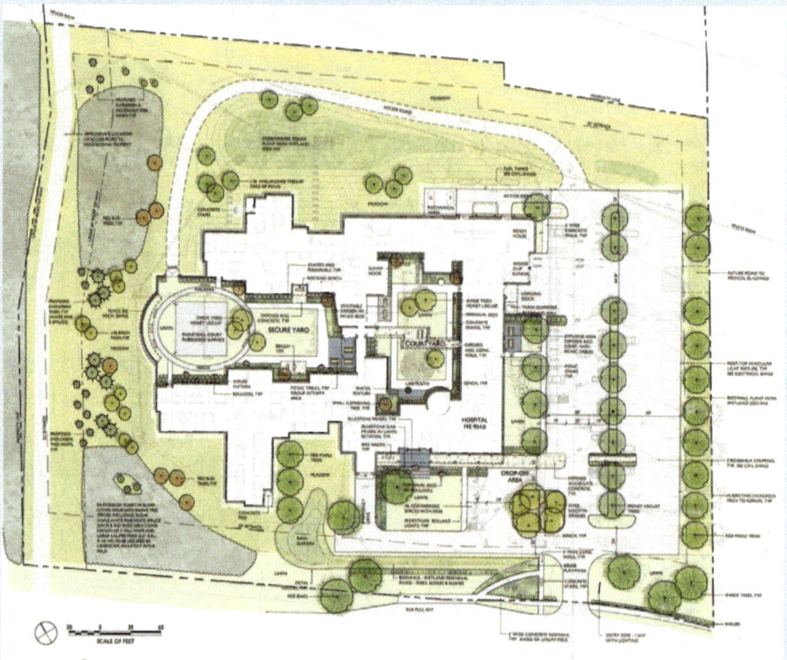

Figure 2.26: *Vermont Psychiatric Care Hospital – site plan (Architects: architecture+ in collaboration with Black River Design; Plan courtesy of architecture+ and Wagner Hodgson)*

References

Allgemeine Anthroposophische Gesellshaft. (1999). *Anthroposophical society*. Retrieved from www.goetheanum.org/aag.html?&L51

Altman, I. (1975). *The environment and social behavior*. Monterey, CA: Brooks/Cole.

Andes, M., & Shattell, M. M. (2006). An exploration of the meanings of space and place in acute psychiatric care. *Issues in Mental Health Nursing*, *27*, 699–707.

Appleton, J. (1996). *The experience of landscape*. New York: Wiley.

Arneill, B. P. (1959). Award winning design for mental health center. *Psychiatric Services*, *10*(6), 37–39.

Bailey, K. (2002). The role of the physical environment for children in residential care. *Residential Treatment for Children & Youth*, *20*(1), 15–27.

Bakos, M., Bozic, R., Chapin, D., & Neuman, S. (1980). Effects of environmental changes on elderly residents' behavior. *Psychiatric Services*, *31*(10), 677–682.

Baltazar, A. P., Kapp, S., Tugny, A., & Furtado, J. P. (2013). Spaces for differences: Dwelling after deinstitutionalization. *Facilities*, *31*(9/10), 407–417.

Bartlett, S. N. (1997). Housing as a factor in the socialization of children: A critical review of the literature. *Merrill-Palmer Quarterly*, *43*, 169–198.

Benedetti, F., Colombo, C., Barbini, B., Campori, E., & Smeraldi, E. (2001). Morning sunlight reduces length of hospitalization in bipolar depression. *Journal of Affective Disorders*, *62*(3), 221–223.

The Caritas Project. (2014). *2012 Award recipients announced*. Retrieved June 23, 2016, from http://thecaritasproject.info/aplacetoflourish/awardWinner_2012.html

Carpman, J., & Grant, M. (2016). *Design that cares* (3rd ed.). New York: Wiley.

Carr, R. (2011). Psychiatric facility. *Whole Building Design Guide*. Retrieved from www.wbdg.org/design/psychiatric.php

Chen, W., Huang, C., Hwang, J., & Chen, C. (2010). The relationship of health-related quality of life to workplace physical violence against nurses by psychiatric patients. *Quality of Life Research Journal*, *19*, 1155–1161.

Choi, B.-C. (1997). Professional and patient attitudes about the relevance of music therapy as a treatment modality in NAMT approved psychiatric hospitals. *Journal of Music Therapy*, *34*(4), 277–292.

Chou, K., Lu, R., & Mao, W. (2002). Factors relevant to patient assaultive behaviour and assault in acute inpatient psychiatric units in Taiwan. *Archives of Psychiatric Nursing*, *16*, 187–195.

Christenfeld, R., Wagner, J., Pastva, G., & Acrish, W. P. (1989). How physical settings affect chronic mental patients. *Psychiatric Quarterly*, *60*, 253–264.

Chrysikou, E. (2013). Accessibility for mental healthcare. *Facilities*, *31*(9/10), 4–4.

Chrysikou, E. (2014). *Architecture for psychiatric environments and therapeutic spaces*. Amsterdam: IOS Press.

Cliff, B. (2012). The evolution of patient-centered care. *Journal of Healthcare Management*, *57*(2), 86.

Csikszentmihalyi, M., & Rochberg-Halton, E. (1981). *The meaning of things: Domestic symbols and the self*. New York: Cambridge University Press.

Cummings, K. S., Grandfield, S. A., & Coldwell, C. M. (2010). Caring with comfort rooms: Reducing seclusion and restraint use in psychiatric facilities. *Journal of Psychosocial Nursing and Mental Health Services*, *48*(6), 26–30.

Davis, C., Glick, I. D., & Rosow, I. (1979). The architectural design of a psychotherapeutic milieu. *Hospital & Community Psychiatry*, *30*(7), 453–460.

Department of Veterans Affairs. (2010). *Mental health facilities: Design guide*. Washington, DC: Department of Veterans Affairs.

Devlin, A. (1992). Psychiatric ward renovation. *Environment and Behavior*, *24*(1), 66–84.

Devlin, A., & Arneill, A. B. (2003). Health care environments and patient outcomes: A review of the literature. *Environment & Behaviour*, *35*(5), 665–694.

Dilani, A. (2008). Psychosocially supportive design: A salutogenic approach to the design of the physical environment. *Design and Health Scientific Review*, *1*(2), 47–55.

Dix, R. (2001). *Physical environment*. London, UK: Greenwich Medical Media.

Doherty, J., & Sell, J. E. (2011). Deinstitutionalizing design: Strategies to design a more residential environment for psychiatric patients. *Behavioral Healthcare*, *31*, 30–33.

Dvoskin, J. A., Radomski, S. J., Bennett, C., Olin, J. A., Hawkins, R. L., Dotson, L. A., & Drewnicky, I. N. (2002). Architectural design of a secure forensic state psychiatric hospital. *Behavioral Sciences & the Law*, *20*(5), 481–493.

Eklund, M., & Hansson, L. (2001). Ward atmosphere, client satisfaction, and client motivation in a psychiatric work rehabilitation unit. *Community Mental Health Journal*, *37*(2), 169–177.

Evans, G. W. (2003). The built environment and mental health. *Journal of Urban Health*, *80*(4), 536–555.

Evans, M., & Rodger, I. (1992). *Complete healing: Regaining your health through anthroposophical medicine*. Forest Row, UK: Floris Books.

Facilities Guidelines Institute. (2014). *Guidelines for design and construction of health care facilities*. Dallas, TX: Facility Guidelines Institute.

Fairbanks, L., McGuire, M., Cole, S., Shordone, R., Silers, F., & Richards, M. (1977). The ethological study of four psychiatric wards: Patient, staff and system behaviors. *Journal of Psychiatric Research*, *13*, 193–209.

Firth, W. (2004). Acute psychiatric wards: An overview. In P. Campling (Ed.), *From toxic institutions to therapeutic environments: Residential settings in mental health services* (pp. 174–187). London, UK: The Royal Society of Psychiatrists.

Fitzgerald, M. M., Kirk, G. D., & Bristow, C. A. (2011). Description and evaluation of a serious game intervention to engage low secure service users with serious mental illness in the design and refurbishment of their environment. *Journal of Psychiatric and Mental Health Nursing*, *18*(4), 316–322.

Foley, A. R., & Lacy, B. N. (1967). On the need for interprofessional collaboration: Psychiatry and architecture. *American Journal of Psychiatry*, *123*(8), 1013–1018.

Forster, P. L., Cavness, C., & Phelps, M. A. (1999). Staff training decreases use of seclusion and restraint in an acute psychiatric hospital. *Archives of Psychiatric Nursing*, *13*(5), 269–271.

Frampton, S. B., & Charmel, P. A. (2009). *Putting patients first: Best practices in patient-centered care*. San Francisco: Jossey-Bass.

Gibson, J. J. (1979). *The ecological approach to visual perception*. Boston, MA: Houghton Mifflin.

Golembiewski, J. (2010). Start making sense: Applying a salutogenic model to architectural design for psychiatric care. *Facilities*, *28*(3/4), 100–117.

Grosenick, J., & Hatmaker, C. (2000). Perceptions of the importance of physical setting in substance abuse treatment. *Journal of Substance Abuse Treatment*, *18*, 29–39.

Gutkowski, S., Ginath, Y., & Guttmann, F. (1992). Improving psychiatric environments through minimal architectural changes. *Hospital Community Psychiatry*, *43*, 920–923.

Gutkowski, S., & Guttmann, F. (1992). Program and process: Designing the physical space of a day hospital. *Israel Journal of Psychiatry and Related Science*, *29*(3), 167–173.

Hamilton, D. K. (2003). The four levels of evidence-based practice. *Healthcare Design*, *3*(4), 18–26.

Hamilton, D. K., & Watkins, D. H. (2009). *Evidence-based design for multiple building types*. Hoboken, NJ: John Wiley & Sons.

Hamre, H. J., Witt, C. M., Glockmann, A., Ziegler, R., Willich, S. N., & Kiene, H. (2006). Anthroposophic therapy for chronic depression: A four-year prospective cohort study. *BMC Psychiatry*, *6*(1), 1.

Heerwagen, J. H., Heubach, J. G., Montgomery, J., & Weimer, W. C. (1995). Environmental design, work, and well being: Managing occupational stress through changes in the workplace environment. *AAOHN Journal: Official Journal of the American Association of Occupational Health Nurses*, *43*(9), 458–468.

Holahan, C., & Saegert, S. (1973). Behavioral and attitudinal effects of large-scale variation in the physical environment of psychiatric wards. *Journal of Abnormal Psychology*, *82*, 454–462.

Hunt, J., & Sine, D. (2012). *Design guide for the built environment of behavioral health facilities*. Washington, DC: National Association of Psychiatric Health Systems.

Institute for Patient-Centered Care. (n.d.). *About*. Retrieved June 23, 2016, from www.institutepcd.org/about

Izumi, K. (1968). Architectural considerations in the design of places and facilities for the care and treatment of the mentally ill. *Journal of Schizophrenia*, *2*(1), 42–52.

Jeffers, T. (1991). Safety considerations in the psychiatric setting. *The Psychiatric Hospital*, *22*(3), 119–122.

Johansson, I., Skärsäter, I., & Danielson, E. (2006). The health care environment on a locked psychiatric ward and its meaning to patients and staff members. *International Journal of Mental Health Nursing*, *15*, 242–250.

Logsdon, R. (1995). Understanding the application of Lazure painting techniques. *Journal of Healthcare Design*, *7*, 205–212.

Lynch, M. F., Plant, R. W., & Ryan, R. M. (2005). Psychological needs and threat to safety: Implications for staff and patients in a psychiatric hospital for youth. *Professional Psychology: Research and Practice*, *36*(4), 415–425.

MacKinnon, D. (2009). Divine service, music, sport, and recreation as medicinal in Australian asylums 1860s–1945. *Health and History*, *11*(1), 128–148.

Martin, J. H. (1995). Improving staff safety through an aggression management program. *Archives of Psychiatric Nursing*, *9*(4), 211–215.

Middelboe, T., Schjødt, T., Byrsting, K., & Gjerris, A. (2001). Ward atmosphere in acute psychiatric in patient care: Patients' perceptions, ideals and satisfaction. *Acta Psychiatrica Scandinavica*, *103*(3), 212–219.

Nanda, U., Eisen, S., Zadeh, R. S., & Owen, D. (2011). Effect of visual art on patient anxiety and agitation in a mental health facility and implications for the business case. *Journal of Psychiatric and Mental Health Nursing*, *18*(5), 386–393.

Nanda, U., Gaydos, H. L. B., Hathorn, K., & Watkins, N. (2010). Art and posttraumatic stress: A review of the empirical literature on the therapeutic implications of artwork for war veterans with posttraumatic stress disorder. *Environment and Behavior*, *42*(3), 376–390.

New York Presbyterian. (2012). First psychiatric hospital in nation to earn prestigious Planetree designation. *Community Update*. Retrieved from www.nyp.org

Olver, J., Love, M., Daniel, J., Norman, T., & Nicholls, D. (2009). The impact of a changed environment on arousal levels of patients in a secure extended rehabilitation facility. *Australasian Psychiatry*, *17*, 207–211.

Orr, R. (1995). The Planetree philosophy. In S. Marberry (Ed.), *Innovations in healthcare design* (pp. 77–87). New York: Van Nostrand Reinhold.

Paget, S., & White, T. (2004). Connecting with the natural environment. In P. Campling (Ed.), *From toxic institutions to therapeutic environments: Residential settings in mental health services* (pp. 79–87). London, UK: The Royal Society of Psychiatrists.

Perkins, N. (2013). Including patients, staff and visitors in the design of the psychiatric milieu: Notes from the field. *Facilities*, *31*(9/10), 379–390.

Planetree. (2014). *Planetree designated sites*. Retrieved from http://planetree.org/planetree-designated-sites/

Planetree. (2015). Stamford hospital: Bringing Planetree through the locked doors of an inpatient psychiatric unit. *Planetree Planetalk*. Retrieved from http://planetree.org/planetalk/stamford-hospital-inpatient-psychiatric-unit/

Porter, W., & Easter, J. (1980). *Architecture for the next generation of state hospitals*. Proceedings of Humanistic Architecture for Mental Health: A Special Symposium, Kaplan/McLaughlin/Diaz, San Francisco, CA.

Potthoff, J. (1995). Adolescent satisfaction with drug/alcohol treatment facilities: Design implications. *Journal of Alcohol and Drug Education*, *41*, 62–73.

Remen, S. (1991). Signs, symbols, and the psychiatric environment. *The Psychiatric Hospital*, *22*(3), 113–118.

Rivlin, L., & Wolfe, M. (1979). Understanding and evaluating therapeutic environments for children. In D. Canter & S. Canter (Eds.), *Designing for therapeutic environments* (pp. 29–61). Sussex, UK: John Wiley & Sons.

Ruga, W. (2008). Your general practice environment can improve your community's health. *British Journal of General Practice*, *58*(552), 460–462.

Ruga, W. (2010). Applied "generative space": Improving health and wellbeing through your practice environment. *Journal of Holistic Healthcare*, *7*(1), 36–39.

Sackett, D. L., Rosenberg, W. M. C., & Muir Gray, J. A. (1996). Evidence-based medicine: What it is and what it isn't. *British Medical Journal*, *312*, 71–72.

Salerno, S., Forcella, L., Di Fabio, U., Figa Talamance, I., & Boscolo, P. (2012). Ergonomics in the psychiatric ward towards workers or patients? *Work*, *41*, 1832–1835.

Shepley, M. (1995). The location of behavioral incidents in a children's psychiatric facility. *Children's Environments*, *12*(3), 352–361.

Shepley, M. (2006). The role of positive distraction in neonatal intensive care units. *Journal of Perinatology*, *26*, S34–S37.

Shepley, M. (2016). *Defining the next generation's focus: National Institute of Building Science*. Washington, DC: The Academy of Healthcare Infrastructure.

Shepley, M. (2017, in press). The healthcare environment. In J. Rollins (Ed.), *Meeting children's psychosocial needs across the healthcare continuum*. Gaithersburg, MD: Aspen Publishers.

Shepley, M. M., Pasha, S., Ferguson, P., Huffcut, J. C., Kiyokawa, G., Martere, J., . . . Malone, E. (2013). *Design research and behavioral health facilities*. Concord, CA: The Center for Health Design. Retrieved from www.healthdesign.org/system/files/chd428_researchreport_behavioral health_1013-_final_0.pdf

Shepley, M. M., & Watson, A. (2012). Evidence-based design: Medical and design researcher collaboration. *Evidence Based Medicine*, *18*(1), 2–4.

Sidman, J., & Moos, R. (1973). On the relation between psychiatric ward atmosphere and helping behavior. *Journal of Clinical Psychology*, *29*(1), 74–78.

Sommer, R. (2008). *Personal space: Updated, The behavioral basis of design*. Bristol, UK: Bosko Books.

Spivak, M. (1984). *Institutional settings*. New York: Human Sciences Press.

Stichler, J. F., & Hamilton, D. K. (2008). Evidence-based design: What is it? *HERD: Health Environments Research & Design Journal*, *1*(2), 3–4.

Timko, C. (1996). Physical characteristics of residential psychiatric and substance abuse programs: Organizational determinants and patient outcomes. *American Journal of Community Psychology*, *24*, 173–192.

Turlington, R. G. (2004). Creating a Planetree inpatient psychiatric unit. *Health Facilities Management*, *17*(6), 12–13.

Ulrich, R. (1999). Effects of gardens on health outcomes: Theory and research. In C. Cooper Marcus & M. Barnes (Eds.), *Healing gardens: Therapeutic benefits and design recommendations* (pp. 27–86). New York: Wiley.

Ulrich, R. (2000). Environmental research and critical care. In D. Kirk Hamilton (Ed.), *ICU 2010* (pp. 195–208). Houston, TX: Center for Innovation in Health Facilities.

Ulrich, R. (2001). Effects of healthcare environmental design on medical outcomes. In A. Dilani (Ed.), *Design and health – The therapeutic benefits of design* (pp. 49–60). Proceedings of the Second International Conference on Design & Health, 2000. Stockholm, Sweden: Svenskbyggtjanst.

Ulrich, R., Berry, L. L., Quan, X., & Parish, J. T. (2010). A conceptual framework for the domain of evidence-based design. *HERD: Health Environments Research & Design Journal*, *4*(1), 95–114.

Ulrich, R., Bogren, L., & Lundin, S. (2012). Towards a design for reducing aggression in psychiatric facilities. In *Arch 12: Architecture/Research/Care/Health*. Gothenberg: Chalmers. Retrieved from http://vbn.aau.dk/files/71203129/FINAL_pdf_UlrichBogren_Lundin_Toward_a_design_theory_for_reducing_aggression_Oct_2_.pdf

Ulrich, R., Zimring, C., Zhu, X., DuBose, J., Seo, H.-B., Choi, Y.-S., . . . Joseph, A. (2008). A review of the research literature on evidence-based healthcare design. *HERD: Health Environments Research & Design Journal*, *1*(3), 61–125.

Visionesse. (2008). *Anthroposophic architecture: Organic architecture and design*. Retrieved from https://visionesse.workpress.com/category/anthroposophic/

Von Sommaruga Howard, T. (2004). The physical environment and use of space. In P. Campling, S. Davies, & G. Farquharson (Eds.), *From toxic institutions to therapeutic environments: Residential settings in mental health services* (pp. 69–78). Glasgow, UK: The Royal College of Psychiatrists.

Whitehead, C., Polsky, R., Crookshank, C., & Fik, E. (1984). Objective and subjective evaluation of psychiatric ward design. *American Journal of Psychiatry*, *82*, 454–462.

Wilson, M., Soth, N., & Robak, R. (1992). Managing disturbed behavior by architectural changes: Making spaces fit the program. *Residential Treatment for Children and Youth*, *10*(2), 63–74.

Wolfe, M. (1975). Room size, group size, and density behavior patterns in a children's psychiatric facility. *Environment and Behavior*, *7*, 199–224.

Part Two: The settings

Outpatient facilities

3

3.1 Introduction to outpatient facilities

3.1.1 *History of outpatient psychiatric care*

New developments in Europe in the nineteenth century such as psychotherapy and new physical treatments were precursors to therapeutic ambulatory care. By the twentieth century, these new forms of treatment were employed in short-stay hospitals and outpatient departments for the mentally ill in the United States and European countries such as France, the United Kingdom, and Belgium (Chrysikou, 2014). At that time, early outpatient examination centers were created as part of the mental hospitals that, following the UK's Mental Treatment Act of 1930, could voluntarily admit patients who would benefit from the facility's care program (Hunter & MacAlpine, 1974).

In 1953, an outpatient psychiatric program appeared as a focus-building typology in *Architectural Record* magazine in the United States. Design criteria at that time were based on staff and patient utilization (Guttersen, 1953a). The facilities were designed to schedule 20 patient hours per week per psychiatric care team, consisting of a psychiatrist, a psychologist, two or three social workers, a nurse, and two administrative staff (Guttersen, 1953b).

In the United Kingdom in 1971, Department of Health and Social Security outpatient facilities moved from having a pure triage function to providing patient assessment, care, and follow-up services. In Italy, by 1978, all hospital admissions stopped, and patients were treated in outpatient clinics, community accommodations, or their own homes (Cole, 1980).

The move toward the design of community-based mental health centers began in the United States after 1963 (Public Law, 88–164), which led to the funding of the Community Mental Health Act (CMHA) to create local mental health centers, in an effort to move away from institutionalization. This new service may have benefited by the participation of architects in early programming and planning phases of psychiatric care environments. Although community mental health centers today are formed around a variety of services and programs, the early community mental health centers typically included diagnostic services, rehabilitation, community based pre-care and aftercare, training of professionals, and research and evaluation (Dorsett & Brown, 1965) and the provision of both inpatient and outpatient care (Ashton, 1976).

While development of psychotherapy and discovery of effective psychopharmacological treatment facilitated the move toward outpatient care in the early to mid-twentieth century, the methods of care changed as medical science grew. Olfson and Marcus (2010) compared rates of psychotherapy use among the U.S. psychiatric outpatients and found that between 1998 and 2007, use of psychotherapy remained stable; however, it lost its prominence to psychotropic medication.

3.1.2 Data regarding the outpatient psychiatric population

Centers for Disease Control and Prevention (CDC) visit data from 2009–2010 segregates psychiatric outpatients in 10 different groups: schizophrenic disorders, major depressive disorders, other psychoses, anxiety states, acute reaction to stress, neurotic depression, depressive syndrome, alcohol dependence syndrome, drug dependence and abuse, and attention deficit disorder (CDC, 2011a). In medical specialty offices the primary populations are schizophrenic disorders, anxiety, and major depressive disorders. Primary care offices were visited most commonly by people with attention deficit disorders and depressive disorders. Patients with anxiety state disorders visited primary care offices and medical specialty offices in equivalent numbers (Figure 3.1). Hospital emergency departments and outpatient departments together represented less than 18% of the total number of MBH patient visits and mostly responded to cases of drug abuse, anxiety, and other categories of psychoses (CDC, 2011b).

In addition to type of diagnosis, age, gender, and comorbidities impact service use trends among patients. For example, research shows differences between men and women in outpatient service use. A nationally representative Canadian survey of 36,984 respondents was conducted by Statistics Canada in 2002. Male and female respondents (53% and 56% respectively) with a major depressive episode in a one-year period had similar patterns for engaging with mental healthcare services. These rates aligned with previous research indicating no significant difference between care seeking of male and female patients once the mental health problem reaches a certain level of severity. The Canadian study, however, found that, at this stage, males are more likely than women to visit a mental health specialist rather than a general physician for their mental care needs. Women, on the other hand, are more likely to continue care with their general physician (Gagne, Vasiliadis, & Preville 2014).

To examine pediatric patterns, Salloum, Johnco, Lewin, McBride, and Storch (2016) recruited 100 children aged 7 to 13 from three community outpatient mental health clinics in Florida. The primary

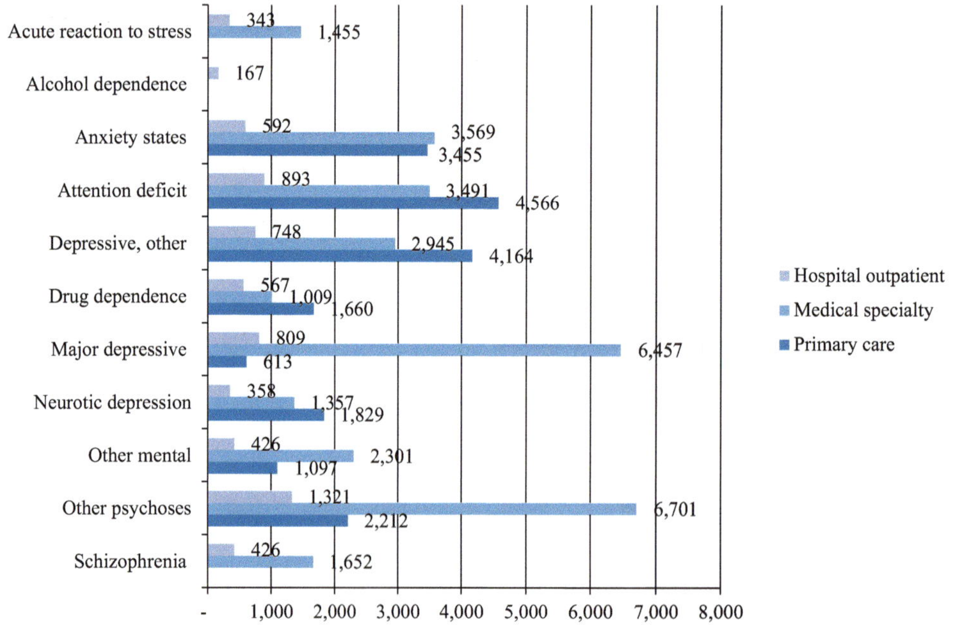

Figure 3.1: *Annual number of ambulatory care visits by setting type according to diagnosis group (Data source: Centers for Disease Control and Prevention, 2011a)*

diagnosis for children included primary anxiety disorders: generalized anxiety (40%), social phobia (26%), separation anxiety (24%), specific phobia (9%), and panic disorder (1%). They found that the most common deterrents to seeking care included undermining or poor recognition of the mental disorder, lack of knowledge regarding available services, stigma, and financial concerns. Stigma and financial concerns were the significant predictors for dropping out of treatment.

Jimenez, Bartels, Cardenas, Daliwal, and Alegría (2012) conducted large-scale surveys of U.S. individuals aged 60 and older (N = 1,658) regarding their medical providers and found differences in outpatient visits among African American, Hispanic, and Caucasian people in the United States. The researchers, as in previous studies, found that older African Americans tended to rely on outpatient visits and counseling rather than medication. Hispanics used a combination of psychotropic medications and counseling, and Caucasians were more likely to use only medications, which translates into a lower number of outpatient visitations.

Data from 2014 among adults aged 18 or older in the United States who had a serious mental illness show that persons without health insurance were twice as likely to not seek the counseling care they needed (SAMHSA, 2015). Data also show that males were less likely than females (62% vs. 72%) and younger adults were less likely than adults 26 and older to seek counseling care (approximately 53% versus 70%). In total, 31.5% of adults 18 years old and older in the United States who had a serious mental disorder and would have benefited from treatment and counseling did not receive treatment.

Physical health conditions and diseases may lead to mental health issues and require attention and access to appropriate providers. Abundant research is available on mental health needs of patients with diabetes (e.g., Polonsky, 1999), cancer (e.g., Institute of Medicine, 2008), and HIV (e.g., American Psychiatric Association, 2000) and their families and their need to access counseling services. For example, research shows that cancer survivors and their spouses are at a higher risk of suffering poor mental health conditions – mostly anxiety and distress. Compared to the general population, a higher percentage of cancer survivors below age 65 made outpatient mental health visits. However, no significant difference was observed between cancer survivors and other adults over 65 years of age. Data also showed that among cancer survivors and their spouses, females and survivors with chronic health conditions were more likely to seek mental healthcare through ambulatory visits and take psychotherapeutic medicines (Punekar, 2010).

Brookman-Frazee, Drahota, Stadnick, and Palinkas (2012) surveyed 100 therapists about their experiences serving children with autism spectrum disorders (ASD) in mental health clinics and followed up with focus groups composed of 17 therapists to clarify and expand survey results. They found that the therapists routinely served school-aged, high-functioning ASD children for behavior or other psychiatric problems. In fact 20.7% of all therapists' caseloads consisted of children with ASD or Asperger's syndrome. The therapists reported that the presenting problems for this population included disruptive behaviors (84.6%), social adjustment issues (82.1%), attention-regulation problems (44.9%), as well as anxiety and fears (39.7%). Therapists displayed negative emotions reflecting on their experience working with this group of children. They believed serving this population was challenging and frustrating because of the children's slow progress or lack of improvement (27.4%), issues with coordinating mental care systems and special education (17.8%), and lack of client insight (12.3%).

Sollie, Mørch, and Larsson (2016) studied parental stress among parents of children with ADHD, and emphasized assessment of parental stress as a prerequisite for family-focused treatment. They studied 214 outpatient children with ADHD symptoms, and compared demographic variables as well as parent and family characteristics of 110 children in the same catchment area with no symptoms. They found that parents of boys under 13 years old experienced more parenting stressors compared to parents of adolescent boys. On the other hand, parents of adolescent girls felt more stressed than parents of younger girls. Parent and family dysfunctions were significantly high among parents of children with both ADHD and oppositional defiant disorder symptoms.

3.2 Characteristics of outpatient psychiatric facilities

3.2.1 *Frequency and duration of visitations*

Psychiatric office visits in the United States compose 3% of annual ambulatory physician office visits (Figure 3.2). However, duration of time spent with the psychiatrist (average 33 minutes per visit) is higher than the average visitation time for any other specialty (national average of 22.6 minutes for all specialties including psychiatry) (Figure 3.3). This is to be expected, as protocols for providing counseling require visits of 30 minutes or longer.

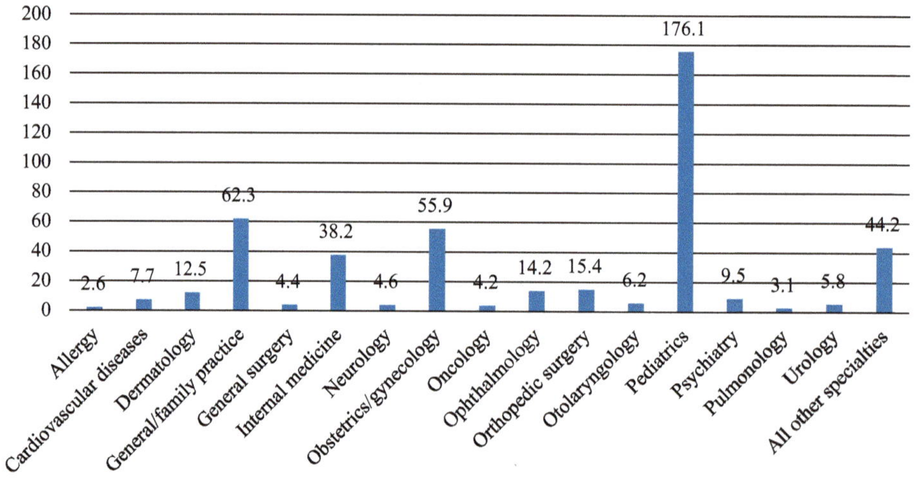

Figure 3.2: *Number of physician office visits per 100 persons per year (Data source: Centers for Disease Control and Prevention, 2012b)*

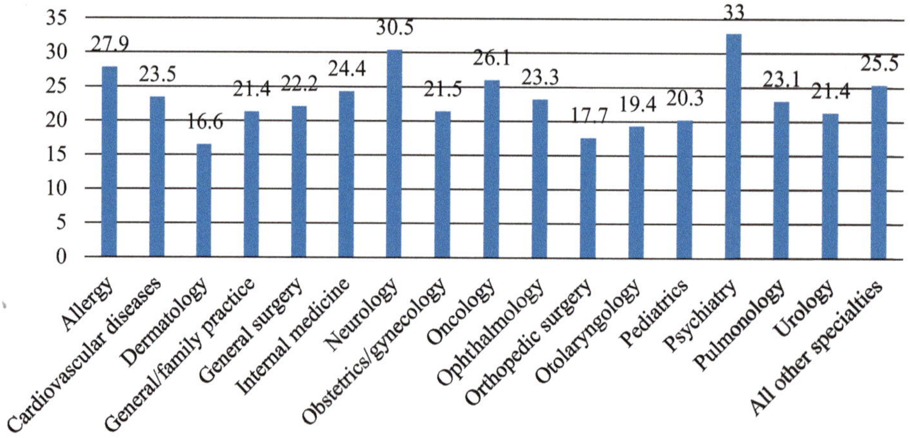

Figure 3.3: *Mean time (minutes) spent with physician (Data source: Centers for Disease Control and Prevention, 2012a)*

While number and frequency of visitations might be impacted by affordability, accessibility, and type of diagnosis, patient dropout is a widely spread issue among mental health outpatients. Dropout is defined as quitting treatment before it is completed. A study of patient dropouts in Canada and the United States showed that patient gender and age was not significantly related to overall risk of treatment dropout (Olfson, Mojtabai, Sampson, Hwang, & Kessler, 2009). College education for patients predicted a lower risk of dropout from services provided by mental health professionals (e.g., psychologists) other than psychiatrists. Most individuals with substance use disorders who dropped out from treatment did so after the first two visits (Olfson et al., 2009).

Several clinical strategies may reduce dropout, including appointment reminders, treatment contracts, case management, and patient education and activation. As one example, primary care physician communications about medication treatment plans and education about side effects may reduce early treatment termination (Olfson et al., 2009).

3.2.2 *Number of psychiatric outpatient facilities*

To provide holistic care to individuals, primary care settings are providing mental health services as well as general healthcare services. Screening and treatment of individuals who visit or receive care in either category takes place through a systematic coordination of general and behavioral healthcare, and can improve patient outcomes for people with multiple healthcare needs (SAMHSA National Council, 2013). According to Peek and the National Integration Academy Council (2013), integrated care may target health behaviors that can contribute to chronic medical illnesses, ineffective patterns of healthcare utilization, as well as mental health and substance abuse conditions.

The integration of mental healthcare services with primary care services was formally initiated in the United States in 2000 and has been on the rise (DATA, 2010). By 2010, almost 70% of primary care clinics were providing mental health services, as shown in Figure 3.4.

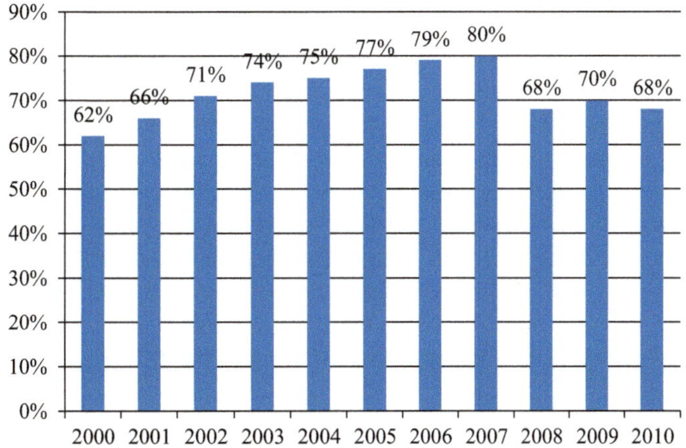

Figure 3.4: *Percentage of primary care facilities that provide mental health treatment (Data source: DATA, 2010, 2011)*

Between 1998 and 2007, the number of community health centers alone – an extensive network of clinics in underserved areas – increased by almost 50% (SAMHSA, 2012). According to the WHO Mental Health Atlas (2011), 6,179 mental health outpatient facilities were providing services to 931.86 persons per 100,000 population in the United States. Among the people receiving the service, 51% are female and 29% are under the age of 18 (WHO, 2011).

3.3 Outpatient psychiatric facility design

3.3.1 *Research on ambulatory psychiatric care design*

There is little research on psychiatric facilities and, of that, a small percentage addresses ambulatory psychiatric care. One group of researchers, however, recently studied the relationship between art displays and patient anxiety in an acute care psychiatric unit. Nanda, Eisen, Zadeh, and Owen (2010) found a significant positive correlation between presence of realistic art displays and anxiety reduction. They measured anxiety levels of patients by measuring the rate of *pro re nata* (PRN) (as the situation arises) incidents as well as nurse feedback in a psychiatric short-stay clinic lounge in an east Alabama hospital. In their study, they displayed visual art on a rotation basis on the walls of a small multipurpose lounge. Results showed significantly lower anxiety and agitation when the visual art was displayed. The positive impact was stronger on days that nature art was displayed instead of abstract art. The researchers translated the results into the time and money saved in management of PRN incidents and medication and reached annual cost savings of $30,000 USD.

Sagha Zadeh, Shepley, and Gartner (2013) investigated the impact of environmental design on therapy from the counseling professionals' perspective using (a) structured and unstructured questionnaires (the Ideal Workspace Survey, and the Workspace Satisfaction Survey), (b) participant interviews, (c) archival and document analysis, and (d) walk-through site evaluation. Critical design characteristics of client interaction spaces and counseling areas were identified.

Designers must consider the needs of outpatient staff as well. Folkins, O'Reilly, Roberts, and Miller (1977) studied the impact of physical environment in an outpatient center on staff job satisfaction. In their study, services were provided at an existing clinic and at a newly built clinic. The new building was designed to be adequately lit and ventilated, was acoustically sound, and had homelike, warm-looking finishes. The old building on the contrary was dimly lighted, poorly ventilated, and noisy. Most walls and floors were composed of painted cement. Staff described the old building as depressing, while they found that the new building helped them to feel freer, lighter, and more positive. They measured staff job satisfaction and overall satisfaction three times over an 18-month period using the Weiss satisfaction survey (Weiss, Dawis, England, & Lofquist, 1967). They found that the staff who moved from the old building to the new one showed an increased satisfaction with their job; however, their overall satisfaction score did not increase significantly. Overall satisfaction of staff can positively impact their ability to inspire hope to the patients and is a critical variable to address (Frank, 1968). However, as the study conducted by Folkins et al. showed, there are several other factors beyond the physical environment that can influence it.

Watkins and Anthony (2007) conducted interviews with 10 psychologists about their office environments. They found two core categories: The first category included therapeutic needs, and the second category consisted of environmental responses that could support the needs. The therapeutic needs can be organized in three major groups consisting of: (1) practicality and adaptability; (2) control, order, comfort, security, and privacy; and (3) cueing of appropriate social roles and empathy. Environmental responses to these therapeutic needs consisted of: color, décor, and plants; proxemics, seating, room size, location; windows, lighting, clocks; and thermal comfort and noise control.

3.3.2 *Outpatient psychiatric care design recommendations and features*

As with research, there are limited resources that provide design recommendations for mental and behavioral health ambulatory care facilities. This section begins with a discussion of a model of care with specific physical implications – Fountain House – which is followed by a discussion of the physical implications of service integration and design goals as outlined by Watkins and Anthony (2007) and Bauzin and Hicks (2014). A proposal for adjacencies between elements is provided in Figure 3.5.

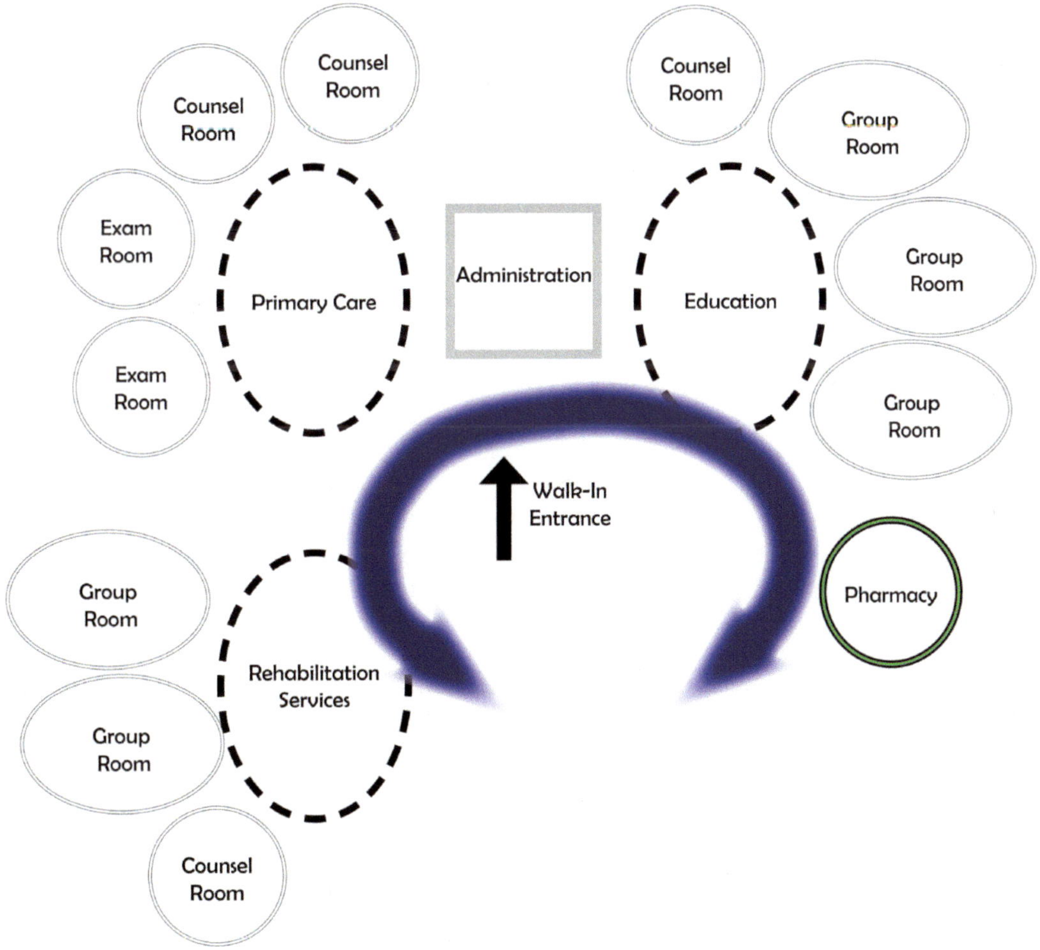

Figure 3.5: *Adjacency diagram for outpatient clinic*

3.3.2.1 Fountain House

Doyle, Lanoil, and Dudek (2013) report that in 1948, prior to inception of the concept of community mental health centers and community residential facilities, patients discharged from a New York psychiatric hospital gathered to discuss an alternative approach to care provided outside of residential facilities. Their goal was to start an alternative support system they referred to as a clubhouse. Since then, many clubhouses have formed around the world, many of them named Fountain House after the original model in New York (Doyle et al., 2013). The initial concept that led to the creation of Fountain House was that engaging in work in a routine daily schedule can bring normalcy into the lives of persons with mental illnesses and help remove the stigma associated with mental illnesses (Doyle et al., 2013, pp. 30–31). For such a concept to be realized, members joining a clubhouse are recognized as persons capable of making contributions, rather than patients in need of repair. In this capacity, members join forces with staff to help deliver the social services they will also use (Doyle et al., 2013, pp. 60–61). Fountain House provides environments for persons with mental illnesses to engage in occupational activities. The physical environment is organized to foster collegiality, voluntarism, and choice through fluidity and openness. The design of the space follows the "person in environment" approach, which is intended to negate feelings of exclusion (Doyle et al., 2013).

Fountain House was designed around the concept of place (Doyle et al., 2013). In Doyle et al.'s terms, this model is "a working community [that] assumes a place. . . where face-to-face collaboration among participants is paramount." Association with a place in society has been hypothesized to be important to people suffering from mental illness (e.g., Whitley, Strickler, & Drake, 2012). Doyle et al. (2013) note that spatial independence is a vital part of the model. Such space needs to be free from rules of a traditional mental health setting and should recognize new roles for members and staff that support creation of a sympathetic environment. The concept of transformational design, with the intent of making activities accessible to the members, was attempted through the following means:

- maintaining a workday structure that kept activities meaningful;
- nourishing the need for being needed; and
- providing opportunities for choice, control, and collaboration.

Doyle et al. (2013) describe the design of the Fountain House, which used space as a means to create meaningful daily tasks. For example, they allocated a small food storage area in the kitchen, which made grocery shopping a required daily task for members. Similarly, they provided a telephone switchboard that could be operated by members. The activity groups work within a defined space. These units are composed of open workspaces with a large board to list activities and assignments. Visual cues are used to advertise and identify each separate work unit and present opportunities to exercise choice for the members.

3.3.2.2 Service Integration

Proximity and collocation are difficult to successfully translate into collaboration and integration. More specifically for the system of care, if traditional roles are maintained, very little flexibility is achieved (SAMHSA National Council, 2013). A similar concept is applicable to design and planning of the space. To achieve goals of integrated primary care, space should be planned and designed to accommodate system integration. For example, design should be responsive to safety needs. SAMHSA (2013) recognizes six levels of collaboration between MBH care and primary care. Level 3 and up are the collocation of services and the areas that need special considerations, depending on level of integration. Bauzin and Hicks (2014) suggest that the current trend, which collocates psychiatric interview rooms with primary units, may be harmful to the physician's safety in two ways: (1) the false sense of safety created by adjacency to other staff, which may not be as effective as perceived, and (2) using medical exam rooms for psychiatric interview rooms without taking necessary safety measures into consideration. However, many feel that by mixing the populations care becomes less stigmatized.

3.3.2.3 Design strategies

Therapists who served as subjects in the Watkins and Anthony study (2007) mentioned several design strategies:

- Support patient ability to control visibility of personal objects, such as clocks and family pictures.
- Provide diffuse lighting to focus the session and facilitate sharing of sensitive information.
- Select furniture and decoration that will reflect the guiding philosophy from therapy sessions. For example, warm and comforting chairs were used in reflection of humanistic philosophy, or seating of therapist and patient was arranged to imply their work as a team. In this regard the therapist should be able to face the client, at the same height and in a chair with similar characteristics, and not block the client's exit route.
- Allow for lighting and view control. While the therapists favored window views and daylight, privacy issues had led them to lower the curtains or blinds and create dimly lit interior space. Some psychologists had solved this problem by using reflective glass or clerestory windows.
- Provide privacy in the waiting room by dedicating an adjoining waiting room for each individual office or by staggering appointment times, so the clients would not run into each other.
- Provide individualized control of thermal conditions.
- Use neutral colors such as creams and whites, which are thought to produce a calming effect.
- Use radios and indoor water features to generate white noise and support audio privacy.
- Provide offices that support psychologists and clients. The researchers noted that psychologists and clients had dramatically different perspectives of the same office. While the therapists had views of "bookshelves and framed images," clients faced "a blinking computer screen and a desk cluttered with paper." In addition, the design of the office was only focused on visual cues and underused tactile, auditory, and olfactory components that can affect the experience of the space and effectiveness of treatment.

Bauzin and Hicks (2014) described design goals for a new outpatient facility for mental and behavioral health patients in West Michigan and provided design recommendations. The clinic was intended to be used by people with mild to severe mental illness who might be low- or high-risk probationers, have substance use disorders, have a recent history of imprisonment, or be homeless. To accommodate the needs of this population, the new facility offered a mix of scheduled and drop-in services. The main goals of the facility pursued by the design team included:

- delivering compassionate care;
- creating a safe and secure environment;
- creating a welcoming, comfortable, and pleasant place; and
- achieving quality and cost-effectiveness.

Bauzin and Hicks recommend several features:

- General ambience. The use of a versatile warm color palette as well as comfortable furniture that is too heavy to be used as weapons are recommended. They also recommend providing window views in public areas. Overall, the quality of design should tell the service users that "you matter."
- Staff spaces. A safe environment should also be created for the receptionists, through the incorporation of locking doors, glass sections for visibility to all the public areas, and alarms. Lockable storage rooms or lockers are recommended to be provided at the entrance of the facility since several service users arrive carrying duffel bags and backpacks.
- Consultation and therapy rooms. The authors specifically advise against use of small 6-foot by 8-foot consultation rooms, because to many service users with a history of imprisonment, this can be reminiscent of incarceration, which can subsequently undermine goals of therapeutic care. A therapy room that is spacious enough to provide space for the service user to walk and talk, store some belongings, or invite a family member, patient advocate, or translator is recommended. In each facility, it is recommended to provide a couple of individual therapy rooms that are slightly larger, to be used when proximity between therapist and client can be a safety issue. Although current trends encourage standardizing room types, providing options (office-like vs. lounge-like) can cater to a variety of preferences. Sound dampening is desirable for confidentiality and creating a quiet environment; however, it should not stop transfer of raised voices for safety reasons. Similarly, visibility into the rooms should be provided to allow monitoring without threatening privacy. Shah (1994) advised the physician's seat to be located closer to the door. With this simple adjustment, if the patient becomes violent, there is lower risk for the physician regarding being cornered and trapped in the room.
- Group rooms. Group rooms should also be designed and located so they can be monitored from the reception and registration area. Since most group sessions take place during the evening hours, making arrangements for security staff to be present at that time may be needed.

3.4 Case study

3.4.1 The Peter B. Lewis and Adam Lewis Wellness Center

Location:	New York, NY
Designer/Architect:	Elskop Scholz Architecture and Design
Client:	Fountain House
Date of Completion:	October 2011
Area:	6,210 gross square feet

Awards: Boston Society of Architects; Behavioral Healthcare Design Showcase

Client, service users, and services

Fountain House provides psychosocial rehabilitation services, housing support, family support and training, pre-vocational services, transitional employment, and supported employment. Many Fountain House members have experienced homelessness in the past. Over 500 members annually take advantage of varied levels of supported housing in New York and can access 24/7 reach-out services.

In collaboration with Mount Sinai St. Luke's and Mount Sinai Roosevelt, the center provides integrated medical, psychiatric, and social care. The Young Adult Program is geared toward individuals ages 18 to 30 and provides them with the support of a community of people who recognize their challenges and address them through education, connecting the individuals with nonprofits, community centers, and schools, and organizing recreational activities.

As the largest supported education program for people living with mental illness in the United States, Fountain House was awarded the First Prize for Excellence in Education by the National Council on Behavioral Health in 2013.

Mission and goals

Since 1948, Fountain House has been a not-for-profit social service organization located in New York City, the purpose of which is to allow members (clientele) to achieve "normal and productive lives within the community." The goal of the Peter B. Lewis and Adam Lewis Wellness Center, an addition to the existing Fountain House program, is to improve the wellness of Fountain House members by encouraging a healthy lifestyle in a noninstitutional environment. The intention is to mitigate side effects of psychotropic medications and improve patients' overall health status through this program.

Since close coordination with psychiatrists and general practitioners can be beneficial to the success of the program, a special group practice of physicians was created that operates at a nearby location. This proximity allows formation of a team-based approach in which the member, as the leader of this team, chooses participants in treatment planning meetings. The concept of a "medical home" is applicable to this setting in that psychiatric and medical needs can be met through a coordinated effort of care. The facility is anticipating the expansion of Fountain House's capacity to provide these services for up to 500 members.

Site

The expanded facility is located on the top two floors of the existing Fountain House building, which is located near mid-town Manhattan. These floors were renovated to house the wellness center. The existing facility, a 57,000-square-foot complex, is nested in a typical New York residential neighborhood and composed of a purpose-built, six-story structure and adjacent renovated four-story brownstone buildings.

Program

The wellness center is designed to provide large open areas with modular furniture that can support a variety of functions including meetings between staff and members, exercise classes, and social gatherings. The physical elements of the program include:

- a multipurpose meeting and teaching space;
- a commercial-grade teaching kitchen space equipped with an integrated audio-visual system that hosts cooking and nutrition classes;
- an exercise loft equipped with gym equipment with views to a green roof and to the city beyond;
- a glass-walled fitness space where yoga, stretching, ballet barre classes, and fitness exams are held; and
- member lockers and showers.

The therapeutic elements integrated into the program include:

- provision of healthy foods for a nominal price;
- low-cost membership at local gyms to support continuation of members' exercise routines;
- a three-day immersion program at a farm where a small group of members learn together and explore practical, healthy choices for their daily lives;
- workshops on a variety of necessary skills and knowledge including preventative testing and stress management; and
- a smoking cessation program.

Configuration and construction

The open floor plan interiors are configured to take advantage of daylighting on the eastern and southern façades. A curved acoustical ceiling, following the existing building ceiling line, connects the two floors of the interlocking space. New windows include thermal breaks and low-emissivity glass. Windows are positioned to permit natural ventilation. The interlocked ventilation system automatically stops HVAC when the windows are open to avoid energy waste. Dimmable, high-efficiency LED and fluorescent lighting fixtures are incorporated to allow greater lighting control. The green roof system installed on the southern exposure is intended to provide positive distraction, as well as cooling and drainage. Sustainably sourced, post-consumer aluminum is used in all the new furniture.

Case study bibliography

Elskop Scholz Architecture and Design. (2015). Project information and other in-house publication materials. Christopher Scholz, AIA & Ines Elskop AAIA.

Fountain House. (2015). Retrieved from organization website at www.fountainhouse.org/

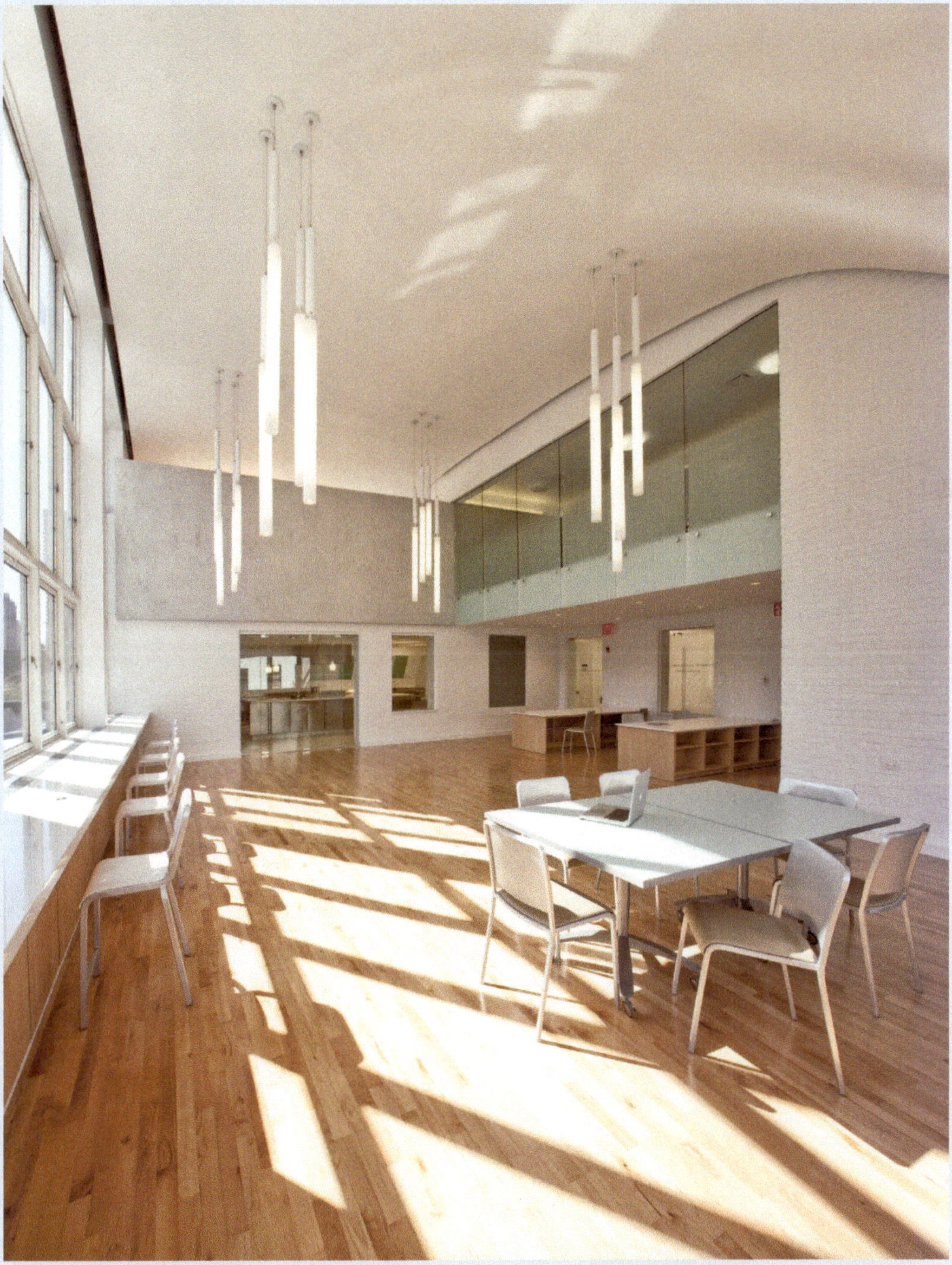

Figure 3.6: Fountain House – wellness meeting space (Architects: Elskop Scholz Architecture and Design)

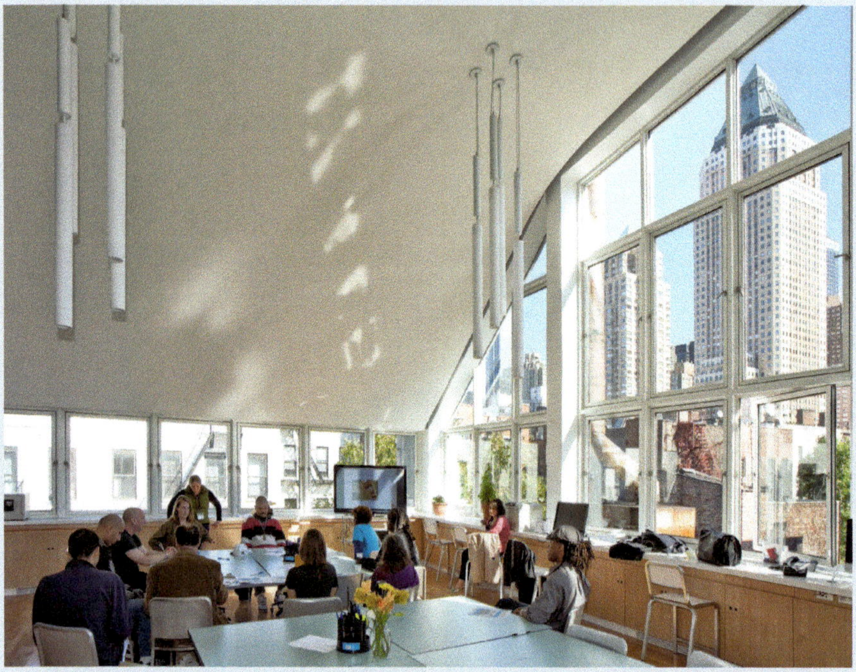

Figure 3.7: *Fountain House – wellness meeting space (Architects: Elskop Scholz Architecture and Design)*

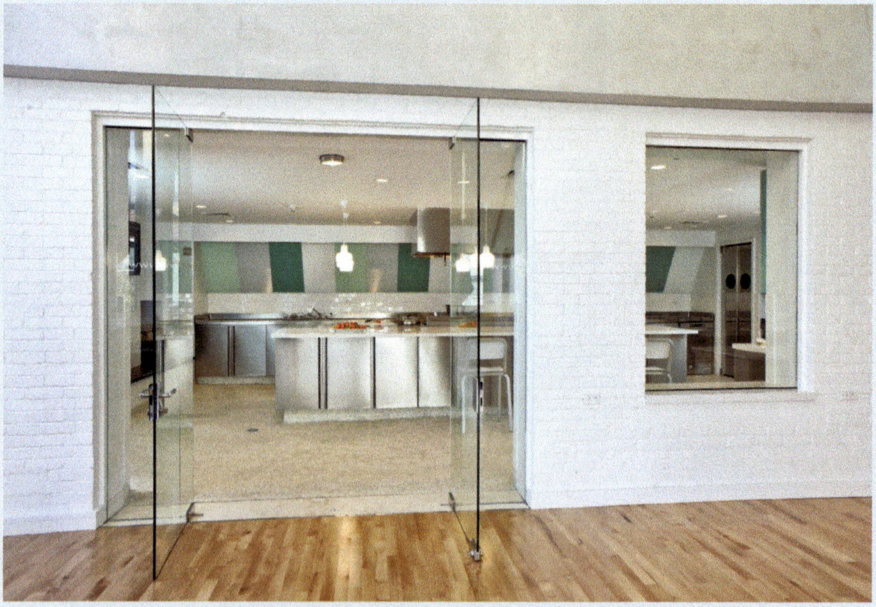

Figure 3.8: *Fountain House – wellness teaching kitchen (Architects: Elskop Scholz Architecture and Design)*

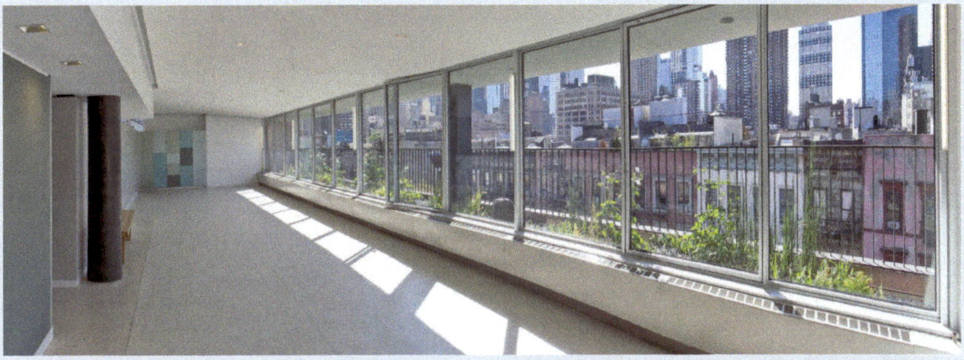

Figure 3.9: *Fountain House – wellness exercise loft (Architects: Elskop Scholz Architecture and Design)*

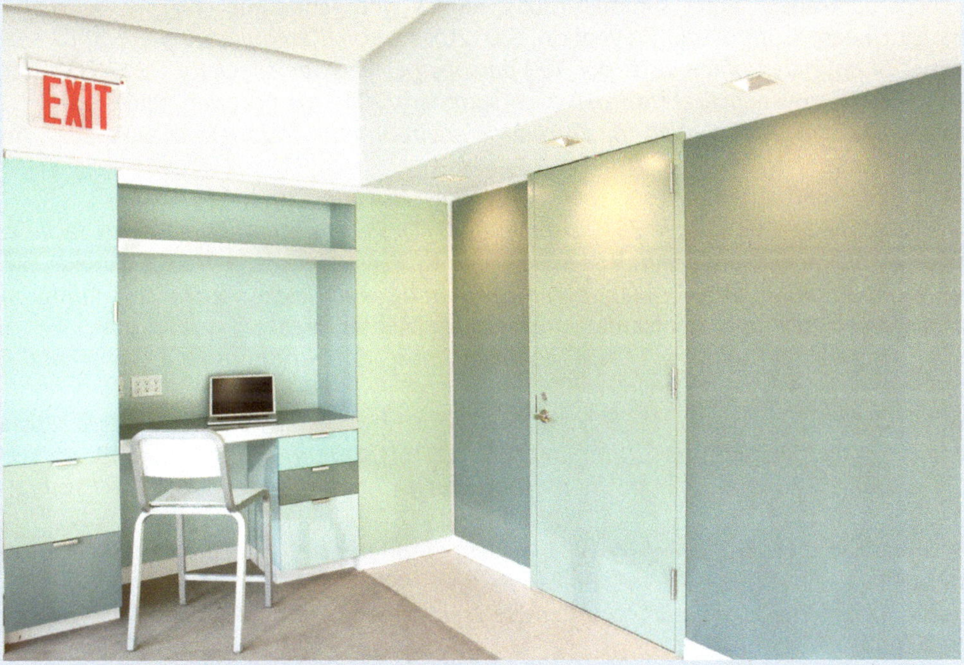

Figure 3.10: *Fountain House – wellness room (Architects: Elskop Scholz Architecture and Design)*

References

Adler, N.E. & Page, A. (2008). Cancer care for the whole patient: Meeting psychosocial health needs. Washington, DC: The National Academies Press.

American Psychiatric Association. (2000). Practice guideline for the treatment of patients with HIV/AIDS. *American Journal of Psychiatry*, *157*(11 Suppl.), 1–62.

Ashton, J. (1976). Community mental health in Britain and the USA. *Update*, 1083–1087.

Bauzin, D., & Hicks, C. (2014). Design recommendations for behavioral health outpatient facilities. *Behavioral Healthcare*. Retrieved from www.behavioral.net/article/design-recommendations-behavioral-health-outpatient-facilities

Brookman-Frazee, L., Drahota, A., Stadnick, N., & Palinkas, L. A. (2012). Therapist perspectives on community mental health services for children with autism spectrum disorders. *Administration and Policy in Mental Health*, *39*(5), 365–373.

Centers for Disease Control and Prevention. (2011a). *Annual number of ambulatory care visits by setting type according to diagnosis group 2009–2010 US*. Retrieved from www.cdc.gov/nchs/data/ahcd/combined_tables/AMC_2009-2010_combined_web_table01.pdf

Centers for Disease Control and Prevention. (2011b). *Annual number and percent distribution of ambulatory care visits by setting type according to diagnosis group: United States, 2009–2010*. Retrieved June 26, 2016, from www.cdc.gov/nchs/data/ahcd/combined_tables/2009–2010_combined_web_table01.pdf

Centers for Disease Control and Prevention. (2012a). *National ambulatory medical care survey: Mean time (minutes) spent with physician, by specialty, 2012 US*. Retrieved from www.cdc.gov/nchs/data/ahcd/namcs_summary/2012_namcs_web_tables.pdf

Centers for Disease Control and Prevention. (2012b). *National ambulatory medical care survey: Number of physician office visits per 100 persons per year, by specialty, 2012 US*. Retrieved from www.cdc.gov/nchs/data/ahcd/namcs_summary/2012_namcs_web_tables.pdf

Chrysikou, E. (2014). *Architecture for psychiatric environments and therapeutic spaces*. Amsterdam: IOS Press.

Cole, A. (1980, April). Alternatives to mental hospitals. *Nursing Times*, 673–674.

DATA. (2010). *The healthy people 2010 database (2011). Percentage of primary care facilities that provide mental health treatment*. Retrieved from http://wonder.cdc.gov/scripts/broker.exe

Dorsett, C., & Brown, B. (1965). *Planning, programming, and design for the community mental health center*. Pittsburgh, PA: National Institute for Mental Health.

Doyle, A., Lanoil, J., & Dudek, K. (2013). *Fountain house: Creating community in mental health practice*. New York: Columbia University Press.

Folkins, C., O'Reilly, C., Roberts, K., & Miller, S. (1977). Physical environment and job satisfaction in a community mental center. *Community Mental Health Journal*, *13*(1), 24–30.

Frank, J. (1968). The role of hope in psychotherapy. *International Journal of Psychiatry*, *5*, 383–395.

Gagné, S. Vasiliadis, H., & Préville, M. (2014). Gender differences in general and specialty outpatient mental health service use for depression. *BMC Psychiatry*, *14*, 135.

Guttersen, A. G. (1953a). Design of intensive treatment building. *Architectural Record*, *204*, 189–203.

Guttersen, A. G. (1953b). Psychiatric service in the general hospital. *Architectural Record*, *204*, 204–212.

Hunter, R., & MacAlpine, I. (1974). *Psychiatry for the poor: 1851 Colney Hatch Asylum-Friern Hospital 1973. A medical and social history*. Kent: Dawsons of Pall Mall.

Jimenez, D., Bartels, S. J., Cardenas, V., Daliwal, S. S., & Alegría, M. (2012). Cultural beliefs and mental health treatment preferences of ethnically diverse older adult consumers in primary care. *American Journal of Geriatric Psychiatry*, *20*(6), 533–542.

Nanda, U., Eisen, S., Zadeh, R. S., & Owen, D. (2010). Effect of visual art on patient anxiety and agitation in a mental health facility and implications for the business case. *Journal of Psychiatric and Mental Health Nursing*, *185*, 386–393.

Olfson, M., & Marcus, S. (2010). National trends in outpatient psychotherapy. *The American Journal of Psychiatry*, *167*(12), 1456–1463.

Olfson, M., Mojtabai, R., Sampson, N. A., Hwang, I., & Kessler, R. C. (2009). Dropout from outpatient mental health care in the United States. *Psychiatric Services*, *60*(7), 898–907.

Peek, C. J., & The National Integration Academy Council. (2013). *Lexicon for behavioral health and primary care integration: Concepts and definitions developed by expert consensus* (AHRQ Publication No.13-IP001-EF). Rockville, MD: Agency for Healthcare Research and Quality.

Polonsky, W. H. (1999). *Diabetes burnout: What to do when you can't take it anymore*. Alexandria, VA: American Diabetes Association.

Punekar, R. (2010). *Mental health, ambulatory mental health visits, and psychotherapeutic medications of U.S. cancer survivors and their spouses*. University Park: The Pennsylvania State University, College of Health and Human Development.

Sagha Zadeh, R., Shepley, M., & Gartner, M. (2013). *Important characteristics of counseling environments: Evaluation of an academic counseling center*. Unpublished manuscript.

Salloum, A., Johnco, C., Lewin, A., McBride, N., & Storch, E. (2016). Barriers to access and participation in community mental health treatment for anxious children. *Journal of Affective Disorders*, *196*, 54–61.

SAMHSA. (2012). *Behavioral health United States, 2012*. U.S. Department of Health and Human Services. Retrieved from www.samhsa.gov/data/sites/default/files/2012-BHUS.pdf

SAMHSA. (2015). *Behavioral Health Barometer United States, 2015*. U.S. Department of Health and Human Services. Retrieved from http://store.samhsa.gov/shin/content//SMA16-BARO-2015/SMA16-BARO-2015.pdf

SAMHSA National Council for Community Behavioral Healthcare. (2013). *A standard framework for levels of integrated healthcare*. SAMHSA-HRSA Center for Integrated Health Solutions. Retrieved from www.integration.samhsa.gov/integrated-care-models/A_Standard_Framework_for_Levels_of_Integrated_Healthcare.pdf

Shah, A. K. (1994). Psychiatric interview rooms and violence. *Medicine Science and the Law*, *34*(3), 247–249.

Sollie, H., Mørch, W., & Larsson, B. (2016, April). Parent and family characteristics and their associates in a follow-up of outpatient children with ADHD. *Journal of Child and Family Studies*, 1–14.

Watkins, N., & Anthony, K. (2007, November). The design of psychologists' offices: A qualitative evaluation of environment-function fit. *AIA Academy Journal*. Retrieved from www.aia.org/groups/aia/documents/pdf/aiab090825.pdf

Weiss, D., Dawis, R., England, G., & Lofquist, L. (1967). *Manual for Minnesota Satisfaction Questionnaire (Bulletin 45)*, Minneapolis: University of Minnesota, Industrial Relations Center.

Whitley, R., Strickler, D., & Drake, R. E. (2012). Recovery centers for people with severe mental illness: A survey of programs. *Community Mental Health Journal*, *48*(5), 547–556.

World Health Organization. (2011). *Mental health Atlas 2011*. Department of Mental Health and Substance Abuse, World Health Organization. Retrieved from www.who.int/mental_health/evidence/atlas/profiles/usa_mh_profile.pdf

Emergency psychiatric facilities 4

4.1 Introduction to emergency facilities

4.1.1 History of psychiatric emergency care in the United States

The first psychiatric emergency department in the United States may have evolved from a specialized variation on a traditional psychiatric hospital. At the turn of the twentieth century, Mosher proposed the creation of a psychiatric pavilion at Albany General Hospital to compensate for lack of mental and behavioral health hospitals in the area (Mosher, 1900). Opened in 1902, this 12-bed pavilion had a triage unit and was intended to admit psychiatric patients with mild symptoms who were perceived to recover without need of long-term psychiatric hospitalization (Lipsitt, 2003). The ward also had capacity to provide emergency care to patients in medical and surgical care who developed psychiatric conditions such as delirium or reacted undesirability to surgical anesthesia. Substance use patients could also be treated in this ward (Mosher, 1900).

For the remainder of the century, psychiatric emergency medicine in the United States evolved along three lines of delivery: (1) psychiatric emergency care in the general hospital emergency department (ED), (2) aftercare services in the psychiatric hospital, and (3) community mental health programs (Wellin, Slesinger, & Hollister, 1987). However, these models expanded in response to increased demand. During the 1960s, due to deinstitutionalization trends both in Europe and the United States, the number of severely mentally ill people living in communities was on the rise. Subsequently, the demand for emergency psychiatric care witnessed a rapid growth, especially in urban areas (Bassuk & Birk, 1984). The number of facilities providing emergency psychiatric care rose from 160 prior to the community care movement in 1963 to over 2,000 by the early 1980s (Wellin et al., 1987). During the first decade of the twenty-first century in the United States, the number of emergency units has shown a decline due to low profit margins (Hsia, Kellermann, & Shen, 2011); however, the number of community-based facilities, despite a 50% growth at the same time, is not still compatible with demand (SAMHSA, 2012).

4.1.2 Data regarding the psychiatric emergency population

In the United States, emergency department visits for psychiatric conditions comprise a substantial share of all ED visits. Of the 95 million adult visits made to U.S. hospital emergency departments in 2007, 12 million of them, or one in eight, involved cases of mental health (MH), substance abuse (SA), or both (MHSA) (Owens, Mutter, & Stocks, 2010). Mental illness and substance abuse as the primary reason for an ED visit accounted for 3% of visits in 2011, with 0.5% of visits resulting in admission to a psychiatric hospital (CDC, 2011).

As Sills and Bland 2002 had predicted the growth of psychiatric visits at times exceeding other patients population in ED, impacting the overall waiting time as ED mental health patients are typically triaged ahead of nonpsychiatric patients. Sills and Bland note that the stress and supervisory impact on staff of high-risk patients presents additional challenges. Most individuals who commit suicide have seen a healthcare professional prior to the event, so the pressure on staff to provide appropriate treatment is high (Sills & Bland, 2002).

Substance use alone imposes a great burden to hospital emergency departments. The Drug Abuse Warning Network (DAWN) categorizes substance abuse in six major categories: illicit drugs, alcohol, nonmedical use of pharmaceuticals, underage drinking, suicide attempts, and seeking detox (SAMHSA, 2013). (See Figure 4.1.) According to national data, during the past decade, the number of ED visits were on the rise almost proportionately to the number of reports of drug use. (See Figure 4.2.)

In every major category of MHSA patients that visit emergency departments in the United States, patients aged 18–44 years comprise the highest percentage in that category, with rates being significantly higher in intentional self-harm, drug-related conditions. (See Figure 4.3.)

In the United States, 41% of ED psychiatric patients are hospitalized, which is more than 2.5 times the rate of hospitalization for other ED visits (Owens et al., 2010). In Germany, analysis of data from the emergency department of Medical University of Hanover in 2002 showed that 51.4% of ED psychiatric patients were hospitalized. Patients who were potentially suicidal or showed symptoms of dementia were more frequently admitted, and patients who had companions were less likely to be admitted (Ziegenbein, Anreis, Brüggen, Ohlmeier, & Kropp, 2006). (See Figure 4.4.)

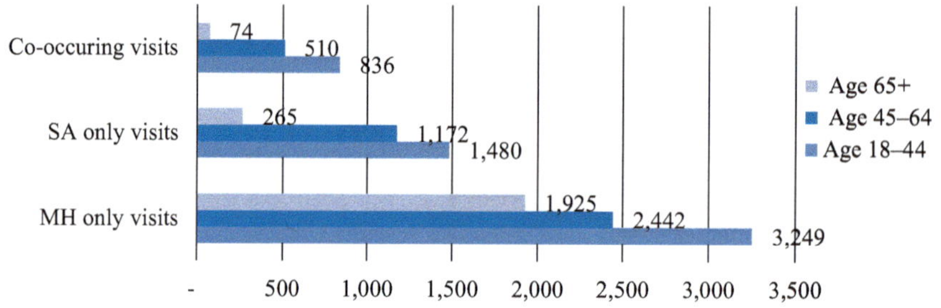

Figure 4.1: *Number of mental health/substance abuse related ED visits (in thousands) (Data source: Nationwide Emergency Department Sample, 2007)*

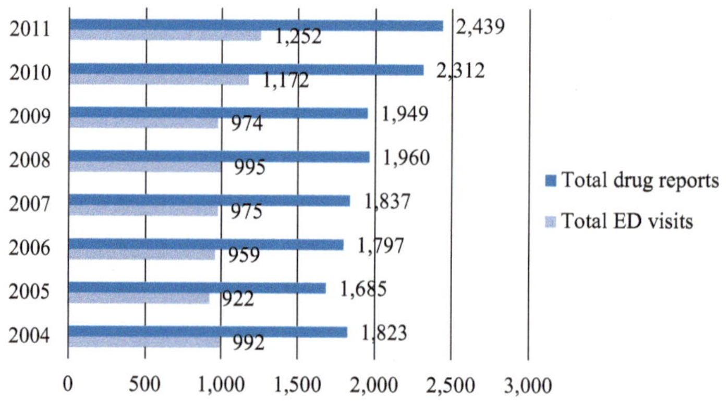

Figure 4.2: *Drug abuse related ED visit weighted estimates, 2004–2011 (in thousands) (Data source: Drug Abuse Warning Network [DAWN], 2011)*

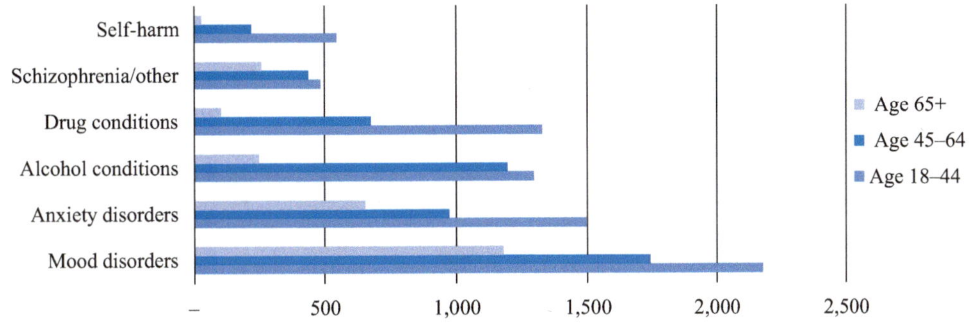

Figure 4.3: *Most common all-listed MHSA conditions seen during an ED visit, 2007 (in thousands) (Data source: Nationwide Emergency Department Sample, 2007)*

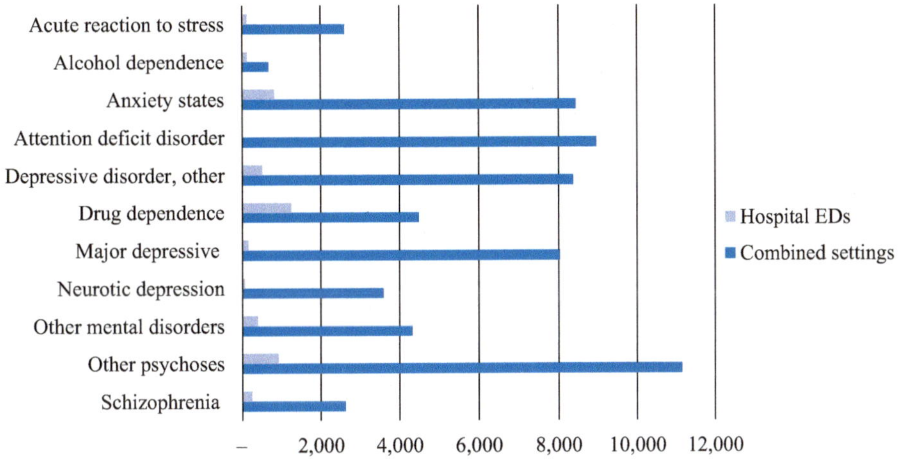

Figure 4.4: *Annual number of ambulatory care visits by setting type according to diagnosis group (Data source: Centers for Disease Control and Prevention, 2011)*

Data have been collected regarding specific subpopulations, primarily for children and adolescents. A summary of conditions with which pediatric ED patients present is provided in Figure 4.4. Of the cases, 10.8% resulted in diagnoses of psychosis and 13.6% were the result of suicide attempts. Pediatric mental health patients represent 1.6% of all ED visits in the pediatric age group (Sills & Bland, 2002). More recently (Pittsenbarger & Mannix, 2013), from 2001 to 2010, of the 28.3 million pediatric visits, there were 560,000 visits (2.0% of all ED visits).

There were approximately 434,000 ED pediatric mental health visits between 1993 and 1998, or approximately 33 visits per 1,000 people. Pediatric ED data from the National Hospital Ambulatory Medical Care Survey (NHAMCS) by Pittsenbarger and Mannix, (2013) show an increase in pediatric psychiatric ED visits – an estimated 491,000 in 2001 to 619,000 in 2010. Seventy-six percent of these patients had primary psychiatric diagnoses, including anxiety states/panic disorder, depression, drug abuse, and conduct disorders. The analysis also showed that teenagers and pediatric patients with public insurance are the most frequent users of emergency departments for psychiatric care. Current practices regarding initial assessment of agitated ED patients recognize five categories of patients: delirium, chronic cognitive disorder, intoxication or withdrawal, psychosis, or other conditions. Patients diagnosed with delirium need a detailed medical evaluation and treatment, while others require only a brief medical evaluation (Stowell, Florence, & Harman, 2012).

Data from North America suggest a reduction in inpatient days, increasing non-urgent ED visits, and lack of child psychiatrists (Carlisle, Mamdani, Schachar, & To, 2012). Case, Case, Olfson, Linakis, and Laska (2011) noted that mental health visits to pediatric ERs were more likely to arrive by ambulance, admitted or transferred. The median length of stay (LOS) was 169 minutes, longer than other visits (108 minutes), thereby placing significant demands on emergency departments.

When comparing the demographics of pediatric nonpsychiatric ED visits to pediatric psychiatric ED visits, we note that the demographics (location, insurance, race and ethnicity, gender, and age) are relatively similar between the two with the exception of age range. The largest percentage of children in the overall population presenting at an emergency department is children less than 5 years of age (46%); adolescents 13–17 years only represent 23% of the population. With regard to psychiatric ED admissions, the trend is in the opposite direction; 70% of admissions are 13–17, while only 5% are less than 5 years. (See Figure 4.5.)

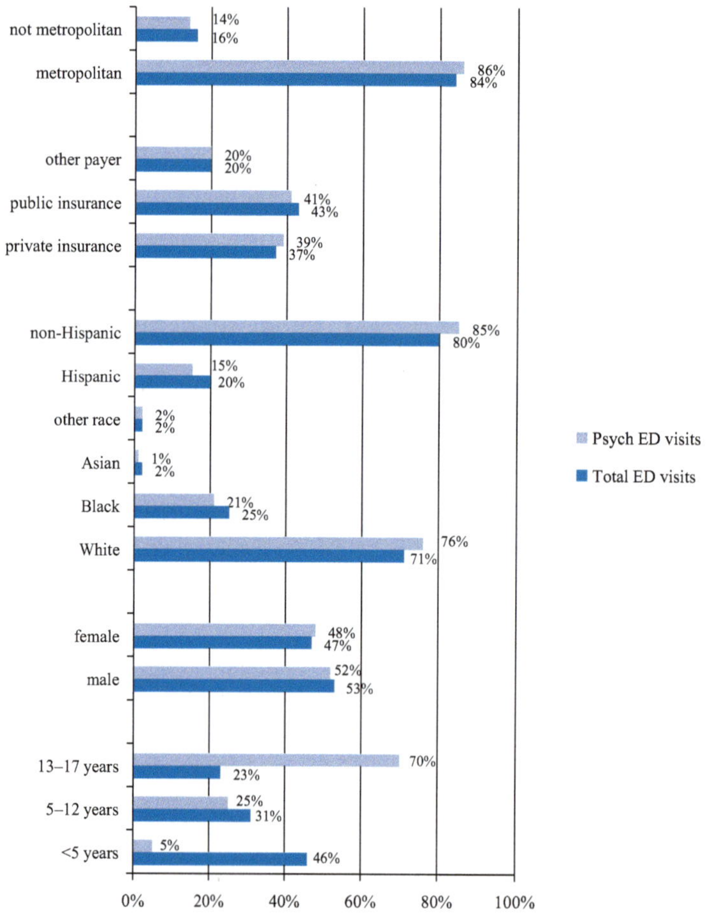

Figure 4.5: *Pediatric nonpsychiatric and psychiatric ER visits by demographic category (percentage) (Data source: Pittsenbarger & Mannix, 2013)*

The 2011 technical report by the American Academy of Pediatrics – *Pediatric and Adolescent Mental Health Emergencies in the Emergency Medical Services System* – states: "The ED has increasingly become the safety net for a fragmented mental health infrastructure in which the needs of children and adolescents, among the most vulnerable populations, have been insufficiently addressed" (p. e1364).

4.2 Characteristics of emergency psychiatric facilities

4.2.1 *Frequency and duration of visitations*

Patients with psychiatric complaints have a longer stay in the emergency department than other patients. Data from U.S. emergency departments between 2001 and 2006 show that the average duration of ED visits for patients with psychiatric complaints was 42% longer than others (Slade, Dixon, & Semmel, 2010). Because psychiatric patients in the United States are underserved, in most cases they use emergency departments for their acute care needs. The consequent overcrowding of the emergency departments negatively impacts emergency care for all patients (ACEP, 2008).

Community health services are intended to reduce the impact on emergency departments and inpatient bed demand. In exploration of this topic, Jespersen et al. (2016) studied a mental health system in Victoria, Australia, that combined the core functions of their services including ambulatory care, consulting, and residential services to help patients and families receive care from the same professionals throughout their use of the system. They conducted surveys with staff, patients, and caregivers, and focus groups with staff, and compared service usage with two other comparable facilities outside of this program. They found that both ED and inpatient use increased in all three facilities, regardless of integration status with community mental health programs. Survey data showed that patients reached out to ED services when in need of help due to urgency of their need, unavailability of community services at the time of need, and perceived shorter wait time. Staff reported that emergency demand was unnecessarily increased because of inappropriate referrals from the community services. However, a comparison of data among the three facilities suggests that population growth may have produced the increased ED use rather than integration of crisis team members into community mental health services.

The boarding time, or the waiting time for admitted psychiatric patients in an emergency department before they can occupy an inpatient hospital bed or be transferred to another inpatient facility, is high, ranging from hours to days for both adults and children (Bender, Pande, Ludwig, & Group, 2008; Case et al., 2011). The Joint Commission recommends that boarding in emergency departments should not exceed four hours (JCR, 2012). According to a 2008 survey conducted by the American College of Emergency Physicians (ACEP), more than 60% of psychiatric patients are boarded more than four hours, one in three wait over eight hours, and 6% wait more than 24 hours after admission before a hospital bed is available. In addition to low capacity for patient intake, screening tests can lengthen the boarding time (Korn, Currier, & Henderson, 2000; Weiss et al., 2012). Zun (2012) found that 70% of facilities board psychiatric patients for more than 24 hours, 10% of which exceed boarding for a week or more. Park, Park, and Siefert (2009) reported lack of insurance, public insurance, use of restraints, and high alcohol levels as predictors of long boarding time.

The Emergency Medicine Practice Group at the American College of Emergency Physicians (2014) summarizes the best practices for reduction of boarding as follows:

- Have a psychiatrist available either in person or via telemedicine to begin a treatment regimen.
- Incorporate treatment protocols, if a psychiatrist can't be available.
- Dedicate a quiet environment as an observation unit separate from the main emergency department to psychiatric patients.
- Involve ED case management and coordinate between emergency departments, community mental health services, and public mental health departments
- Increase reimbursement for psychiatric services to encourage providers to increase supply.

Other recommendations have been made regarding means of managing ED load and wait times. Little-Upah, Carson, and Williamson (2013) advocate use of regional psychiatry centers, staffed by psychiatrists 24 hours a day, seven days a week, supported by a dedicated and standardized regional transfer center with an active directory of available beds and services in the region as a means of managing the load. Abello, Brieger, and Dear (2012) studied efforts of three Texas hospitals servicing approximately one million people in Central Texas. The intention of the hospitals was to determine frequent ED users through a community database and create a care plan for them. ED visit frequency dropped from 8.9 to 5.9; however, due to study limitations, the authors suggest this finding cannot be readily translated to most ED populations.

Alakeson, Pande, and Luswig (2010) proposed a seven-step plan to reduce emergency room boarding needs that reflects some of the previously discussed approaches. Their plan consisted of:

1. Quantifying and monitoring the problem: The extent of psychiatric boarding issues needs to be studied nationwide.
2. Improving quality of care for psychiatric ED service users: High-quality care in ED can reduce the need for inpatient admission and will reduce demand for hospital beds.
3. Increasing efficiency of service delivery: Better communication, computerized bed management, and more efficient admission and discharge plans can create a more efficient patient flow.
4. Implementing low-cost collaborations: Instead of reaching out for costly hospitalization services, some patients can be referred to outpatient or community mental health centers.
5. Collaboration with law enforcement: This involves training of law enforcement officers about psychiatric crisis management, or including crisis management mental health professionals in the law enforcement teams.
6. Developing community crisis services: Provide psychiatric assessment and interventions outside of emergency departments.
7. Ensuring continuity of care: Guarantee the presence of effective and accessible community mental health services.

Satisfaction with psychiatric emergency departments is directly tied to availability and accessibility of services. O'Regan and Ryan (2009) conducted a survey study of 55 psychiatric ED patients to assess their post-service satisfaction. Almost 65% of respondents showed medium to low satisfaction with the service they received. Patients were mostly dissatisfied with unavailability of beds and long waiting time for assessment. Other areas of concern were poor communication, lack of information, and absence of care delivery at home. The authors concluded that this feedback has implications for development of community care to reinforce home-based interventions for adult mental healthcare.

4.2.2 *Number of emergency facilities*

According to data from the American Hospital Association, between 1998 and 2008, there was a 27% decline in the number of non-rural, hospital-based emergency departments in the United States, from 2,446 to 1,779. Hsia et al. (2011) analyzed data associated with 2,814 urban acute care hospitals over an 18-year study interval (1990–2007), and suggested that for-profit hospitals and those with low profit margins were more likely to shut down their emergency departments. Currently, psychiatric emergency services are handled primarily through walk-in emergency departments with psychiatric services and crisis intervention teams. Figure 4.6 describes the patterns by state.

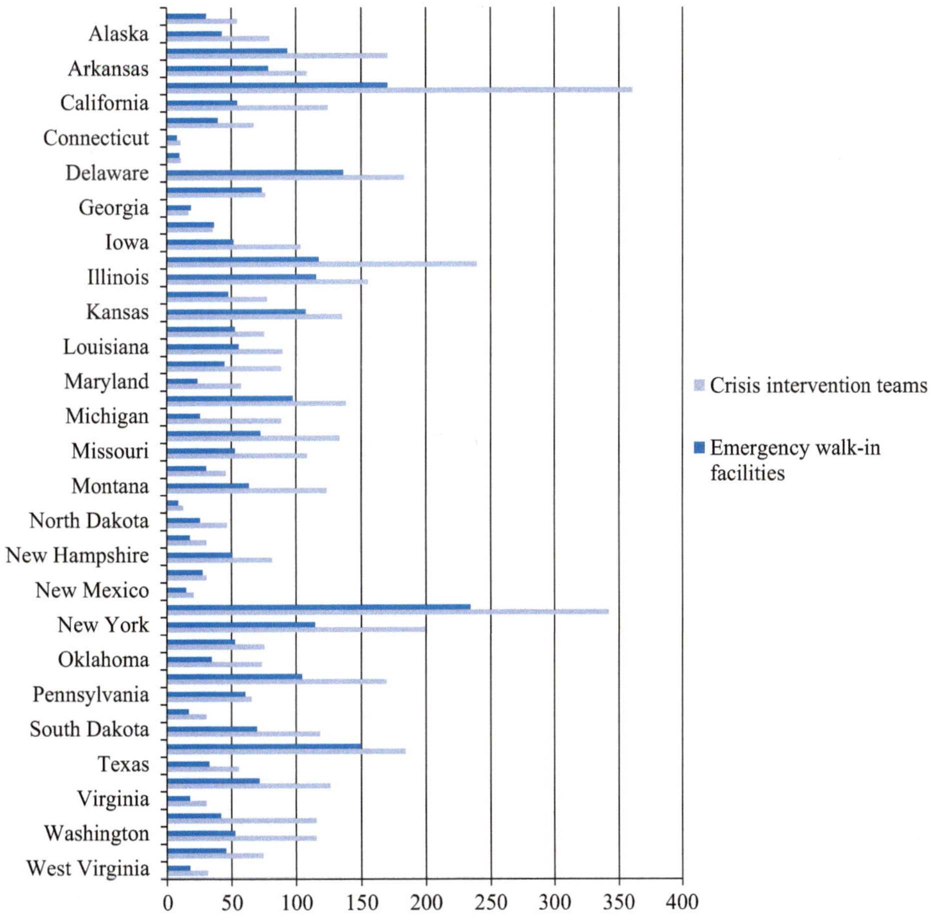

Figure 4.6: *Number of emergency psychiatric services per state (Data source: SAMHSA, 2016)*

4.3 Emergency psychiatric facility design

4.3.1 *Research on emergency psychiatric care design*

While there is limited research on the design of psychiatric emergency facilities, there are several studies the outcomes of which have clear physical environmental implications – studies regarding the need for dedicated spaces, the impact of creating regional facilities, and facility collocation.

4.3.1.1 Dedicated spaces

From psychiatric patients' perspective, emergency departments may fail in treating them at a status level equal to other patients. Clarke, Dusome, and Hughes (2007) found that psychiatric patients felt labeled and triaged regardless of the health concerns that motivated the ED visitation. For these reasons, the patients did not welcome the idea of separate emergency departments. As a result, the Emergency Nurses Association recommends defining and arranging a section of the emergency department for psychiatric patients and developing psychiatric nursing positions within the emergency departments (Manton et al., 2013).

Quick access to mental health assessment by specialized staff was identified as a major benefit to mental and behavioral health patients. The patients who needed short-term assessment would ideally be placed in a small admission area located within the psychiatric emergency department to eliminate the need for inpatient admission. Despite the benefits, the authors admit that psychiatric emergency centers can only be financially justified if they are collocated with large emergency departments, as they can be very expensive to staff (Frank, Fawcett, & Emmerson, 2005).

4.3.1.2 Regional services

To solve the long boarding time issue, two solutions have been explored: increasing available hospital inpatient beds or providing alternative emergency care facilities with the capacity to provide prompt treatment. In both cases prompt treatment is possible and might actually reduce the need for extended hospitalizations. A 2010 cost estimate by Doherty showed that a 20-hour stay at a regional psychiatric emergency service (at $110 per hour) would cost slightly less than the average ED boarding ($2,264) while eliminating the burden on emergency departments, as well as securing savings on avoiding expenses associated with psychiatric hospitalization and delayed treatment. This solution, however, requires a tightly knit network of hospitals and regional health services planning. In addition to capacity increases, better coordination and integration between the systems can help facilities make better use of available resources.

4.3.1.3 Collocation

In an Australian study, the efficiency of service delivery was investigated in a psychiatric emergency center that was collocated with the emergency department at a women's hospital. The psychiatric emergency center was intended to take referrals from the hospital emergency department, in addition to intakes from the police, ambulance and interhospital transfers, self-presentation, general practitioners and psychiatrists, drug and alcohol services, and community mental health centers associated with the hospital. In addition, a psychiatric emergency nurse would attend morning rounds on the acute patient units to identify likely referrals. Several benefits were realized after incorporation of this model, including direct access to specialized mental care, a better quality of care, and shorter wait times. The most important benefit is early involvement of mental health care services in cases of patients with a mental illness (Frank et al., 2005).

Gutkowski, Davis, and Ghinea (2000) followed changes in location and capacity of a psychiatric emergency department over a 20-year period. The changes, described in four distinct phases, included:

- Phase 1: Emergency department added to a psychiatric hospital to fill the void between inpatient and outpatient services.
- Phase 2: Services were added to the emergency department to enable stronger interaction with the surrounding community. These services included 24-hour services, telephone consultations, patient's family involvement, social services, the police, and other community services.
- Phase 3: Reorganization and downsizing of psychiatric inpatient services due to external forces and policies led to moving the emergency department to a psychiatric open ward.
- Phase 4: With the closure of the hospital, the emergency department was moved to a standalone facility, providing a full range of assistance, consultation, education, and hospitalization services.

They found that diversity and number of service users was increased in Phase 4. The authors suggest that the increase is due to reduced stigma and fear of being locked away due to the communal form of service delivery.

4.3.2 *Emergency psychiatric care design recommendations and features*

Design recommendations for emergency mental and behavioral health facilities are broken into the following subheadings in this section: general recommendations, entry, waiting areas, assessment rooms, seclusion rooms, and public/private space, the latter of which addresses risk assessment.

4.3.2.1 General recommendations

The functions of the psychiatric emergency center include triage, mental health and substance use assessments, admission and bed coordination, holding, and assessment. Admission, intake, and triage; referral to other community providers; resource information; and community, child and youth extended hours' services can take place by phone and in person (Frank et al., 2005). Spaces include indoor waiting and outdoor non-secure and semi-secure spaces, three interview/physical examination rooms, seclusion room, staff workstation, team room and offices, four-bed dormitory area for patient holding and observation, toilets/showers, and direct access to resuscitation area, short stay, security, and trauma entrance in the medical emergency department (Frank et al., 2005).

Controlled access, camera monitoring, metal detectors, and bulletproof glass are some of the design and physical provisions intended to enhance the security of emergency departments, according to the available literature (e.g., ENA, 2011; Pati, Harvey, & Pati, 2014). Pati, Pati, and Harvey (2016) suggested providing dedicated areas away from entrance or exit points in the emergency department for psychiatric patients. It is recommended these spaces be separated from other patients while having a nurse station nearby for supervision.

Similarly, Hunt and Sine recommend using a separate room for emergency admissions to the psychiatric unit. The room can be strategically positioned to protect the unit and emergency admitted patient from interrupting each other. Preferably this room should be welcoming, minimally furnished, and spacious enough to allow for several staff to physically manage the patient if necessary (Hunt & Sine, 2014). Strike et al. (2008) also recommend a psychiatric emergency area that is separated from the general emergency department to avoid exposure to noise and stress in the general ED, which can exacerbate the mental health condition of psychiatric patients.

4.3.2.2 Entry

Huddy (2014) proposes positioning a separate psychiatric zone in the emergency department that is directly accessible from both the walk-in entrance and ambulance entrance. In their proposed diagram (see Figure 4.7), this zone is easily accessible and visible by staff from other zones as well as security, to ensure added flexibility and safety. Huddy (2014) challenges the clinicians' desire for dedicating only one entrance/exit to the behavioral health zone as a means of reducing elopement. He argues that such layouts will create dead ends and unsafe situations for staff trapped by aggressive patients. Instead he proposes use of door-locking mechanisms to reduce chances of elopement while keeping staff safe.

4.3.2.3 Waiting areas

Pati et al. (2014) identified entry areas and the waiting/lobby area to be the most challenging security issues in an emergency department. Patient flow through the emergency department is a source of agitation among the patients. For example, patients who had to wait longer than more acute patients perceived that prioritization as discriminatory, and patients who had to return to the main waiting area after being triaged felt they were neglected or sent back (Pati et al., 2014). To address this negative impression, Pati and colleagues proposed sequencing of waiting areas in such a way that it matches the patient's movement through the care process as well as separating fast-track patients with higher levels of acuity.

Long waiting times have led facility administrators to think of new interventions to make waiting more manageable for the patients. Some studies have investigated the impact of therapeutic activities on patients and visitors. Miller and Spence (2013) used breathing exercises (abdominal yogic breathing as instructed by a yoga therapist) and music intervention (a compilation of calming music on a CD) on different days in a psychiatric emergency department. Pre- and post-intervention stress was measured using a survey with a 10-point Likert scale. From a total of 142 respondents, 63% endorsed breathing exercises and 51% supported music intervention. However, there were no significant differences between the interventions in terms of perceived stress reduction.

4.3.2.4 Assessment rooms

Psychiatric assessment rooms have been created to cater to the needs of a growing psychiatric ED population. Strike et al. (2008) conducted semi-structured interviews with 25 substance use male service users and staff in the emergency department at a large urban general hospital in Canada. They found that although the psychiatric assessment rooms were designed for patients requiring a quiet environment, the collocation of the room with general ED treatment rooms created a stressful environment for behavioral health patients, which according to staff "was not appropriate for patients in need of a calm environment." The staff also criticized lack of furnishings and art and felt

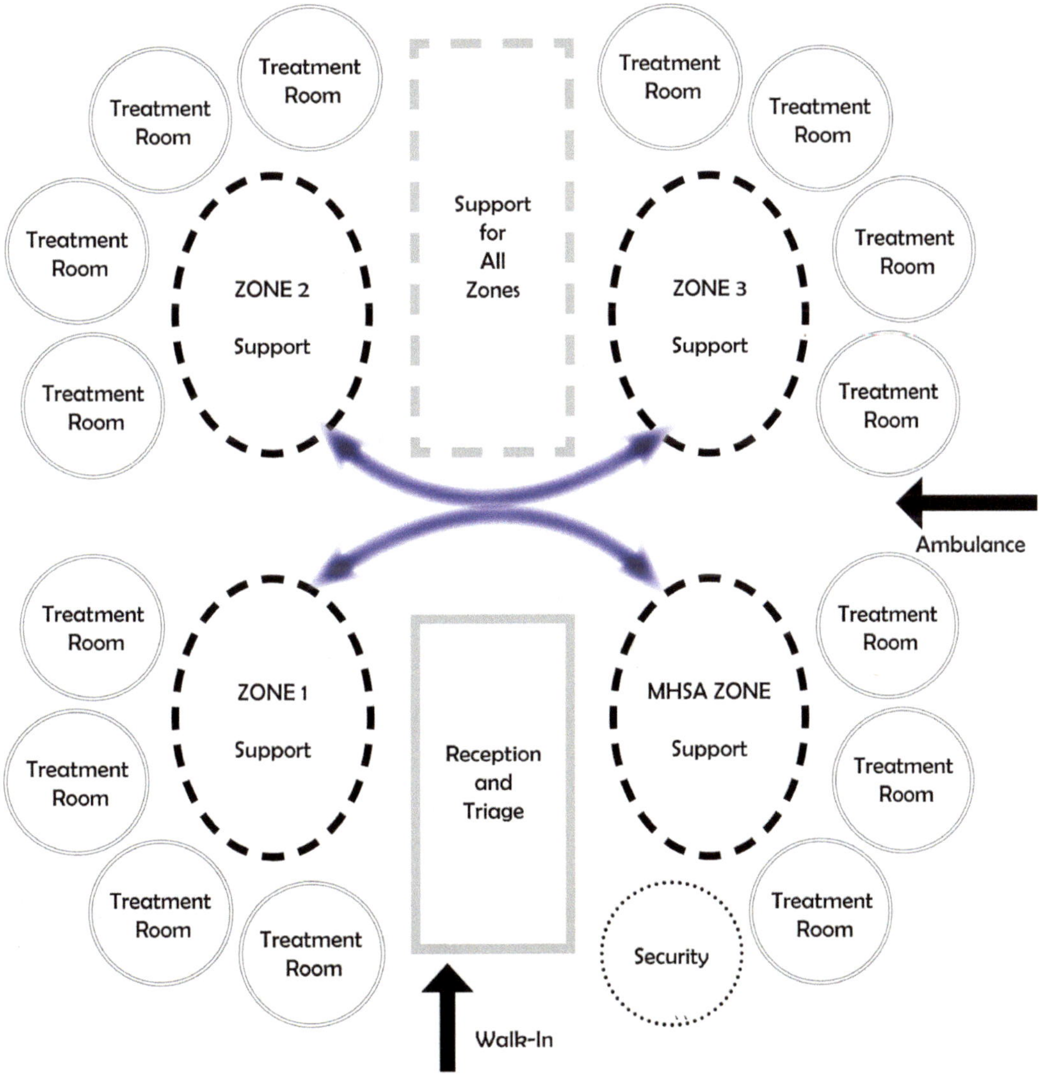

Figure 4.7: *Adjacency diagram of emergency department with a separate zone for mental health/substance abuse cases (Based on: Huddy, 2014)*

the rooms were isolated, claustrophobic, and jail-like. Patients described the rooms with the same qualities often used to describe seclusion rooms. Strike et al. (2008) suggest that such an environment can result in negative experiences that lead to patients avoiding or delaying visits, which can have fatal consequences. They recommend distancing assessment or seclusion rooms from staff socialization areas because patients might perceive that they are the subject of conversation and laughter they hear.

In behavioral health screening rooms or assessment areas, patients' reactions and behaviors are unknown to staff. Moreover, the patients might become agitated and violent regarding decisions for their admission. Consequently, such spaces should be minimally furnished, with equipment and supplies kept as far from the patients as possible. Arrangement of the space should grant a short and uninterrupted escape route to staff, in case the patient becomes violent. Duress alarms are also recommended to be used in these places (Hunt & Sine, 2015).

4.3.2.5 Seclusion rooms

Conflicts exist regarding various parts of programs and treatment in psychiatric emergency departments, the most important of which is the use of seclusion rooms. Nelstrop et al. (2006) conducted an exhaustive literature search, including systematic reviews, before and after studies, and qualitative studies from 1985 to 2002. The study was focused on safety and effectiveness of restraint and seclusion for the short-term management of psychiatric patients in emergency departments with destructive behavior. Nelstrop et al.'s (2006) review of the literature showed that seclusion rooms created feelings of anger, injustice, suppression, powerlessness, and degradation among the service users and can create long-lasting anxiety, trauma, and mental upset. Among the 36 studies identified, none were randomized controlled trials and most of them included many limitations that overall undermined the strength of the evidence produced. Consequently, the authors concluded that restraints and seclusion rooms should be used only as a last resort once other methods have failed. Some of the studies, however, suggest staff need for safety and control, which creates a conflict of interest for staff when making decisions about use of a seclusion room or restraints (Marangos-Frost & Wells, 2000). This need must be placed in the context of federal regulations in the United States (2003) that state that patients have the right to be free from seclusion or restraints and such interventions are only allowed to ensure the patient's physical safety in emergency situations.

4.3.2.6 Public and private space

McCurdy et al. (2015) examined seclusion rates before and after a design intervention that restricted patient movement between the waiting area and the unit. They documented a significant decline in number of seclusions, from 67 in 2,277 patients to 44 per 2,431 patients (approximately half the rate). The door that was added limited patient movement through the unit, which consequently limited the number of patients finding opportunities to act out outside of staff view. The authors also argued that limiting patient movement throughout the unit helped staff maintain a lower level of agitation in general, hence feeling less frustrated, more secure, and in control when the crisis arises. In closing, the authors note that although open accessible spaces can be therapeutic elements of design and promote staff-patient communication, there may be benefits to limiting patient access to clinical areas.

Building on the topic of surveillance, a matrix developed by Hunt and Sine (2014) categorizes spaces based on patients' degree of aloneness or privacy in the ED space. Design and operational decisions can be made based on the level of risk:

- Level I: Areas with no patient access or constant staff presence (mostly staff areas)
- Level II: Areas where patients are almost constantly supervised and escorted
- Level III: Areas where patients are less often supervised or escorted
- Level IV: Areas where patients have minimal or no supervision

Based on this definition, areas with Level I and II risk levels have more potential to take advantage of a homelike and residential design, while Level IV and III, due to higher risk of self-harm or violence, have more often than not assumed an institutional look.

Although the risk matrix was initially developed for inpatient units (Hunt & Sine, 2014), its principles may apply to any healthcare or residential setting that serves patients with mental and behavioral health diagnoses.

4.4 Case studies

4.4.1 Behavioral Healthcare Center of Excellence – Erie County Medical Center

Location:	Buffalo, NY
Designer/Architect:	Kideney Architects, P.C., in association with architecture+
Client:	Erie County Medical Center
Completion:	2014
Area:	18,000 square feet (outpatient programs)

Awards: Best Medical Complex – Buffalo Business First "Brick by Brick" Award

Client, service users, and services

Behavioral Healthcare Center of Excellence at Erie County Medical Center offers a comprehensive psychiatric emergency program (CPEP), as well as outpatient and inpatient mental healthcare to patients across western New York. The center is an expansion of the existing emergency behavioral health program, expanding from 6,500 to 18,000 square feet.

Mission and goals

The mission of the ECMC is to address the needs of patients and their families from across western New York and provide the best patient experience.

Site

The emergency department is located in the 36,000-square-foot behavioral health building on the ECMC campus and is one of three additions to the campus between 2011 and 2014. The building includes a 162-bed inpatient psychiatric program.

Program

The Behavioral Healthcare Center provides mental and behavioral health services including chemical dependency evaluations. The ED is composed of four areas: fast track, children's CPEP, adults' CPEP, and extended-stay observation beds.

Configuration

The fast-track and extended-stay units are located between the children's and adults' CPEPs, so they can be conveniently divided between the two populations. These four units form a U-shape that wraps around a central waiting and reception area. This central zone includes separate secure waiting zones for children and adults and one holding room for each, and a central spine that is dedicated to staff areas including reception, security, and triage. A locker room is also located along the secure spine, which patients can use to store their belongings. Two additional nurse stations are located inside the units and are connected through a staff corridor, which allows for both staff security and flexibility in staffing.

Case study bibliography

architecture+. (2015). Project information and other in-house publication materials.

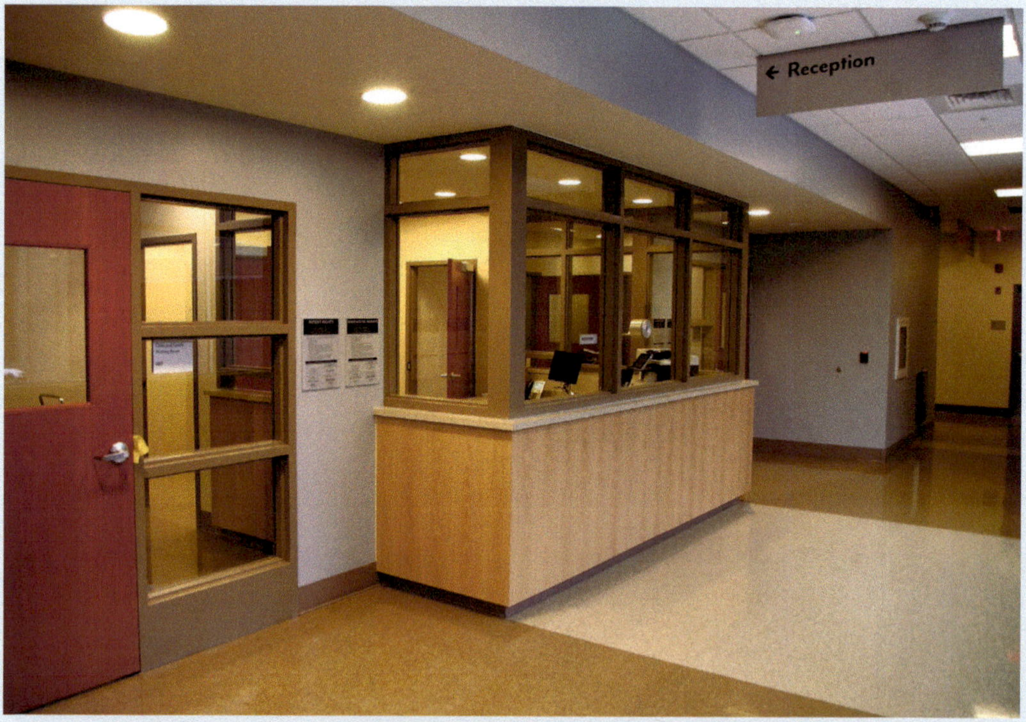

Figure 4.8: *Erie County Emergency Department – reception (Architects: Kideney Architects, P.C., in association with architecture+; Photo credit: Kideney Architects)*

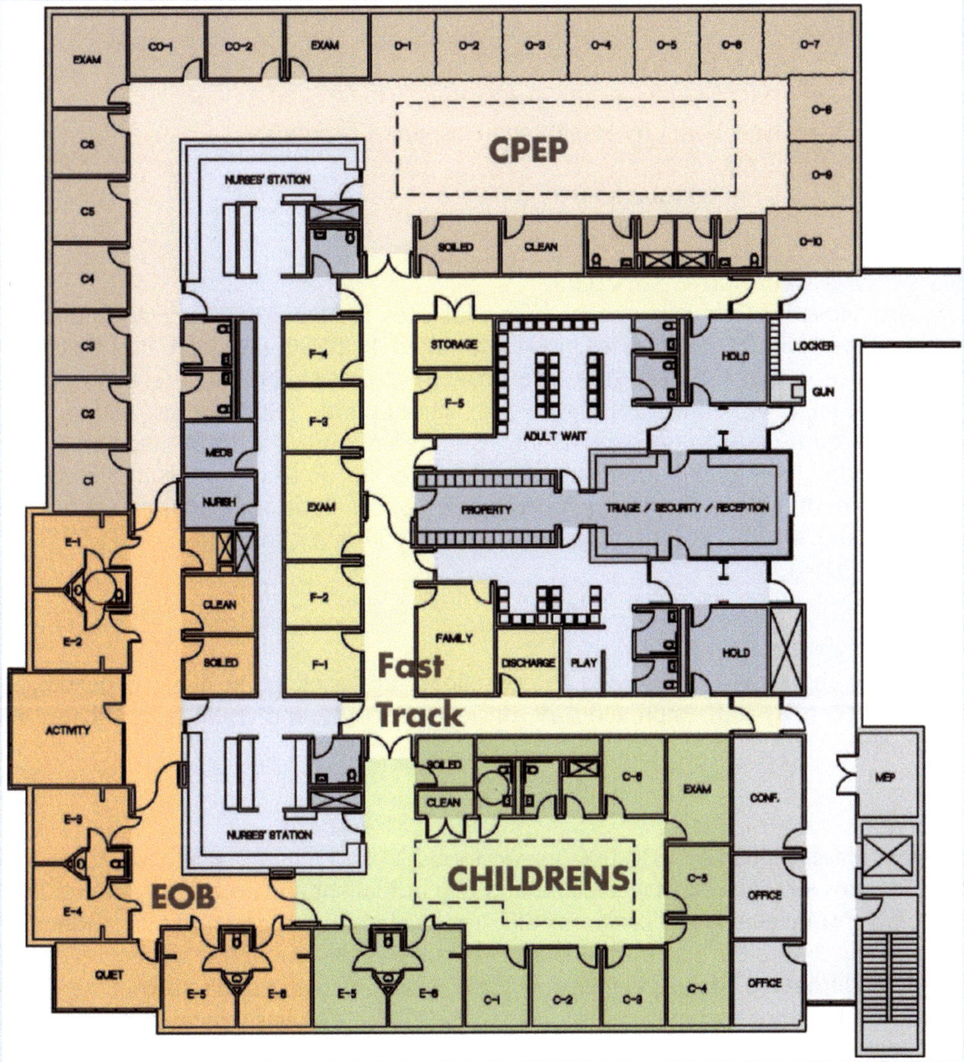

Figure 4.9: *Erie County Emergency Department – floor plan (Architects: Kideney Architects, P.C., in association with architecture+; Plan courtesy of Kideney Architects and architecture+)*

4.4.2 Emergency Department at Kings County Behavioral Health Center

Location:	Brooklyn, NY
Designer/Architect:	RBSD Architects and architecture+
Client:	New York City Health and Hospitals Corporation
Completion:	2008
Area:	314,000 square feet

Client, service users, and services

Kings County Hospital Center is one of four pilot sites in New York State to implement the "OnTrackNY" program that addresses individuals aged 16 to 30 who have had their first psychotic experience within the past year. The program provides tools to these individuals and their families to cope with stress associated with school, work, relationships, and identity, and to successfully reintegrate these persons into the community. The tools associated with this effort are intended to engage patients and their families for up to two years and include medication management, employment and educational support, substance abuse treatment, illness management, and suicide prevention, as well as family intervention and support (NYC Health and Hospitals, 2014).

Mission and goals

The mission for the overall center was to consolidate all functions in a single building. Goals included easy access by staff, improved staff efficiency, security, and visual compatibility with the site and context.

Site

The emergency facility is part of a 314,000-square-foot, 227-bed center that includes acute adult and pediatric programs including substance abuse and two outpatient and ambulatory clinics. The comprehensive psychiatric emergency program (CPEP) is located on the ground floor of Kings County Hospital, and adjacent to the intake area. The location allows for emergency admissions while being accessible to and from the intake and interview programs. This adjacency also allows the emergency department to serve more patients in peak hours. The intake area has secure vertical circulation to access the inpatient units on the upper levels. The entrance is in the back of the facility.

Program

The program has four zones: CPEP intake (sallyport, security, waiting, triage, secure holding, and seclusion), CPEP treatment (offices and exam rooms), CPEP observation (six rooms with direct access to shared restrooms), and CPEP administration (medical director, administrator, assistant administrator, and staff and secretarial spaces).

Configuration

The CPEP area has separate spaces dedicated for waiting and examination of children and adults. A triage area is strategically located with visual access to waiting areas, and immediate access to a secure holding room, exam room corridors, and a central observation unit. The central observation area includes three changeable zones for maximum flexibility based on day-to-day needs and demands. The CPEP also includes extended-stay observation beds located further away from the triage area.

Case study bibliography

architecture+. (2015). Project information and other in-house publication materials.

NYC Health and Hospitals. (2014). Kings County Hospital Center opens new mental health services to better care for adolescents in crisis. *News*. Retrieved August 25, 2016, from http://64.251.41.89/hhc/html/news/press-release-20140506-kchc-mental-health-adolescents.shtml

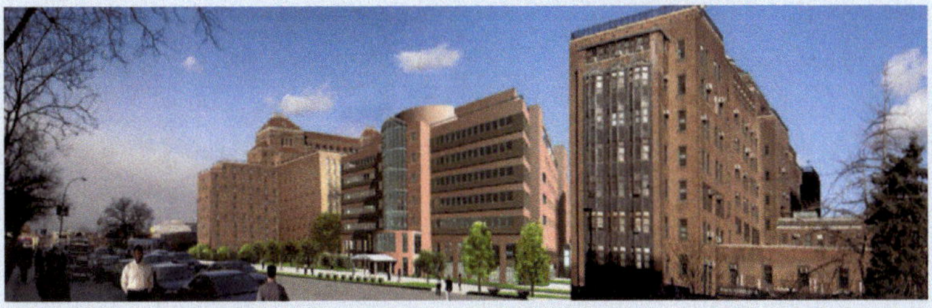

Figure 4.10: *Kings County Emergency Department – exterior (Architects: RBSD Architects and architecture+; Rendering by Alkhayer courtesy of RBSD Architects)*

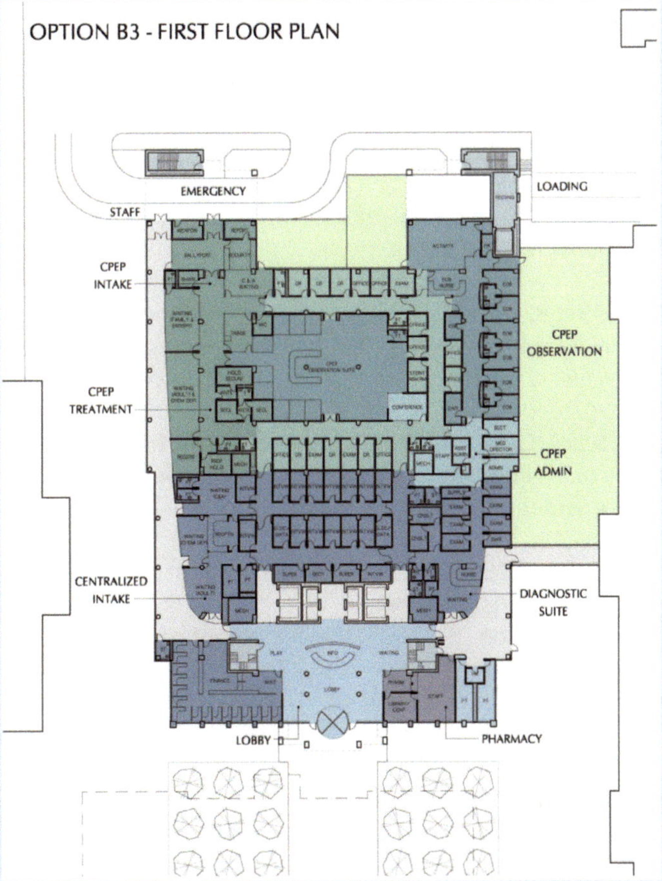

Figure 4.11: *Kings County Emergency Department – first floor plan (RBSD Architects and architecture+; Plan courtesy of RBSD Architects and architecture+)*

References

Abello, A., Brieger, B., & Dear, K. (2012). Care plan program reduces the number of visits for challenging psychiatric patients in the ED. *American Journal of Emergency Medicine*, *30*(7), 1051–1067.

Alakeson, V., Pande, N., & Luswig, M. (2010). A plan to reduce emergency room boarding of psychiatric patients. *Health Affairs*, *9*, 1637–1624.

American Academy of Pediatrics. (2011). *Pediatric and adolescent mental health emergencies in the emergency medical services system*, *127*(5), 1356–1366.

American College of Emergency Physicians. (2008). *ACEP psychiatric and substance abuse survey*. Irving, TX: ACEP.

Bassuk, E. L., & Birk, A. W. (1984). *Emergency psychiatry: Concepts, methods, and practices*. New York: Plenum Press.

Bender, D., Pande, N., Ludwig, M., & Group, T. L. (2008). *A literature review: Psychiatric boarding: Office of disability, aging and long-term care policy*. Washington, D.C.: Office of the Assistant Secretary for Planning and Evaluation. U.S. Department of Health and Human Services.

Carlisle, C. E., Mamdani, M., Schachar, R., & To, T. (2012). Predictors of psychiatric aftercare among formerly hospitalized adolescents. *Canadian Journal of Psychiatry*, *57*(11), 666–676.

Case, S. D., Case, B. G., Olfson, M., Linakis, J. G., & Laska, E. M. (2011). Length of stay of pediatric mental health emergency department visits in the United States. *Journal of the American Academy of Child & Adolescent Psychiatry*, *50*(11), 1110–1119.

Centers for Disease Control and Prevention. (2011). *National hospital ambulatory medical care survey: 2011 Emergency department summary tables*. Retrieved from www.cdc.gov/nchs/data/ahcd/nhamcs_emergency/2011_ed_web_tables.pdf

Clarke, D. E., Dusome, D., & Hughes, L. (2007). Emergency department from the mental health client's perspective. *International Journal of Mental Health Nursing*, *16*(2), 126–131. doi:10.1111/j.1447–0349.2007.00455.x

Doherty, R. B. (2010). The certitudes and uncertainties of health care reform. *Annual Internal Medicine*, *152*(10), 679–682.

Drug Abuse Warning Network (DAWN). (2011). *National estimates of drug related emergency department visits, 2004–2011*. Retrieved from www.samhsa.gov/data/emergency-department-data-dawn/reports

Emergency Medicine Practice Group. (2014). Care of the psychiatric patients in the emergency department – A review of the literature. *American College of Emergency Physicians*. Retrieved from https://www.ena.org/practice-research/research/Documents/ENAEDVSReportNovember2011.pdf

Emergency Nurses Association. (2011). *Emergency department violence surveillance study*. Des Plaines, IL: Emergency Nurses Association.

Frank, R., Fawcett, L., & Emmerson, B. (2005). Development of Australia's first psychiatric emergency centre. *Australian Psychiatry*, *13*(3), 266–272.

Gutkowski, S., Davis, H., & Ghinea, C. (2000). The wandering psychiatric emergency room, design, location and transformations. *Israel Journal of Psychiatry and Related Sciences*, *37*(4), 297–301.

Hsia, R. Y., Kellermann, A. L., & Shen, Y. C. (2011). Factors associated with closures of emergency departments in the United States. *JAMA*, *305*(19), 1978–1985.

Huddy, J. (2014). Behavioral health suites: Locations can support safe environment. *Huddy Healthcare Solutions*. Retrieved July 2, 2016, from http://huddyhealthcare.com/behavioral-health-suites-location-can-support-a-safe-environment/

Hunt, J., & Sine, D. (2014). Design guide for the built environment of behavioral health facilities. *National Association of Psychiatric Health Systems*. Retrieved from www.naphs.org

Hunt, J., & Sine, D. (2015). Common mistakes in designing psychiatric hospitals, an update. *Facility Guidelines Institute*. Retrieved from www.fgiguidelines.org/resource/common-mistakes-in-designing-psychiatric-hospitals-an-update/

Jespersen, S., Lawman, B., Reed, F., Hawke, K., Plummer, V., & Gaskin, C. J. (2016). The impact of integrating crisis teams into community mental health services on emergency department and inpatient demand. *Psychiatric Quarterly*. doi:10.1007/s11126-016-9420-8.

Joint Commission Resources. (2012). Approved: Standards revisions addressing patient flow through the emergency department. *Joint Commission Perspectives, 32*(7), 1–5.

Korn, C. S., Currier, G. W., & Henderson, S. O. (2000). Medical clearance of psychiatric patients without medical complaints in the emergency department. *Journal of Emergency Medicine, 18*(2), 173–176.

Lipsitt, D. (2003). Psychiatry and the general hospital in an age of uncertainty. *World Psychiatry, 2*(2), 87–92.

Little-Upah, P., Carson, C., & Williamson, R. (2013). The banner psychiatric center: A model for providing psychiatric crisis care to the community while easing behavioral health holds in emergency departments. *The Permanente Journal, 17*(1), 45–49.

McCurdy, J., Haliburton, J., Yadav, H., Yoder, A., Norton, L., Froehlich, J., . . . El-Mallakh, R. (2015). Case study: Design may influence use of seclusion and restraint. *Health Environments Research and Design Journal, 8*(3), 116–121.

Manton, A. (2013). *Care of the psychiatric patient in the emergency department*. Des Plaines, IL: Emergency Nurses Association.

Marangos-Frost, S., & Wells, D. (2000). Psychiatric nurses' thoughts and feelings about restraint use: A decision dilemma. *Journal of Advanced Nursing, 31*, 362–369.

Miller, R., & Spence, J. (2013). The impact of breathing and music on stress level of clients and visitors in a psychiatric emergency room. *The Art in Psychotherapy, 40*, 347–351.

Mosher, J. M. (1900). The insane in general hospitals. *American Journal of Insanity, 57*, 325–329.

Nationwide Emergency Department Sample. (2007). Number of mental health/substance abuse related ED visits. *AHRQ, Healthcare Cost and Utilization Project*. Retrieved from www.hcup-us.ahrq.gov/reports/statbriefs/sb92.pdf

Nelstrop, L., Chandrler-Oatts, J., Bingley, W., Bleetman, T., Corr, F., Cronin-Davis, J., . . . Tsuchiya, A. (2006). A systematic review of the safety and effectiveness of restraint and seclusion as interventions for the short term management of violence in adult psychiatric inpatient setting and emergency department. *Worldwide Views on Evidence-Based Nursing, 3*(1), 8–18.

O'Regan, C., & Ryan, M. (2009). Patient satisfaction with an emergency department psychiatric service. *International Journal of Healthcare Quality Assurance, 22*(5), 525–534.

Owens, P., Mutter, R., & Stocks, C. (2010). *Mental health and substance abuse-related emergency department visits among adults, 2007*. Rockville, MD: Agency for Healthcare Research and Quality.

Park, J. M., Park, L. T., & Siefert, C. J. (2009). Factors associated with extended length of stay for patients presenting to an urban psychiatric emergency service: A case-control study. *Journal of Behavioral Health Service and Research, 36*(3), 200–208.

Pati, D., Harvey, T., & Pati, S. (2014). Physical design correlates of efficiency and safety in emergency departments: A qualitative examination. *Critical Care Nursing, 37*(3), 299–316.

Pati, D., Pati, S., & Harvey, T. (2016). Security implications of physical design attributes in the emergency department. *Health Environments Research and Design Journal, 9*(4), 50–63.

Pittsenbarger, Z., & Mannix, R. (2013). Trends in pediatric visits to the emergency department for psychiatric illness. *Academic Emergency Medicine*, *21*(1), 25–30.

SAMHSA. (2012). *Behavioral Health United States, 2012*. U.S. Department of Health and Human Services. Retrieved from www.samhsa.gov/data/sites/default/files/2012-BHUS.pdf

SAMHSA. (2013). *Drug abuse warning network, 2011: National estimates of drug related emergency department visits* (HHS Publication number (SMA) 13–4760, DAWN Series D-39). Rockville, MD: Substance Abuse and Mental Health Services Administration.

SAMHSA. (2016). *Behavioral health treatment facility locator*. Retrieved from www.findtreatment.samhsa.gov

Sills, M. R., & Bland, S. D. (2002). Summary statistics for pediatric psychiatric visits to US emergency departments, 1993–1999. *Pediatrics*, *110*(4), e40–e40.

Slade, E. P., Dixon, L. B., & Semmel, S. (2010). Trends in the duration of emergency department visits, 2001–2006. *Psychiatric Services*, *61*(9), 878–884.

Stowell, K. R., Florence, P., & Harman, H. J. (2012). Psychiatric evaluation of the agitated patient: Consensus statement of the American Association for Emergency Psychiatry Project Beta Psychiatric Evaluation Workgroup. *The Western Journal of Emergency Medicine*, *13*, 11–16.

Strike, C., Rufo, C., Spence, J., Links, P., Bergmans, Y., Ball, J., & Eynan, R. (2008). Unintended impact of psychiatric safe rooms in emergency departments: The experiences of suicidal males with substance use disorders. *Brief Treatment and Crisis Intervention*, *8*(3), 264–273.

Weiss, A. P., Chang, G., Rauch, S. L., Smallwood, J. A., Schechter, M. Kosowsky, J., . . . Orav, E. J. (2012). Patient- and practice-related determinants of emergency department length of stay for patients with psychiatric illness. *Annals of Emergency Medicine*, *60*(2), 162–171.

Wellin, E., Slesinger, D. P., & Hollister, C. D. (1987). Psychiatric emergency services: evolution, adaptation and proliferation. *Social Science Medicine*, *24*(6), 475–482.

Ziegenbein, M., Anreis, C., Brüggen, B., Ohlmeier, M., & Kropp, S. (2006). Possible criteria for inpatient psychiatric admissions: Which patients are transferred from emergency services to inpatient psychiatric treatment? *BMC Health Services Research*, *6*, 150. Retrieved from http://doi.org/10.1186/1472-6963-6-150

Zun, L. S. (2012). Pitfalls in the care of the psychiatric patients in the ED. *Journal of Emergency Medicine*, *43*(5), 829–835.

Substance use disorder treatment settings

5

5.1 Introduction

5.1.1 History of facilities for treatment of substance use disorders in the United States

As early as the nineteenth century, asylums were established as charitable institutions to treat alcoholism. Social reformers of the period, as well as physicians, argued that inebriants were creating chaos in jails and "insane asylums" and needed dedicated facilities to receive proper treatment (Yanni, 2007). The New York State Inebriate Asylum, later known as Binghamton State Hospital, was founded in 1858 based on the theory that inebriety, like insanity, needs medical and moral treatment and was the first of this kind established in the world (Barber & Howe, 1861).

Another prototype, therapeutic communities, was shaped later to help people struggling with drug addiction to recover and return to society. The concept behind a therapeutic community is to use the social interactions of a group of individuals confronted with similar challenges as part of the treatment program. This treatment plan originated in 1958, when psychiatry and general medicine were unsuccessful in treating substance use disorders (Center for Substance Abuse Treatment, 1999). Synanon, a self-supporting community of ex-addicts founded in 1958 in Santa Monica, California, is known as the first therapeutic community established in the United States (Goethals, Soyez, Melnick, Leon, & Broekaert, 2011).

By 1993 the federal government funded each state to provide community mental health services through the Alcohol, Drug Abuse and Mental Health Block Grant (Rochefort, 1993). Since then, the standard therapeutic community model has been modified to create programs for women with children, persons with co-occurring psychiatric disorders, prisoners, or other specific populations (Sacks, Chaple, Sacks, McKendrick, & Cleland, 2012).

Through the work of proponents of deinstitutionalization during the past 50 years, treatment for substance abuse has moved from the hospital to community-based residential facilities. Also, a gradual shift from inpatient care to outpatient care for substance abuse recovery patients was observed in the 1970s and 1980s (Malkin, 1991) and is continually observed through available nationwide data reports (e.g., SAMHSA, 2012).

5.1.2 Characteristics and needs of substance use disorder patients

Privacy and safety are important factors in design for substance abuse patients, as discussed by Malkin (1991). Job security or family status might be threatened by public awareness of an individual's addiction. Similar to any mental health setting, safety issues should be considered, since many service users are dual diagnosis patients. According to NAMI (2016) almost half of people with severe mental illnesses also experience substance abuse. Half of all drug abusers also report a mental illness diagnosis.

As for all patients, environments for patients with substance use disorders must address the various cultural backgrounds and the resultant need for a more universal treatment plan. Dialectical behavior therapy (DBT) is an evidence-based treatment for substance use disorders (e.g., Neacsiu & Linehan, 2014) and considers cultural differences. Because of DBT's emphasis on mindfulness, a concept known to most cultures throughout history, it can be successfully used with people with different backgrounds and demographics. DBT addresses problem behaviors of patients, such as life-threatening behavior including self-injury and suicide, behaviors that interfere with treatment, and behaviors that interfere with quality of life (Beckstead, Lambert, DuBose, & Linehan, 2015).

Efficacy of the treatment is determined by both the program or setting and the social environment. A social network can play a significant role in decreasing support for substance-seeking behavior while increasing support for sobriety that is associated with reduced risk for relapse (e.g., Litt, Kadden, Kabela-Cormier, & Petry, 2009). Another factor that can determine success of treatment programs is continuity of care. Patients in recovery generally experience high levels of anxiety, anger, and hyperactivity (Malkin, 1991). Lack of continuity can be particularly problematic for specific populations. According to Zinbarg, Barlow, and Brown (1997), anxiety sensitivity is an individual's fear of consequences of anxiety-related sensations including physical, mental, and social aspects, and it can be related to treatment dropout among individuals admitted to residential treatment facilities. The physical environment can play a significant role in anxiety reduction.

Continuity of care has multiple definitions. Washington Circle (a group of national experts) measures continuation of care based on outpatient follow-up visitation within 14 days after discharge from residential treatment (Garnick et al., 2012). RAND and the Altarum Institute measure continuity of care by identifying the proportion of patients admitted to residential treatment who are discharged or self-discharged within one week (Peterson, Swindle, Phibbs, Recine, & Moos, 1994). Harris et al. (2015) conducted a study to evaluate the validity of these measures and found that they can predict two-year mortality rates, while the early discharge measure can also predict subsequent detoxification episodes. These measures might be useful tools for post-occupancy evaluation.

Technology can be used as a viable platform for supporting patients following treatment completion. For example, Dahne and Lejuez (2015) found that smartphone use among patients who will be admitted to or discharged from residential substance abuse treatment facilities is identical to that of the U.S. general public. Consequently, treatment programs can potentially make follow-up care more successful through use of smartphone applications. Facilities that provide space for staff to privately respond to patient calls would support this activity.

Researchers argue that because shorter treatment plans require less commitment for completion, they are more likely to be successful compared to long treatment plans. However, each group may benefit more from either long or short treatment programs based on their unique needs.

Other demographic variables may have a significant impact on recovery of persons with substance use disorders. Drake et al. (2015) compared two cohorts in two different community mental health centers (one in rural New Hampshire and the other in urban Connecticut), with both substance use disorder and schizophrenia symptoms. The integrated mental health and substance abuse treatment was provided by multidisciplinary teams offering motivational interviewing and access to dual recovery groups (recovery self-help groups for persons with dual diagnosis). The cohorts had differences in terms of demographics. The rural New Hampshire group was predominantly Caucasian and relatively well-educated persons who mostly abused alcohol. The urban Connecticut group was mostly minorities, only half of whom had graduated from high school, and most of whom had experienced homelessness, incarceration, unemployment, and cocaine use.

The majority of participants in both cohorts achieved meaningful clinical recoveries. However, the less advantaged cohort did not attain significant improvements in social and activity measures, such as independent living and working competitively, and were more likely to be hospitalized and incarcerated after the treatment. Challenges to living in inner-city environments compared to rural environments can be responsible for this outcome. However, the greater social disadvantage the inner-city cohort experienced could be the main reason for differences in recovery.

Substance use disorder (SUD) is a condition in which the use of one or more psychoactive drugs leads to a clinically significant impairment or distress. This term encompasses substance abuse and substance dependence (defining social consequences and physiological-behavioral symptoms respectively) (American Psychiatric Association, 2013). Physiological and behavioral consequences of substance use may include paranoia, hallucinations, sleepiness, and violent behavior, among several others (National Institute for Drug Abuse, 2016). Social consequences of substance abuse include persistent or recurrent social or interpersonal problems or impairments that are caused or exacerbated by the physical, financial, or psychological effects of substance abuse.

The National Survey on Drug Use and Health (NSDUH) administered by SAMHSA estimates the percentage of the population aged 12 or older who had SUDs in the past 12 months. This percentage has been growing steadily from 2002 through 2014, primarily by marijuana use and the nonmedical use of prescription pain relievers. In 2014, approximately 21.5 million people aged 12 or older had an SUD in the past year, of which 17.0 million had an alcohol use disorder. In the same year, 7.1 million had an illicit drug use disorder (including marijuana, cocaine, heroin, hallucinogens, inhalants, and the nonmedical use of prescription-type psychotherapeutic drugs), and 2.6 million had both.

Amongst the adults surveyed in 2014, about 3.3% had a mental illness in addition to substance use disorder, of which almost one-third had a severe mental illness. An estimated 340,000 adolescents had an SUD and major depressive episode in 2014 (Center for Behavioral Health Statistics and Quality, 2015).

During the past two decades, co-occurring disorders (CODs) have been the focus of several publications on persons with substance use disorders. COD is attributed to individuals with severe mental illness who are at a higher risk of substance use compared to the general population. The combination makes persons with COD less likely to seek or continue treatment (Priester et al., 2016). The Comprehensive, Continuous, Integrated System of Care (CCISC) recognized by SAMHSA is used in the United States, Canada, and Australia as an integrated COD treatment protocol (Minkoff, 2013). The COD principles are focused on providing individualized, empathic, and recovery-oriented care plans that address both mental health and substance abuse diagnoses as primary concerns. The protocol has shown success; however, researchers are still in quest for a more integrative approach (Moore & Fraser, 2013).

5.2 Characteristics of facilities for persons with substance use disorders

SAMHSA's facility locator identifies available settings as hospital inpatient, day treatment, outpatient, short-term or long-term residential, and computerized treatment. Data from SAMHSA show the number of substance abuse treatment facilities increased slightly between 2003 and 2013 (from 13,623 facilities in 2003 to 14,148 facilities in 2013). The number of service users increased by 14% (from 1,092,546 in 2003 to 1,249,629 in 2013). Newly approved methods of treatment including long-acting injectable medications have been growing more rapidly in the past decade (Rinaldo & Rinaldo, 2013). Available services currently are provided in a wide variety of settings, including hospitals, day hospitals, residential facilities, and outpatient facilities. (See Figure 5.1.)

A successful recovery program will help patients restore confidence and self-esteem and find a reason for living. The program can include group therapy, family counseling, individual therapy, lectures, and exercise (Malkin, 1991). However, several other ancillary services for patients and their families, as well as necessary health screening and testing, are required to create a complete program. Testing and assessment includes screening for substance abuse, substance abuse assessment, mental health disorder screening, tobacco use screening, outreach, comprehensive assessment, drug/alcohol screening, and STD testing. A complete list of screening and support services is provided in Figures 5.2 and 5.3.

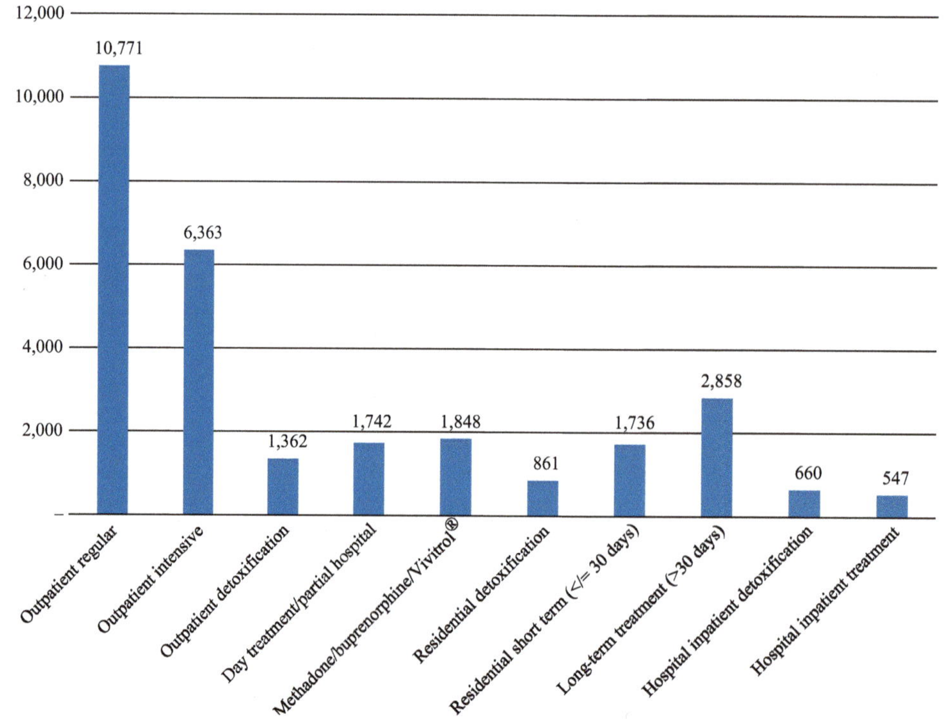

Figure 5.1: *Number of substance abuse treatment facilities (Data source: SAMHSA, 2013)*

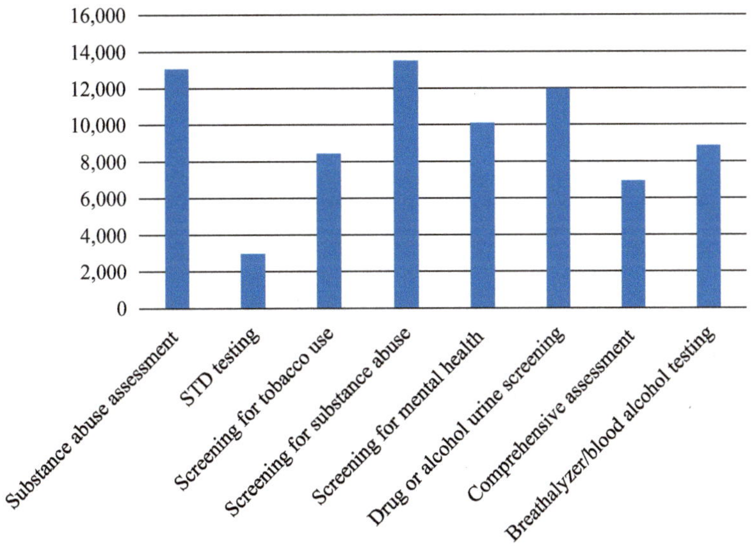

Figure 5.2: *Number of screening services provided, by facility operation, 2013 (Data source: SAMHSA, 2013)*

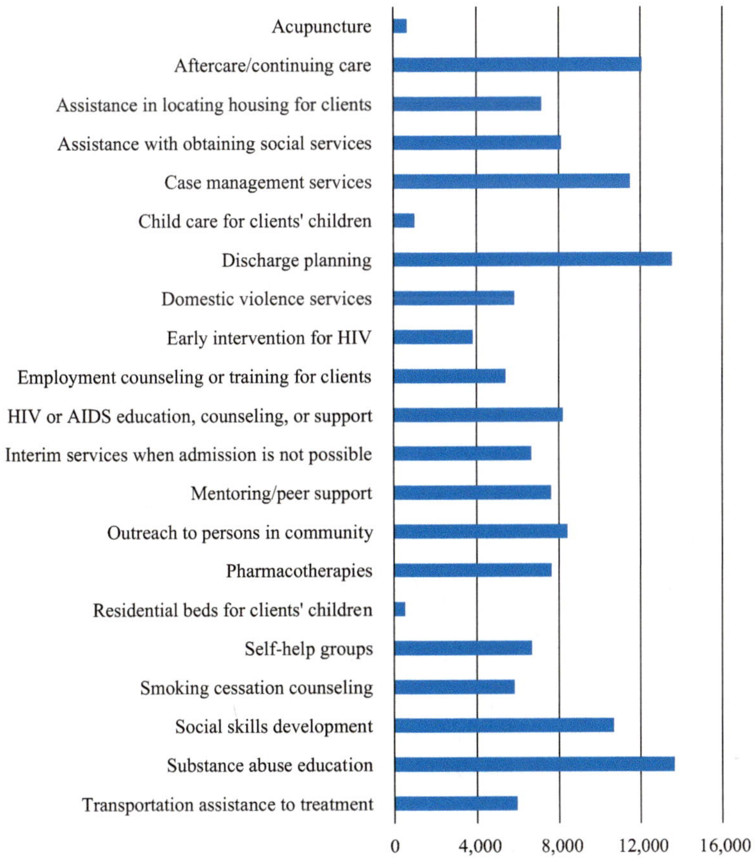

Figure 5.3: *Number of support services provided, by facility operation, 2013 (Data source: SAMHSA, 2013)*

Various programs have been tried in hospitals treating substance use patients. Therapeutic communities focus on personal responsibility reinforced by a supportive community (e.g., Simpson, Joe, & Brown, 1997), psychological rehabilitation via the development of work and social skills to manage high-risk situations (e.g., Platt, 1995), and 12-step programs drawn from Alcoholics Anonymous (e.g., Ouimette, Finney, & Moos, 1997). Moos, Moos, and Andrassy (1999) compared the treatment of substance use disorders in community residential facilities using each of these three approaches to a control group. The control group participants were treated in a facility focused on providing safety and security with treatment limited to counseling and social activities. Patients in all programs showed significant progress, while patients benefiting from any of the three treatment plans had better scores in substance use and symptom outcome.

Therapeutic communities (TC) are resident programs that provide structured daily treatment plans, as well as legal, employment, and psychological support for individuals with severe substance use disorders. Research shows that these programs can achieve best outcomes for individuals who need structure and support in comparison to other interventions (such as outpatient methadone maintenance therapy) when residents stay long enough and continue with the aftercare (Vanderplasschen et al., 2013). TC activities include group discussions, individual counseling, meetings and seminars, confrontation, games, and role-playing. Sometimes TCs take place in prisons or shelters (National Institute on Drug Abuse, 2015). Historically TCs were flexible with regard to length of stay; however, shortened lengths of stay in addiction treatment programs have resulted from increased costs (De Leon, 2012).

According to SAMHSA, the number of persons with substance use disorder as well as the number of facilities treating these persons are the highest in the states of California and New York. However, the numbers show a decreased rate in both states from 2003 to 2013, unlike almost all other states (Figures 5.4 and 5.5). Colorado, Pennsylvania, Minnesota, Connecticut, and Colorado show significant growth in both categories between 2003 and 2013.

5.3 Research on facilities for persons with substance use disorders

Potthoff (1991) surveyed adolescent satisfaction with the interior environment in three settings: a renovated college dormitory, a renovated priest dormitory, and a facility designed for drug treatment for adolescents. Questionnaires were distributed to the children and medical records were examined. The dormitory environments were institutional-appearing, characterized by mismatched furniture, while the environment designed for drug rehabilitation had high-quality finishes, furnishings, and artwork. As might be expected, the overall experience and physical environment was more highly rated.

In a related study, Potthoff (1995) similarly examined the impact of rehabilitation facilities, but this time the settings were a renovated club, a hospital wing, and a facility built for alcohol and drug treatment. Using surveys and patient records, the researcher found that satisfaction decreased with all three facilities over time during the four-week treatment period due to the lack of familiar posters, paintings, photographs, and collectibles. The patients indicated they missed their own bed, chair, and pets from home. Spaciousness, views to the outside, and privacy were the most positively received elements of the new space. Least liked were lack of carpeting, color scheme, lack of comfort, and particularly the quality of the bed. Lack of recreational equipment was also mentioned as problematic.

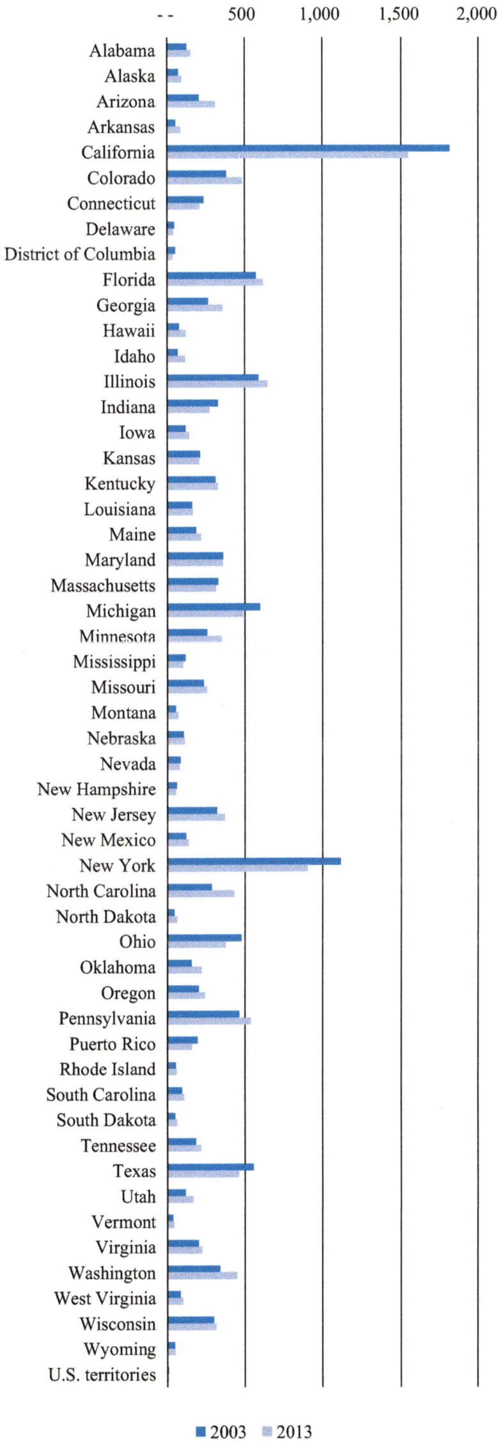

Figure 5.4: *Number of substance abuse treatment facilities by state (2003 and 2013) (Data source: SAMHSA, 2013)*

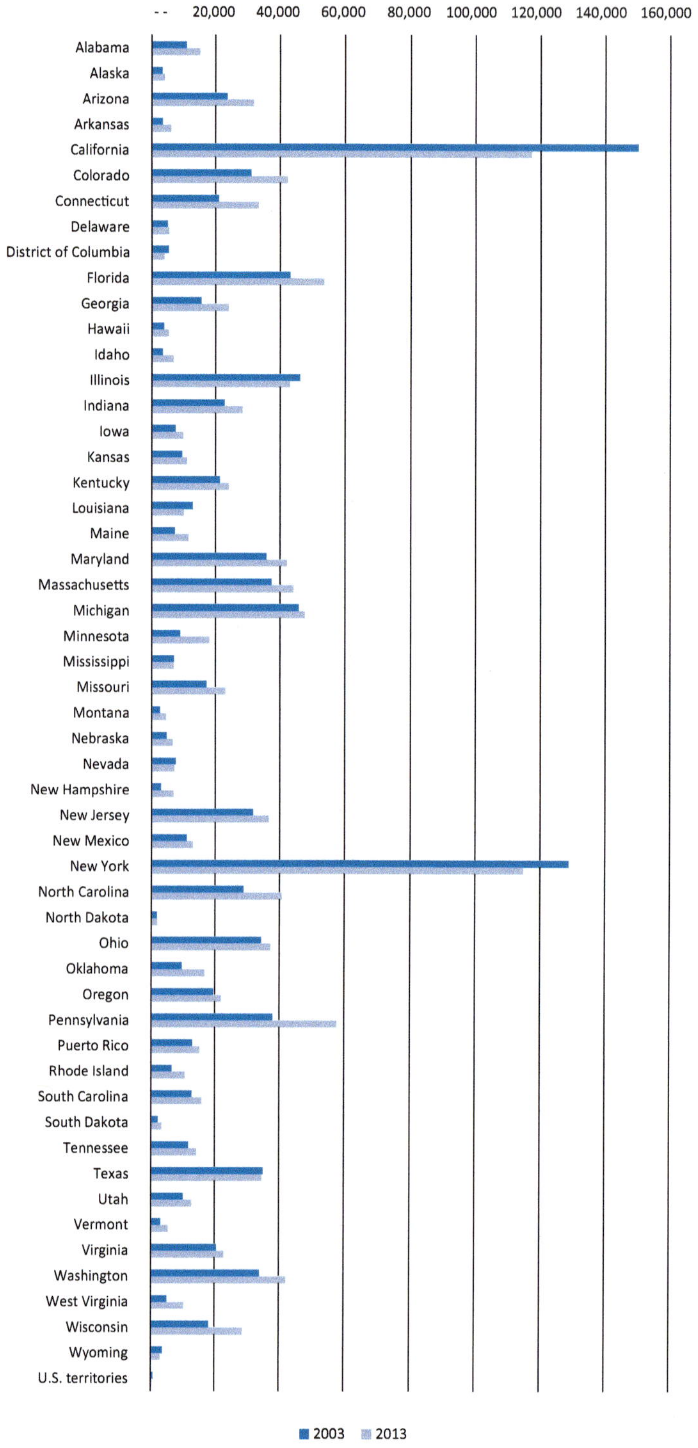

Figure 5.5: *Number of clients by state, 2003, 2013 (Data source: SAMHSA, 2013)*

There is a debate regarding the effectiveness of community integration relative to patient outcomes. The proponents of normalization theory propose that more integration with the community can help patients recover and merge into the community more successfully (Chrysikou, 2014), and new outpatient care methods have made this possible. However, specific groups may actually need protection from the surrounding social environment to fully recover. Stahler, Mennis, and DuCette (2016) noticed that opioid abusers could benefit from a residential treatment setting that provides them with necessary protection from social and environmental triggers that can lead to relapse. Other factors, however, that affected treatment completion in residential facilities included race, gender, education, and employment status, with all data demonstrating better completion rates for persons with more advantageous demographics.

Lipscomb et al. (2012) surveyed 409 staff in 13 residential addiction treatment facilities in the eastern United States. They assessed the adequacy of safety design measures in the physical environment of select facilities with the supervision of an architect who specialized in safety design. Frequency of violent behaviors was measured using staff questionnaires. The various levels of violence were categorized as: raised voice, physically threatening behavior, physical attack, and threatening to cause harm outside the facility. Predictors of occurrence of violent behavior were found to be: client's active resistance toward the treatment program, client's unknown history of violence, and lack of management commitment to violence prevention.

Novotna, Urbanoski, and Rush (2016) evaluated the physical design of a substance use disorder center. The unit was relocated and expanded its medical withdrawal service from 12 to 24 beds, with other programs remaining unchanged. These programs included relapse prevention, stress management, and related skill development. The newly designed residential units had dormitories, with each floor consisting of six private bedrooms with en suite bathrooms, and shared kitchen, dining room, and living areas. The researchers gathered qualitative data on staff (nursing staff, social workers, occupational and recreational therapists, psychologists, and counselors) impressions of service delivery as well as physical and social environment. They also conducted behavior mapping on the unit. Workspace for clinical staff in the residential building was limited to small nurse stations on alternating floors, and most staff offices were located in a separate building. The goal was to encourage staff-client interaction and limit time spent in the clinical and office areas. The clinical spaces located outside of the residential building included offices of social workers, occupational and recreational therapists, and psychologists.

5.4 Substance use disorder facility design goals

5.4.1 Inpatient environments

As a result of the occupancy evaluation conducted by Novotna et al. (2016), several design themes emerged:

- Supporting recovery: The provision of private rooms offers more autonomy and freedom and control.
- Reducing stigma: Attractive exterior and homelike interior were perceived to provide a positive image to the residents, community, family, and other visitors.

From a service delivery standpoint, the following topics were identified:

- Concerns around safety: Limited staff spaces on the units translated into limited surveillance and resulting safety concerns.
- Insufficient therapeutic space: Lack of designated spaces on the residential units for group-based programs or individual consultation posed confidentiality and efficiency issues.
- Communication and therapeutic relationship: Limited staff space on the units, however, served to create a more approachable staff space for the clients, making more informal communications between staff and residents possible.

From a work environment standpoint, the following topics emerged:

- Insufficient space for staff: Lack of staff-designated communal areas and the small size of nurse stations on the units was deemed problematic; in general, it seemed like the move toward creation of a client-friendly environment was aversely accompanied by the move away from staff-friendly design.
- Team cohesion, communication, and greater service integration: The bright and clean physical environment was perceived to promote staff well-being, involvement with care delivery, and teamwork.

Malkin (1991) suggests four primary design guidelines for residential treatment facilities for chemical dependency patients, including the provision of:

- identical patient rooms that suggest all patients are equal,
- semiprivate patient rooms to encourage social support and trust,
- a simple and understated design that is comforting to the restless population, and
- sturdy furniture and finishes that can resist abuse of stressed patients.

Reisdorfer (1996) adds:

- space provisions for personalized service that actively engages clients and their families,
- space for multidisciplinary care teams, and
- co-localization of services.

A potential adjacency arrangement for a rehabilitation facility is provided in Figure 5.6.

5.4.2 *Outpatient environments*

Recommendations are provided by CARF, NCBI, and SAMHSA for the design of rehabilitation facilities.

- Outpatient services for treatment or continuation of care are available and can include various levels of intensity or time investment depending on severity of addiction. Dual diagnosis,

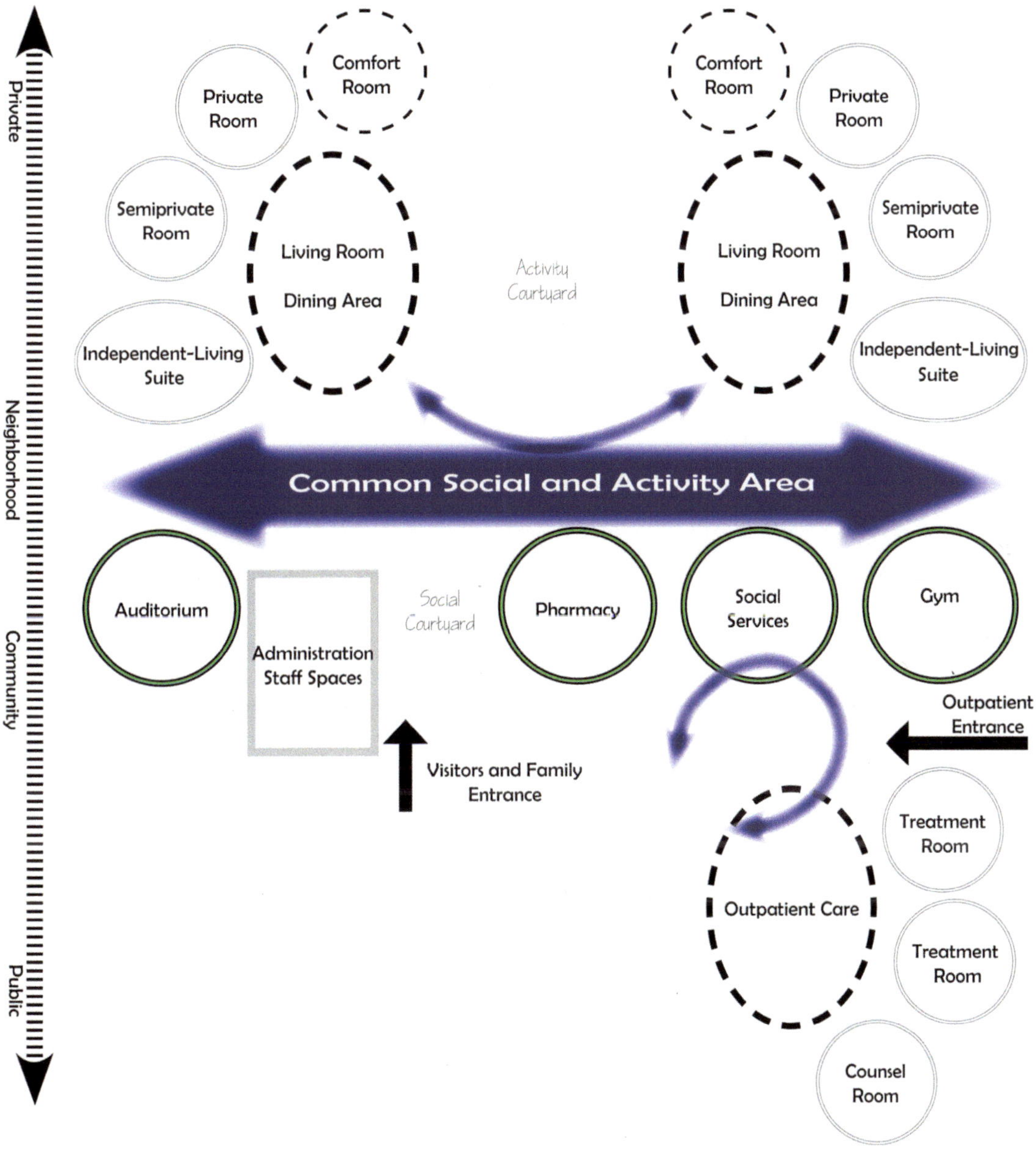

Figure 5.6: *Adjacency diagram for a rehabilitation facility*

partial hospital/day treatment programs work with patients with co-occurring mental health and substance use disorders. These programs are the most intensive and structured type of outpatient treatments and can take four to five days per week for up to six hours per day (CARF, 2016).

- Intensive outpatient plans offer a structured outpatient program that is held three to four days a week but decreases in frequency as clinical milestones are met (NCBI, 2016).

- Individual and group counseling is a relatively less structured outpatient program that is highly focused on the needs and motivation of patients who have maintained sobriety for a period of time. The sessions can be scheduled one to two times a week for one hour (SAMHSA, 2015).

5.5 Case studies

5.5.1 *Margaret and Charles Juravinski Centre for Integrated Care*

Location:	Hamilton, ON
Designer/Architect:	CannonDesign on the basis of an indicative design and output specification developed by Zeidler Partnership Architects and architecture+
Client:	St. Joseph's Healthcare Hamilton
Completion:	2014
Area:	930,000 square feet

Awards: Honor Award, AIA Eastern New York Chapter, 2008

Client, service users, and services

Juravinski Centre for Integrated Care is located at Hamilton's West 5th Campus, which provides regional specialized mental health services for South Central Ontario. The center is a mental health and addiction hospital that employs an integrated approach to providing mental and physical health services in both inpatient and outpatient settings. The majority of patients treated in the center have a diagnosis of schizophrenia, bipolar disorder, or major depression. The integration of services, in addition to attracting the community, will enable behavioral health patients to receive all care in one place. The high prevalence of substance abuse among persons with mental illness serves as justification for this collocation of services.

The center endeavors to serve the community by providing diagnostic imaging services, an expressed need of the region; outpatient medical services; and public access to its gymnasium, auditorium, walking trails, baseball diamond, soccer field, tennis court, labyrinth, gardens, chapel, and cafeteria (Frketich, 2014).

Mission and goals

The center's goal is to destigmatize mental illness by providing medical care to the surrounding community and communicating the idea that poor mental health is an illness that does not require separation from other health services (Frketich, 2014).

Site

The West 5th Campus is located in Hamilton, Ontario. Hamilton is a city 70 kilometers southwest of Toronto, and situated near Lake Ontario. The health campus is located across from the Mohawk College campus in a suburban residential area.

Program

The inpatient program is composed of 305 beds, 110 of which are dedicated to persons with severe mental illness who have committed a criminal offense. A 12-bed unit is dedicated to seniors with mental illness. Each patient has a private bedroom with an adjoining en suite bathroom that together total 188 square feet. All of the units have a courtyard, visitors' lounge, and dining room in addition to a nursing station.

Patients have free movement outside of their units, while remaining in a secure area. The secure area includes a coffee shop, library, hair salon, used-clothing store, game rooms, exercise room, and a gym. Patients have access to a secure perimeter at certain times, as well as their own private room with key card entry. The key card can be programmed for each individual patient based on the patient's recovery status. Four apartments, 1,200 square feet each, are provided and can be occupied by patients who are prepared to be discharged for a trial period of a few weeks to develop and improve their independent living skills (Frketich, 2014). The facility includes administrative education and research spaces as well.

Configuration and construction

The patient units form four distinct cross forms that are connected through a rectilinear mass, running at an east-west direction to take advantage of sunlight. Five interior courtyards increase daylighting and access to vegetated open spaces. The east-west mass connects to a parallel and slightly curved mass, which houses most of the public, administrative, education, and research functions as well as outpatient clinics.

The center has achieved LEED Gold certification. Sustainable design strategies include access to daylight in more than 70% of interior spaces, use of daylighting sensors, incorporation of recycled, locally sourced and low-emitting building materials, drought-resistant planting, rainwater collection for irrigation, a heat recovery system, and a green roof system (Plenary Group, 2014).

Case study bibliography

architecture+. (2015). Project information and other in-house publication materials.

Frketich, J. (2014). New Hamilton hospital campus designed to destigmatize mental illness. *Hamilton Spectator*. Retrieved August 21, 2016, from www.thespec.com/news-story/4315512-new-hamilton-hospital-campus-designed-to-destigmatize-mental-illness/

Plenary Group. (2014). Margaret and Charles Juravinski Centre for Integrated Health scores LEED gold. *Plenary Group*. Retrieved August 21, 2016, from http://plenarygroup.com/news-and-media/news-articles-and-press-releases/2014/margaret-and-charles-juravinski-centre-for-integrated-health-scores-leed-gold.html

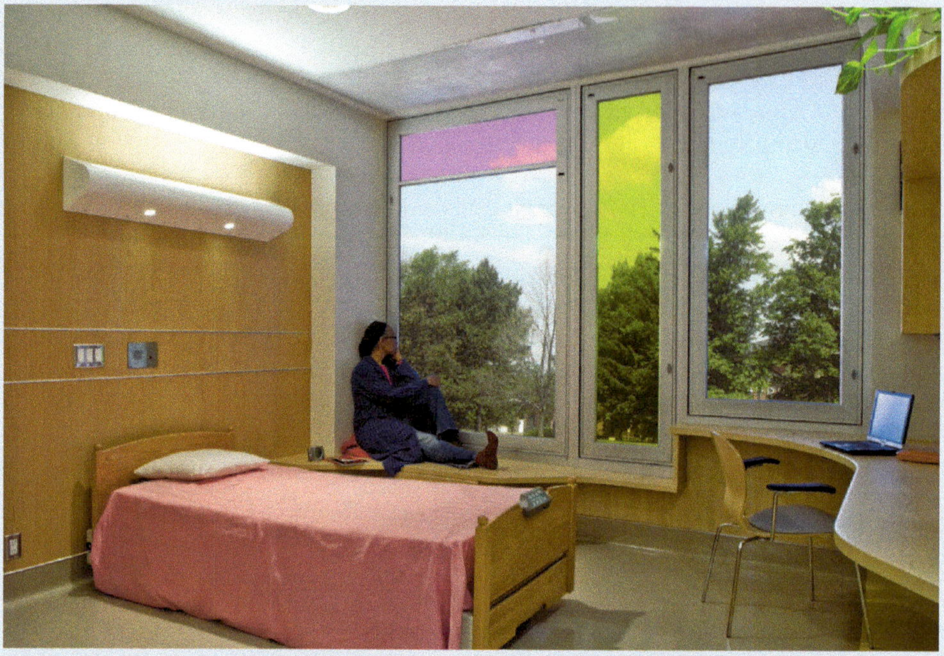

Figure 5.7: *Juravinski Centre for Integrated Care – patient bedroom (Architects: CannonDesign in collaboration with Ziedler Partnership Architects and architecture+; Photo credit Zeidler Partnership Architects)*

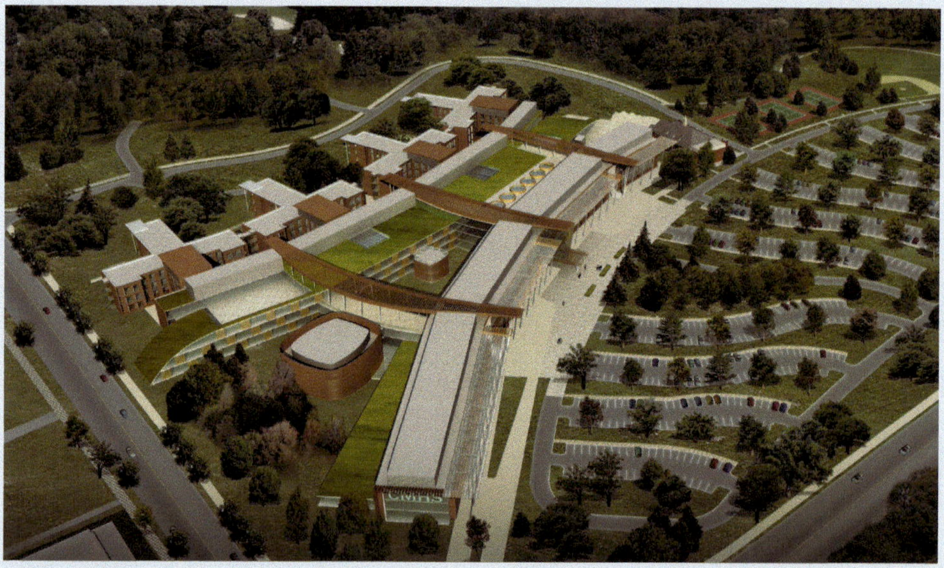

Figure 5.8: *Juravinski Centre for Integrated Care – exterior, bird's-eye view from south (Architects: CannonDesign in collaboration with Ziedler Partnership Architects and architecture+; Photo credit: Zeidler Partnership Architects)*

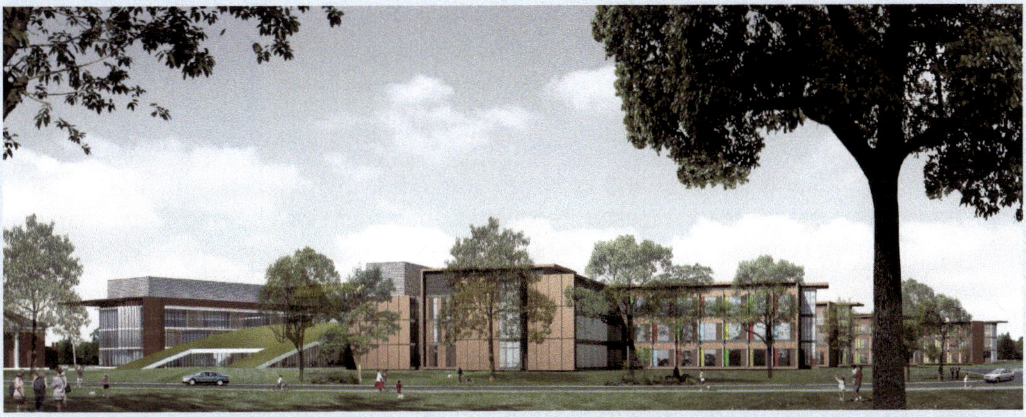

Figure 5.9: *Juravinski Centre for Integrated Care – view from escarpment (Architects: CannonDesign in collaboration with Ziedler Partnership Architects and architecture+; Photo credit: Zeidler Partnership Architects)*

5.5.2 *Worcester Recovery Center and Hospital*

Location:	Worcester, MA
Designer/Architect:	Ellenzweig in collaboration with architecture+
Client:	The Commonwealth of Massachusetts
Completion:	2012
Area:	428,000 square feet

Awards: AIA New England Honor Award; AIA Eastern NY Institutional Merit Award; Citation, Boston Society of Architects/AIA Healthcare Facilities Design Awards, 2014; Merit Award, AIA Eastern NY Chapter, 2013; WAN (World Architecture News) Healthcare Awards Shortlist, 2013; American Society of Interior Designers, Upstate New York/Canada East Chapter, Commercial Project/Large, Design Award, 2013; Merit Award, AIA Eastern NY Chapter, 2006 (unbuilt project)

Client, service users, and services

In a 2004 report by the Department of Mental Health to the General Court, it was recommended that the programs at Worcester State Hospital and Westborough State Hospital be combined into a new recovery center (Commonwealth of Massachusetts, 2016). The facility, completed in 2012, serves 260 adults and 60 adolescents from across the Commonwealth of Massachusetts and promotes recovery and return to community living as soon as possible through treatment, active rehabilitation plans, and medication education. The multidisciplinary care teams are composed of psychiatrists, psychologists, social workers, nurses, and occupational therapists. Therapeutic interventions include individual therapy, group therapy, illness management, and family outreach counseling. Multidisciplinary treatment teams work with patients to develop individualized treatment plans consisting of various elements such as individual and group therapy, rehabilitative services, and psychopharmacology.

Mission and goals

The focus of the facility is recovery and resiliency through living independently in communities of their choice. The goal of the Worcester Recovery Center and Hospital is to foster dignity and respect for service users throughout the continuum of care.

Site

Worcester Recovery Center and Hospital is located on the former Worcester State Hospital campus, in Worcester, Massachusetts. The site is surrounded by the wooded Biotech Park in a suburban area with low-rise commercial functions and detached residential buildings.

Program

The facility is formed around creating "house" to "neighborhood" to "downtown" zones that reflect stages of recovery as well as the various levels of social needs of the residents. The facility houses 320 private inpatient beds in five separate units (two of which are dedicated to adolescents). Units at each level have 15 patient beds as well as a dining area, laundry room, seclusion room, visiting room, and activity area. The two adolescent units and the three adult units are connected to separate "neighborhood" zones. The neighborhood zones serving adolescent and adult units are separated by a segment of downtown functions. Community areas or "downtown" include a bank, gym, chapel, café, social center, store, social workers' office, and a common therapy area. The "neighborhood" zones consist of classrooms, group meeting rooms, and social workers' offices and consult rooms.

Configuration and construction

The "downtown" zone wraps around a central courtyard or "village green." The low-rise scale of the buildings resembles residential buildings. The neighborhood zone, in addition to facilitating group activities and fostering the concept of community, provides a mix of professional specialties and skills among the staff. Several sustainable design strategies have been incorporated into the design, construction, and operation of the facility, including waste recycling; low-maintenance, long life materials; and water conservation.

Case study bibliography

Commonwealth of Massachusetts. (2016). *Worcester Recovery Center and Hospital*. The Official Website of the Executive Office of Health and Human Services (EOHHS). Retrieved from August 20, 2016, from www.mass.gov/eohhs/docs/dmh/services/wrch-brochure.pdf

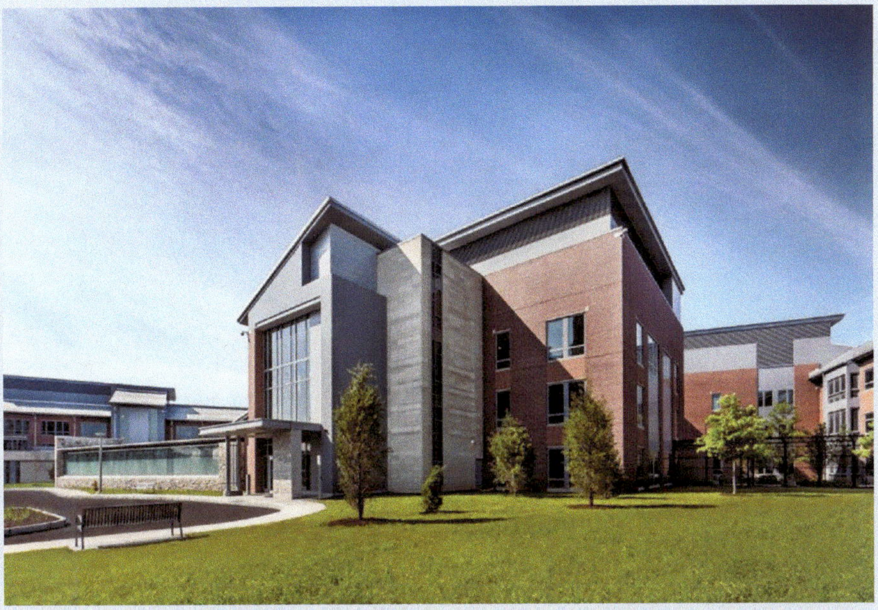

Figure 5.10: *Worcester Recovery Center – exterior (Architects: Ellenzweig in collaboration with architecture+; Photo credit: Ellenzweig)*

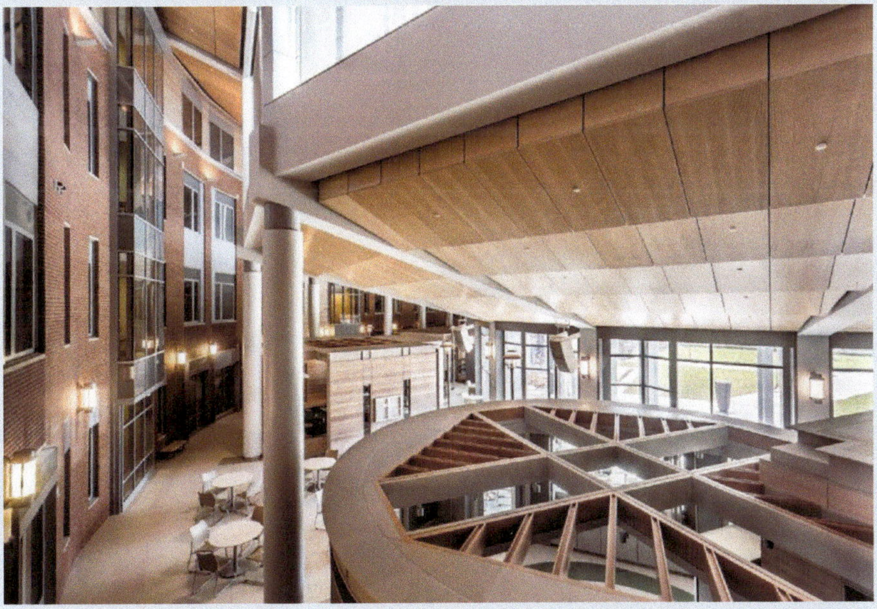

Figure 5.11: *Worcester Recovery Center – overhead view of activity pavilion (Architects: Ellenzweig in collaboration with architecture+; Photo credit: Ellenzweig)*

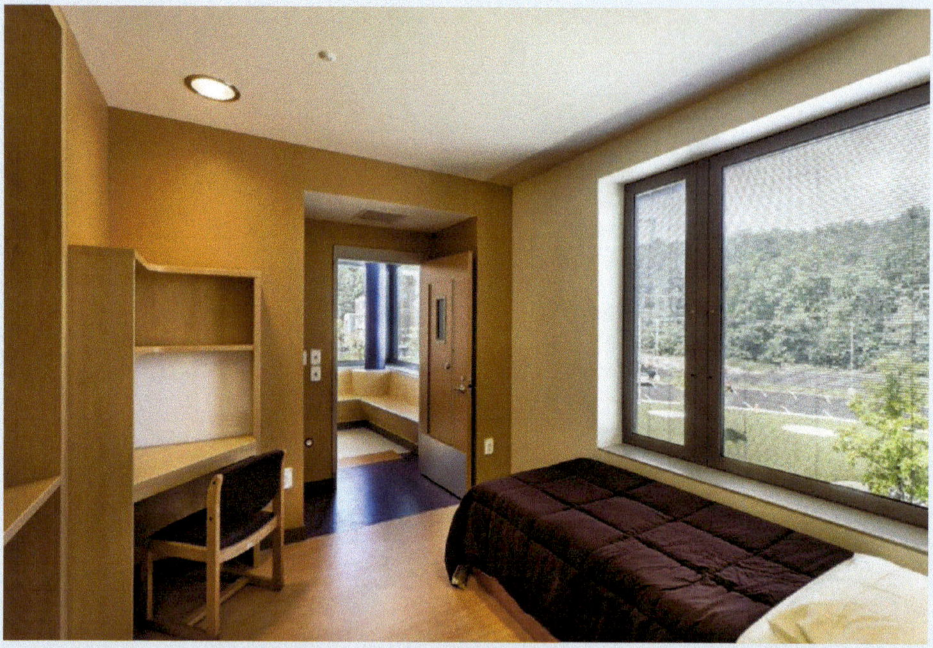

Figure 5.12: *Worcester Recovery Center – patient bedroom (Architects: Ellenzweig in collaboration with architecture+; Photo credit: Ellenzweig)*

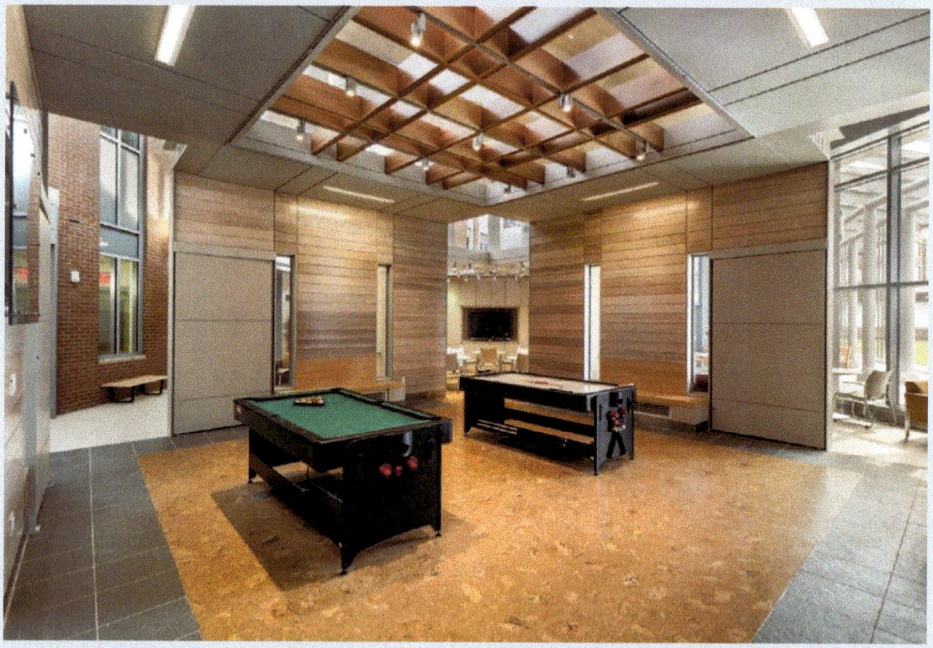

Figure 5.13: *Worcester Recovery Center – activity pavilion (Architects: Ellenzweig in collaboration with architecture+; Photo credit: Ellenzweig)*

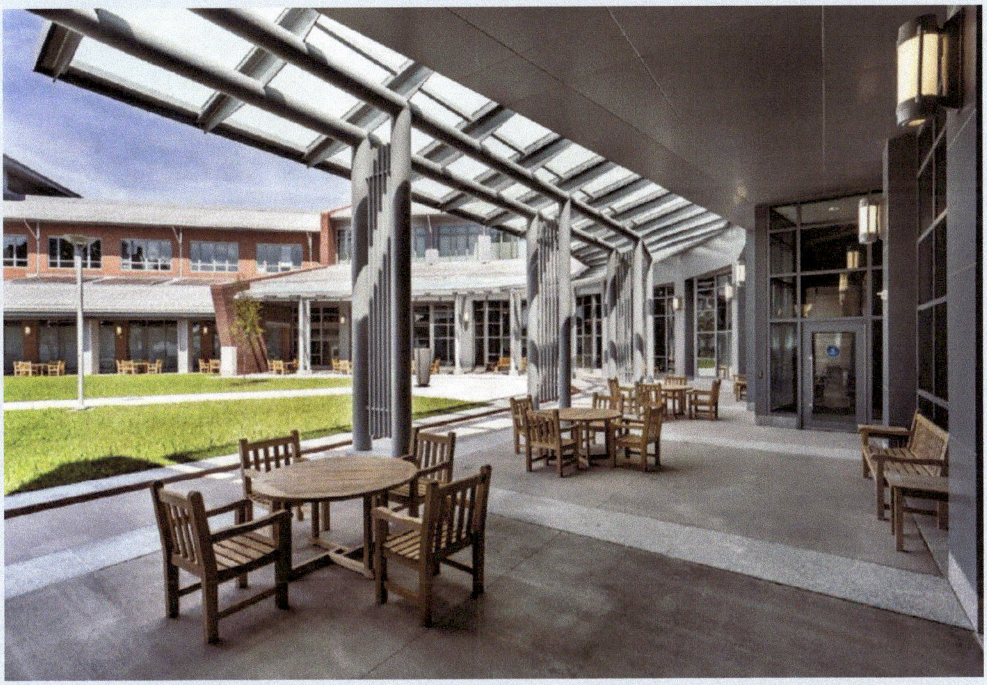

Figure 5.14: *Worcester Recovery Center – village green (Architects: Ellenzweig in collaboration with architecture+; Photo credit: Ellenzweig)*

References

American Psychiatric Association. (2013). *Diagnostic and statistical manual of mental disorders: DSM-5*. Washington, DC: American Psychiatric Association.

Barber, J. W., & Howe, H. (1861). *Our whole country: Or the past and present of the United States, historical and descriptive*. New York: George F. Tuttle and Henry Mcauley.

Beckstead, D. J., Lambert, M. J., DuBose, A. P., & Linehan, M. (2015). Dialectical behavioral therapy with American Indian/Alaska native adolescents diagnosed with substance use disorders: Combining an evidence based treatment with cultural, traditional, and spiritual beliefs. *Addictive Behaviors, 51*, 84–87.

CARF. (2016). *Partial hospitalization*. CARF International. Retrieved from www.carf.org/Programs/ProgramDescriptions/BH-Partial-Hospitalization/

Center for Behavioral Health Statistics and Quality. (2015). *Behavioral health trends in the United States: Results from the 2014 National Survey on Drug Use and Health* (HHS Publication No. SMA 15–4927, NSDUH Series H-50). Retrieved from www.samhsa.gov/data/sites/default/files/NSDUH-FRR1-2014/NSDUH-FRR1-2014.pdf

Center for Substance Abuse Treatment. (1999). *Treatment of adolescents with substance use disorders – Therapeutic communities* (Treatment Improvement Protocol (TIP) Series, 32). Rockville, MD: Substance Abuse and Mental Health Services Administration (US). Retrieved from www.ncbi.nlm.nih.gov/books/NBK64342/

Chrysikou, E. (2014). *Architecture for psychiatric environments and therapeutic spaces*. Amsterdam: IOS Press.

Dahne, J., & Lejuez, C. W. (2015). Smart phone and mobile application utilization prior to and following treatment among individuals enrolled in residential substance use treatment. *Journal of Substance Abuse Treatment, 58*, 95–99.

De Leon, G. (2012). *Therapeutic communities: Today and tomorrow*. Presentation to Drugs and Society Seminar, Columbia University.

Drake, R. E., Luciano, A. E., Mueser, K. T., Covell, N. H., Essock, S. M., Xie, H., & McHugo, G. J. (2015). Longitudinal course of clients with co-occurring schizophrenia spectrum and substance use disorders in urban mental health centers: A 7-year prospective study. *Schizophrenia Bulletin, 42*(1), 202–211.

Garnick, D. W., Lee, M. T., O'Brien, P. L., Panas, L., Ritter, G. A., Acevedo, A., . . . Godley, M. D. (2012). The Washington Circle engagement performance measures' association with adolescent treatment outcomes. *Drug and Alcohol Dependence, 124*(3), 250–258.

Goethals, I., Soyez, V., Melnick, G., Leon, G. D., & Broekaert, E. (2011). Essential elements of treatment: A comparative study between European and American therapeutic communities for addiction. *Substance Use and Misuse, 46*(8), 1023–1031.

Harris, A., Gupta, S., Bowe, T., Ellerbe, L., Phelps, T., Rubinsky, A., . . . Trafton, J. (2015). Predictive validity of two process-of-care quality measures for residential substance use disorder treatment. *Addictive Science & Clinical Practice, 31*, 10–22.

Lipscomb, J. A., London, M., Chen, Y. M., Flannery, K., Watt, M., Greiger-Brown, J., . . . McPhaul, K. (2012). Safety climate and workplace violence prevention in state-run residential addiction treatment centers. *Work, 42*, 47–56.

Litt, M. D., Kadden, R. M., Kabela-Cormier, E., & Petry, N. M. (2009). Changing network support for drinking: Network support project 2-year follow-up. *Journal of Consult Clinical Psychology, 77*, 229–242.

Minkoff, K. (2013). Treating comorbid psychiatric and substance use disorders. *Psychiatric Times, 30*(4), 44–47.

Moore, D., & Fraser, S. (2013). Producing the "problem" of addiction in drug treatment. *Qualitative Health Research, 23*, 916–923.

Moos, R., Moos, B., & Andrassy, J. (1999). Outcomes of four treatment approaches in community residential programs for patients with substance use disorders. *Psychiatric Services, 50*(12), 1577–1583.

NAMI. (2016). Dual diagnosis. *National Alliance for Mental Health*. Retrieved from www.nami.org/Learn-More/Mental-Health-Conditions/Related-Conditions/Dual-Diagnosis#sthash.97jKwhDT.dpuf

National Institute on Drug Abuse. (2015). *What are the fundamental components of therapeutic communities?* Retrieved from www.drugabuse.gov/publications/research-reports/therapeutic-communities/what-are-fundamental-components-therapeutic-communities

National Institute for Drug Abuse. (2016). *Commonly abused drugs*. Retrieved from www.drugabuse.gov/sites/default/files/commonly_abused_drugs_final_02292016.pdf

NCBI. (2016). Services in intensive outpatient treatment programs. *Substance Abuse: Clinical Issues in Intensive Outpatient Treatment*. Retrieved from www.ncbi.nlm.nih.gov/books/NBK64094/

Neacsiu, A. D., & Linehan, M. M. (2014). Borderline personality disorder. In D. H. Barlow (Ed.), *Clinical handbook of psychological disorders* (5th ed., pp. 394–461). New York: Guilford Press.

Novotna, G., Urbanoski, K. A., & Rush, B. R. (2016). Client centered design of residential addiction and mental healthcare facilities: Staff perception of the work environment. *Qualitative Health Research, 21*(11), 1527–1538.

Ouimette, P., Finney, J., & Moos, R. (1997). Twelve-step and cognitive-behavioral treatment for substance abuse: A comparison of treatment effectiveness. *Journal of Consulting and Clinical Psychology*, *65*, 220–234.

Peterson, K. A., Swindle, R. W., Phibbs, C. S., Recine, B., & Moos, R. H. (1994). Determinants of readmission following inpatient substance abuse treatment: A national study of VA programs. *Med Care*, *32*(6), 535–550.

Platt, J. J. (1995). Vocational rehabilitation of drug abusers. *Psychological Bulletin*, *117*, 416–433.

Potthoff, J. (1991). Young adult male satisfaction with drug and alcohol rehabilitation facilities: Interior design implications. *Journal of Alcohol and Drug Education*, *37*(1), 38–45.

Potthoff, J. (1995). Adolescent satisfaction with drug/alcohol treatment facilities: Design implications. *Journal of Alcohol and Drug Education*, *41*, 62–73.

Priester, M. A., Browne, T., Iachini, A., Clone, S., DeHart, D., & Seay, K. D. (2016). Treatment access barriers and disparities among individuals with co-occurring mental health and substance use disorders: An integrative literature review. *Journal of Substance Abuse Treatment*, *61*, 47–59.

Reisdorfer, J. T. (1996). Building a patient-focused care unit. *Nursing Management*, *27*(10), 38–42.

Rinaldo, S., & Rinaldo, D. (2013). *State Medicaid coverage and authorization requirements for opioid dependence medications*. Final report prepared for the American Society of Addiction Medicine. The AVISTA Group. Retrieved from http://www.asam.org/docs/default-source/advocacy/aaam_implications-for-opioid-addiction-treatment_final

Rochefort, D. A. (1993). *From poorhouses to homelessness: Policy analysis and mental healthcare*. Westport, CT: Auburn House.

Sacks, S., Chaple, M., Sacks, J. Y., McKendrick, K., & Cleland, M. (2012). Randomized trial of a re-entry modified therapeutic community for offenders with co-occurring disorders: Crime outcomes. *Journal of Substance Abuse Treatment*, *42*(3), 247–259.

SAMHSA. (2012). *Behavioral health United States, 2012*. U.S. Department of Health and Human Services. Retrieved from www.samhsa.gov/data/sites/default/files/2012-BHUS.pdf

SAMHSA. (2013). National survey of substance abuse treatment services: 2013. *Data on Substance Abuse Treatment Facilities*. Retrieved from www.samhsa.gov/data/sites/default/files/2013_N-SSATS_National_Survey_of_Substance_Abuse_Treatment_Services/2013_N-SSATS_National_Survey_of_Substance_Abuse_Treatment_Services.pdf

SAMHSA. (2015). *Treatment for substance use disorders*. Rockville, MD: Substance Abuse and Mental Health Services Administration.

Simpson, D. D., Joe, G. W., & Brown, B. S. (1997). Treatment retention and follow-up outcomes in the Drug Abuse Treatment Outcome Study (DATOS). *Psychology of Addictive Behaviors*, *11*, 294–307.

Stahler, G. J., Mennis, J., & DuCette, J. P. (2016). Residential and outpatient treatment completion for substance use disorders in the U.S.: Moderation analysis by demographics and drug of choice. *Addictive Behaviors*, *58*, 129–135.

Vanderplasschen, W., Colpaert, K., Autrique, M., Rapp, R., Pearce, S., Broekaert, E., & Vandevelde, S. (2013). Therapeutic communities for addictions: A review of their effectiveness from a recovery-oriented perspective. *The Scientific World Journal*, Article ID 427817.

Yanni, C. (2007). *The architecture of madness: Insane asylums in the United States*. Minneapolis: University of Minnesota Press.

Zinbarg, R., Barlow, D. H., & Brown, T. (1997). The hierarchical structure and general factor saturation of the anxiety sensitivity index: Evidence and implications. *Psychological Assessment*, *9*, 277–284.

Mental health facilities for veterans of war

6

6.1 Introduction

6.1.1 History of mental and behavioral health facilities for veterans in the United States

The origin of the U.S. Veterans Administration (VA) can be traced back to colonial times. As early as 1776, the Continental Congress provided pensions to enlistees, and the first domiciliary and the first VA medical facility were opened in 1811. In 1917 programs were expanded to accommodate veterans of World War I, and the Veteran's Bureau was founded in 1921. The various components serving veterans were consolidated into the VA in 1930. Following World War II the sudden increase in veterans served as the impetus for the 1944 GI Bill (Department of Veterans Affairs, 2015), which provided a range of benefits to veterans such as tuition and low-cost mortgages.

In 1918 Congress tasked the Bureau of War Risk Insurance and Public Health Service to operate hospitals specifically for World War I veterans. Today, the Veterans Health Administration (VHA) is a national healthcare delivery system and the largest of the three administrations that constitutes the Department of Veterans Affairs (VA). The VA has evolved from 54 hospitals in 1930 to approximately 152 hospitals today. There are currently 800 outpatient clinics, 126 nursing homes, and 35 domiciliaries (Department of Veterans Affairs, 2015). The VHA is an integrated healthcare system employing approximately 53,000 licensed healthcare practitioners and serves more than 8,300,000 veterans annually (Department of Veterans Affairs, 2015).

The initial attempt to establish the VHA's residential mental healthcare programs followed 1860s legislation of the Domiciliary Care Program to provide a home for soldiers of the Civil War (Department of Veterans Affairs, 2009). During the 1980s, domiciliary programs started to admit veteran patients with mental health disorders including PTSD, schizophrenia, and substance use disorders, in addition to homeless veterans. This step created a need for a convergence of the provision of medical care and the domiciliary program into one Domiciliary Residential Rehabilitation and Treatment Program (DRRTP) (Department of Veterans Affairs, 2009). In 1995, the Psychosocial Residential Rehabilitation Treatment Program (PRRTP) was established for veterans with mental health problems or addictive disorders who were in need of additional support for addressing multiple and severe psychosocial dilemmas including unemployment and homelessness (Department of Veterans Affairs, 2009). Due to the convergence of rehabilitative and therapeutic objectives of existing therapy programs, the Office of Residential Rehabilitation and Treatment Programs section of the Office of Mental Health Services unified them under a Mental Health Residential Rehabilitation Treatment Program (MH RRTP) (Department of Veterans Affairs, 2009).

6.1.2 Data regarding war veterans population

When designing VA hospitals, it is useful to be aware of the demographics and diagnoses presented by this population. According to the most recent data from the U.S. Department of Veterans Affairs regarding analysis of VA healthcare utilization among OEF (Operation Enduring Freedom), OIF (Operation Iraqi Freedom), and OND (Operation New Dawn) veterans from October 1, 2001, to March 31, 2015, over 61% of all separated OEF/OIF/OND veterans have accessed VA healthcare since 2001. Regarding the frequency and percentages of most common health diagnoses, mental disorders are the third most prevalent with 57.6%, after musculoskeletal ailments (61.8%) and "symptoms, signs, and ill-defined conditions" (58.1%) (Epidemiology Program Post-Deployment Health Group, 2015).

Seal, Bertenthal, Miner, Sen, and Marmar (2007), in studying the impact of mental health disorders among 103,788 veterans returning from Iraq and Afghanistan who were examined at VA facilities, reported that 31% were diagnosed with mental health and/or psychosocial conditions. Sixty percent of the initial detections and diagnoses of mental health disorders were made in primary care settings at VA facilities (Seal et al., 2007).

The single most prevalent mental health disorder – representing 52% of veterans who received a mental illness diagnosis – was identified as post-traumatic stress disorder (Seal et al., 2007). The most recent report by the U.S. Department of Veterans Affairs (September 2015) regarding analysis of VA healthcare utilization among OEF/OIF/OND veterans confirms that PTSD is the most commonly diagnosed mental health disorder among veterans, followed by depressive disorders, neurotic disorders, affective psychoses, alcohol dependence syndrome, nondependent abuse of drugs, special symptoms (not elsewhere classified), drug dependence, and sexual deviations and disorders (Department of Veterans Affairs, 2015). (See Figure 6.1.)

Seal, Maguen, and Cohen (2015) assessed data from VA national administrative databases on the entire population of OEF/OIF/OND veterans who visited VA healthcare nationwide and reported that the burden of mental health diagnosis continued to escalate since the initial conflicts in 2001. Seal, Maguen, and Cohen (2015) also summarized several key findings with regard to the occurrence of mental health disorders and stated that:

- PTSD and depression account for as many as 70% of the comorbidity diagnoses among veterans who suffer from multiple conditions.
- From 2002 to 2011, the rate of overall PTSD among veterans increased by 100-fold; the most dramatic increase in PTSD followed the Iraq invasion in 2003.
- One factor that contributed to increased diagnostic complexity and complications in treatment was identified as co-occurring mental health diagnoses among OEF/OIF/OND veterans who were diagnosed with two or more mental health disorders.
- Substance use disorder was diagnosed among 11% of OEF/OIF veterans, and among those diagnosed for substance use disorders, 55%–57% had comorbid depression or PTSD diagnosis.
- Female veterans had less than half the risk for substance use disorder as male veterans. However, they are at higher risk for depression, anxiety disorders, and eating disorders than men. Thirty-one percent of female veterans with PTSD, compared to 1% of male veterans with PTSD, were tested positively for military sexual trauma (MST). PTSD was over four times more likely to develop in women veterans with MST than female veterans without MST.

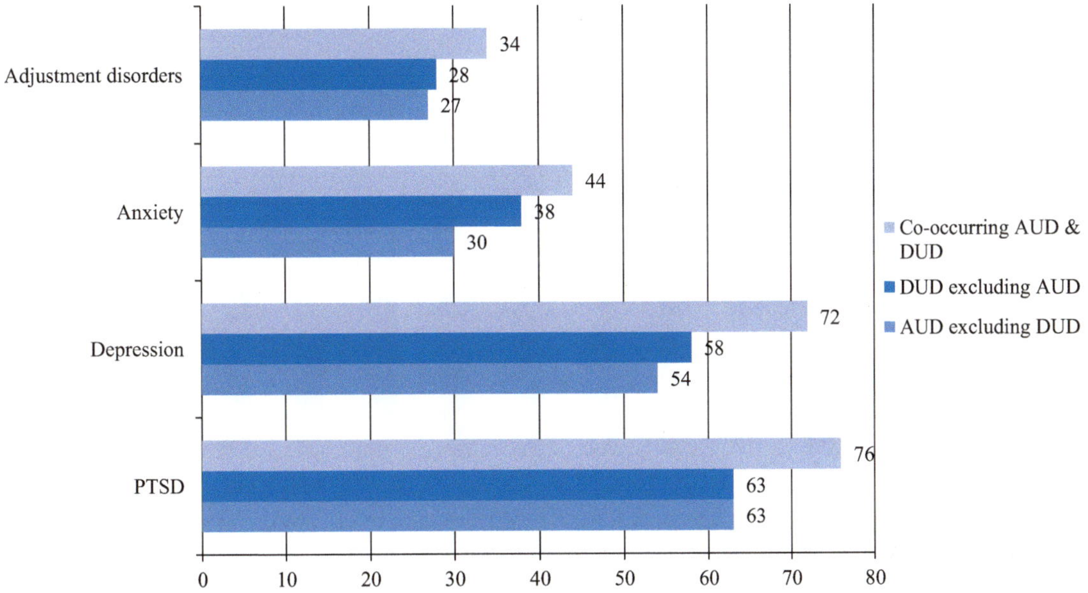

Figure 6.1: *Percent of unadjusted prevalence of comorbid military service-related mental health diagnoses associated with alcohol use disorders (AUD), drug use disorders (DUD), and both among active duty and National Guard and Reserve veterans of Iraq and Afghanistan (Data source: Seal, Maguen, & Cohen, 2015)*

6.1.3 Characteristics and needs of war veterans

Challenges faced by military personnel include pain management, post-traumatic stress disorder, traumatic brain injury, drug addiction, and suicide. The number of suicides by U.S. military personnel has more than doubled since 2004 (Bryan, Rudd, & Wertenberger, 2013). Only two studies were found addressing completed and attempted suicides while in VA hospital settings (i.e., Mills, King, Watts, & Hemphill, 2013; Watts et al., 2012). While many of these suicides take place outside of MBH settings, they are an indicator of the increased need for mental health treatment facilities for veterans.

Now that more women are involved as war veterans, data is available regarding their exposure to traumatic experiences and PTSD outcomes. Butterfield, Forneris, Feldman, and Beckham (2000) investigated hostility and health outcomes in women veterans with and without PTSD and found higher levels of hostility in the former. Women with PTSD were also more likely to have poorer health outcomes. In spite of a few recent studies, increased deployment and frontline activities by women and notable differences between men and women with regard to PTSD suggest that future research is required to better understand women veterans' mental health needs (Street, Vogt, & Dutra, 2009).

According to the population tables published by National Center for Veterans Analysis and Statistics (2015), veterans between the ages of 65 and 69 comprise more than 14% of the total population of veterans (Figure 6.2). The most recent data from U.S. Department of Veterans Affairs regarding service utilization among 1,189,709 OEF/OIF/OND veterans from October 1, 2001, through March 31, 2015, demonstrates that over 48% of all OEF/OIF/OND veterans utilizing VA healthcare since 2001 were born between 1980 and 1989 (see Figure 6.3).

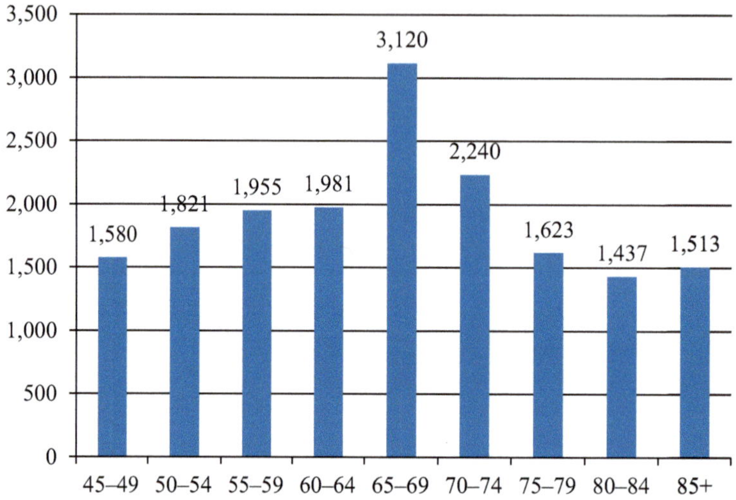

Figure 6.2: *Distribution of veteran population by age (Total N = 21,680,534) (in thousands) (Data source: National Center for Veterans Analysis and Statistics – Veteran Population, 2015)*

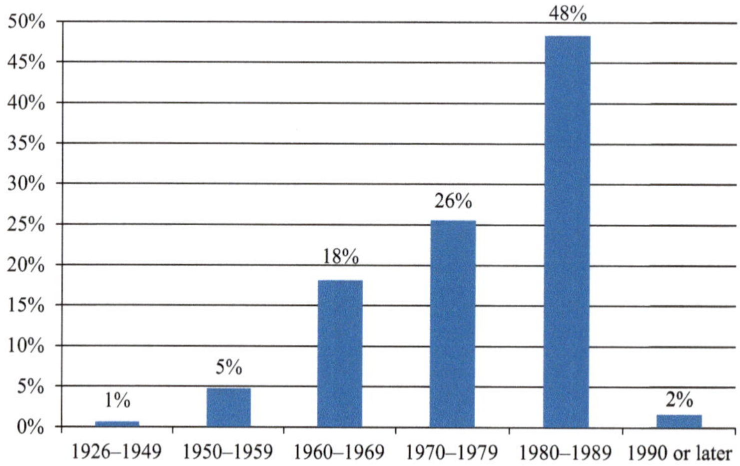

Figure 6.3: *Percentage of age distribution among OEF/OIF/OND veterans (N = 1,189,709) (Data source: Department of Veterans Affairs, 2015)*

Seal et al. (2015) noted that age and unit type (active duty vs. reserve/guard) played an important role in prevalence of mental health disorders among veterans. Younger active duty veterans (less than 25 years old) had 2–5 times higher rates of PTSD due to higher combat exposure and alcohol and drug use disorder diagnoses compared to active duty veterans over 40. However, National Guard/Reserve veterans over 40 had a higher risk for PTSD and depression than their counterparts under 25 years of age (Seal et al., 2015).

Regarding race/ethnicity of veterans, White race/ethnicity represents 82% of the total population followed by 12% African Americans (Figure 6.4). Male veterans make up 91% of the total veteran population.

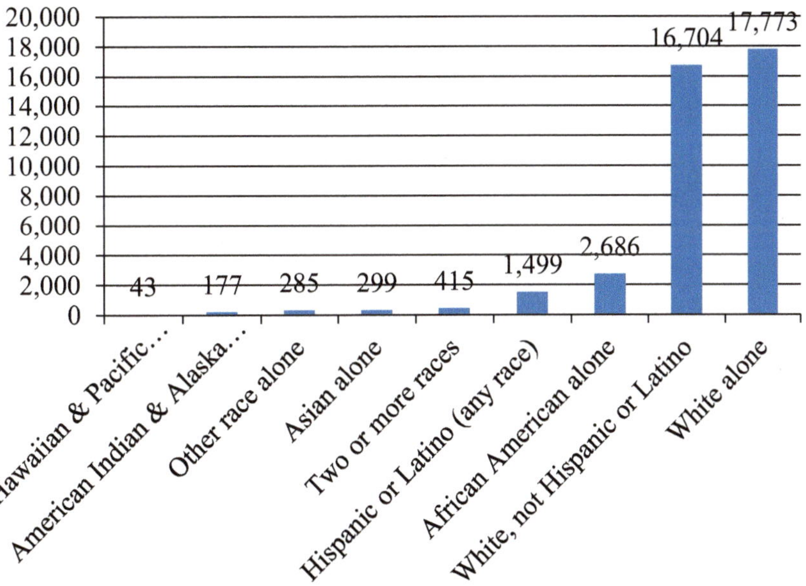

Figure 6.4: *Distribution of veteran population by race/ethnicity (Grand total, N = 21,680,534) (in thousands) (Data source: Department of Veterans Affairs, 2015)*

6.2 Characteristics of residential mental health facilities for war veterans

Due to the convergence of rehabilitative and therapeutic objectives of the DRRTP and PRRTP programs, the Office of Residential Rehabilitation and Treatment Programs section of the Office of Mental Health Services unified the DRRTP and PRRTP programs under a Mental Health Residential Rehabilitation Treatment Program (MH RRTP) and specified a common set of procedures and requirements related to VHA residential programs (Department of Veterans Affairs, 2009). Care models that were incorporated in the MH RRTP include:

- Domiciliary Residential Rehabilitation and Treatment Program (General DRRTP),
- Psychosocial Residential Rehabilitation Treatment Program (General PRRTP),
- Domiciliary Care for Homeless Veterans (DCHV),
- Substance Abuse Residential Rehabilitation Treatment Program (SARRTP),
- Posttraumatic Stress Disorder Residential Rehabilitation Treatment Program (PTSD-RRTP), and
- Compensated Work Therapy-Transitional Residence (CWT-TR).

The mental health component of the VHA is guided by eight principles, all of which are significantly impacted by the physical environment:

1. Focus on recovery
2. Coordinated care
3. Provision of treatment in the context of primary care

4. Provision of a treatment coordinator
5. 24/7 service
6. Gender and culturally sensitive care
7. Evidence-based medicine
8. Couples and family services (*Mental Health Facilities Design Guide*, 2010)

The following sections describe current facility data regarding length of stay, average daily census, and number of beds.

6.2.1 Length of stay

According to Bowersox, Szymanski, and McCarthy (2013), the average length of stay for inpatient psychiatric facilities decreased from 33.1 days for fiscal year 1999 to 19 days in fiscal year 2007 (Figure 6.5). Figure 6.6 illustrates that the number of inpatient psychiatric admissions lasting over 7 days decreased significantly between 1999 and 2007, whereas length of stays of less than 7 days remained approximately the same (Bowersox et al., 2013).

Regarding the length of stay in residential facilities, the *Mental Health Facilities Design Guide* (2010) published by the Department of Veterans Affairs mentions that the average length of stay at MH RRTP facilities is approximately two to three months.

Cook and colleagues (2013) studied the clinical challenges and distinctive issues in 38 VA PTSD residential treatment programs and reported that Afghanistan and Iraq veterans have higher levels of anger-related problems and acute PTSD indications than veterans from other time periods when admitted to residential programs. Fontana and Rosenheck (2008) reported that Afghanistan/Iraq veterans differed from Vietnam veterans in that they were younger, more likely to be female, less likely to have spent time incarcerated, less frequently married, more often working, and less likely to indicate "exposure to atrocities."

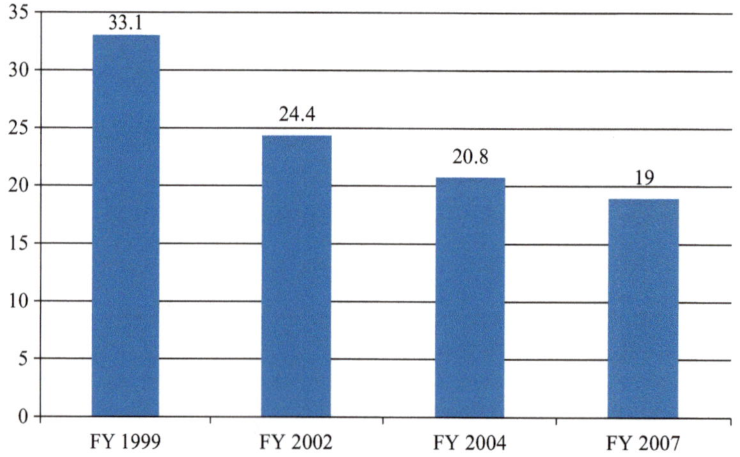

Figure 6.5: *Trends in Veterans Affairs inpatient psychiatric facilities' average length of stay for FY 1999 to FY 2007 (Data source: Bowersox et al., 2013)*

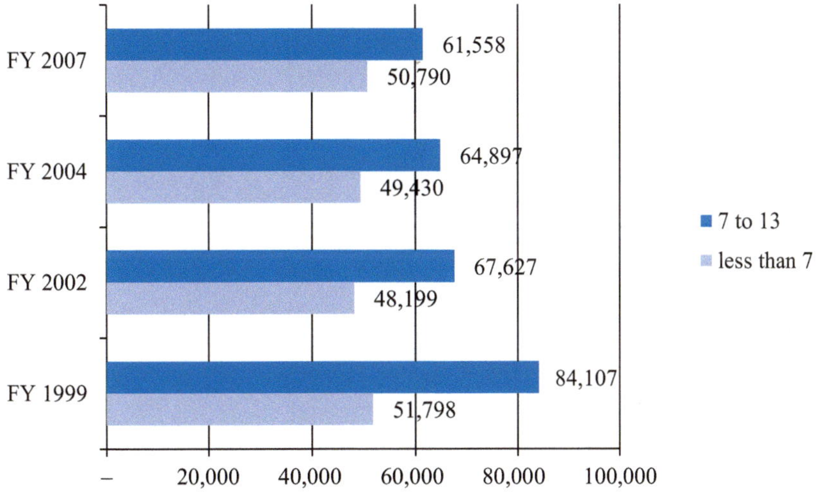

Figure 6.6: *Trends in Veterans Affairs inpatient psychiatric facilities' admissions and length of stay for FY 1999 to FY 2007 (Data source: Bowersox et al., 2013)*

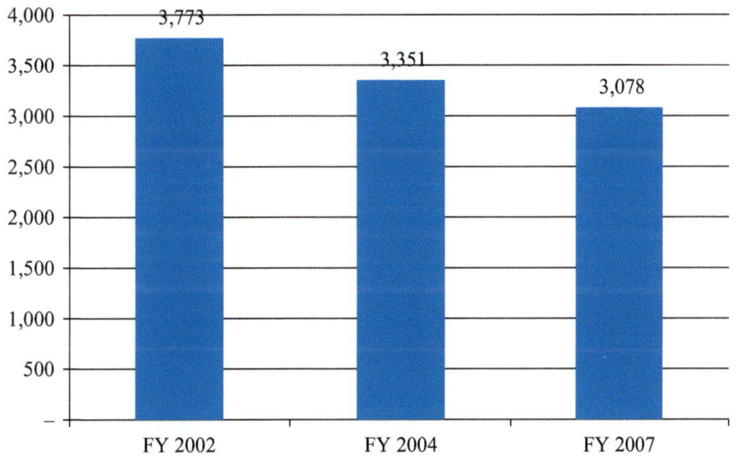

Figure 6.7: *Trends in Veterans Affairs inpatient psychiatric facilities' average daily census for FY 2002 to FY 2007 (Data source: Bowersox et al., 2013)*

Shorter length of stay and decreased treatment satisfaction and adherence to treatment are distinct characteristics of veterans assigned to Afghanistan and Iraq (Cook et al., 2013). Five to 98 days was reported as the targeted length of stay for these 38 residential programs (Cook et al., 2013). The authors further state that commitment to a length of stay of five to eight weeks is particularly challenging for young veterans, as they are trying to build relationships with their families and find or maintain employment (Cook et al., 2013). As a result, more residential programs are trying to adopt veteran-centered and recovery-oriented care models that offer greater flexibility in length of stay for meeting veterans' various and distinct needs (Cook et al., 2013).

6.2.2 *Average daily census*

Figure 6.7 illustrates a decrease in average daily census of inpatient psychiatric facilities from 3,773 in fiscal year 2002 to 3,078 in fiscal year 2007 (Bowersox et al., 2013).

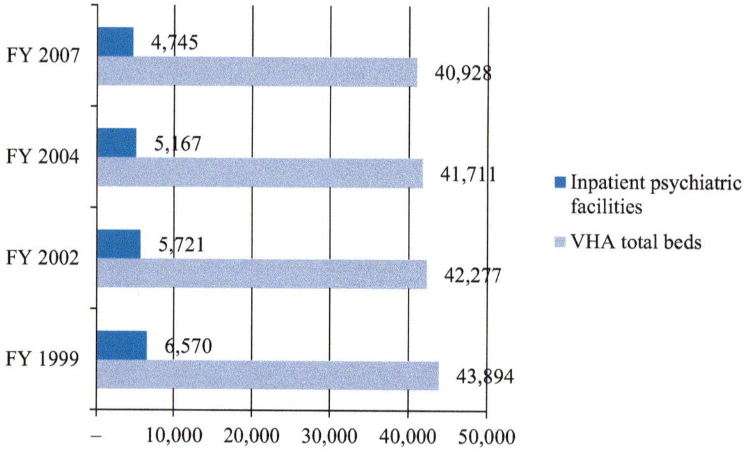

Figure 6.8: *Trends in Veterans Affairs inpatient psychiatric bed availability for FY 1999 to FY 2007 (Data source: Bowersox et al., 2013)*

6.2.3 *Number of beds and facilities*

Bowersox et al. (2013) assessed the number of beds in VHA inpatient psychiatric facilities and observed a decline from 1999 to 2007 both in VHA total number of beds (43,894 down to 40,928) and inpatient psychiatric beds (6,570 down to 4,745) (see Figure 6.8).

6.3 Research on mental and behavioral health facilities for war veterans

Research in VA hospitals is some of the earliest. As early as the 1950s, VA facilities have served as sites for design research. In 1963, Rice and colleagues tested the Ward Atmosphere Scale (WAS) tool at three VA psychiatric hospitals: a new 100-bed hospital with a small number of patients per ward, a somewhat older hospital with 1,800 beds, and a considerably older hospital with 2,000 beds. The WAS evaluation asks 69 questions, the first 22 of which relate to the physical environment (see Figure 6.9). Researchers found that patients from the VA hospitals evaluated the wards differently, particularly with regard to physical facilities. The WAS tool has been used frequently to understand the implications of the environment (Klett, Berger, Sewall, & Rice, 1963; Rice, Berger, Klett, Sewall, & Point, 1966).

In another study, Fairbanks et al. (1977) collected data on four inpatient wards, two at a university hospital and two at a VA hospital. Researchers used direct observation to record the following activities: social, noninvolvement, movement, entertainment, task-oriented, self-maintenance, and deviant behavior. (See Figures 6.10 and 6.11.) The primary difference between the sets of units was the policy in the VA facility of allowing patients to leave the unit to eat. Researchers concluded that the social organization was similar across the units; the probability of patients engaging in conversation was highest when only two were in the room or a staff member was present, and deviant behavior was most common when an individual was alone. In subsequent related research in a VA hospital setting, McGuire et al. (1977) noted via mapping that patient behavior, more than staff behavior, was responsive to social and physical environmental changes. Of particular note was the impact of modifications to seating arrangements, which resulted in increased social interaction.

Figure 6.9: *Environmental questions in the WAS tool (Rice, Berger, Klett, Sewall, & Lemkau, 1963)*

1. It's noisy on the ward.
2. The beds on your ward are not comfortable.
3. The patients' beds on your ward are too close together.
4. The halls and offices on your ward are kept clean.
5. It's often too hot or too cold on your ward.
6. There are plenty of toilets for the number of patients on your ward.
7. Some of the patients on your ward have to sleep on mattresses on the floor.
8. The smell on your ward is very bad.
9. The floors on your ward are usually clean and orderly.
10. The furniture on your ward is in good condition
11. The dormitory in which the patients on your ward sleep is too drafty.
12. The place where patients on your ward eat is often hot and stuffy.
13. Your ward is kept free of bugs and insects.
14. There's too much talking on the ward.
15. There are enough mirrors in the washroom on your ward.
16. There are plenty of ashtrays on your ward.
17. The bed area on your ward is well lighted.
18. Every patient on the ward has his own chest of drawers or locker by his bed.
19. There are attractive pictures on the walls.
20. The temperature on your ward is generally comfortable.
21. Your ward is painted a cheerful color.
22. The nurses and nursing aides are generally able to keep your ward quiet.

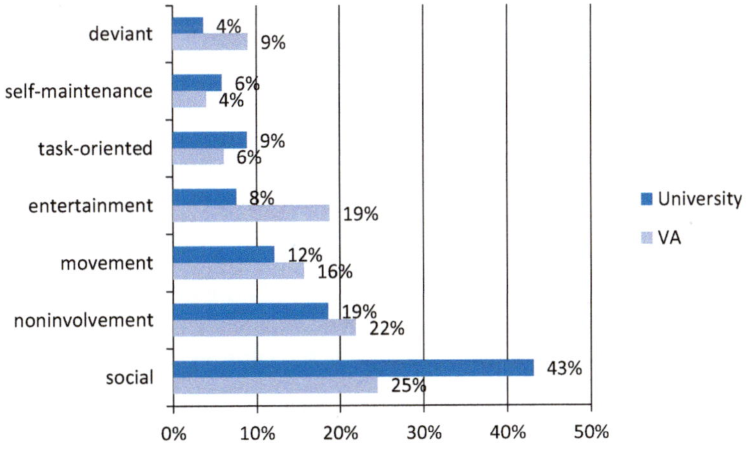

Figure 6.10: *Behavior activities, VA versus university inpatient unit (Data source: Fairbanks et al., 1977)*

Setting-Response Inventory (SRI) is another tool used to obtain staff input regarding psychiatric ward settings. In research on an open-door, 32-patient unit in a VA hospital, Moos and Daniels (1967) asked staff members to describe eight different ward social settings, including individual

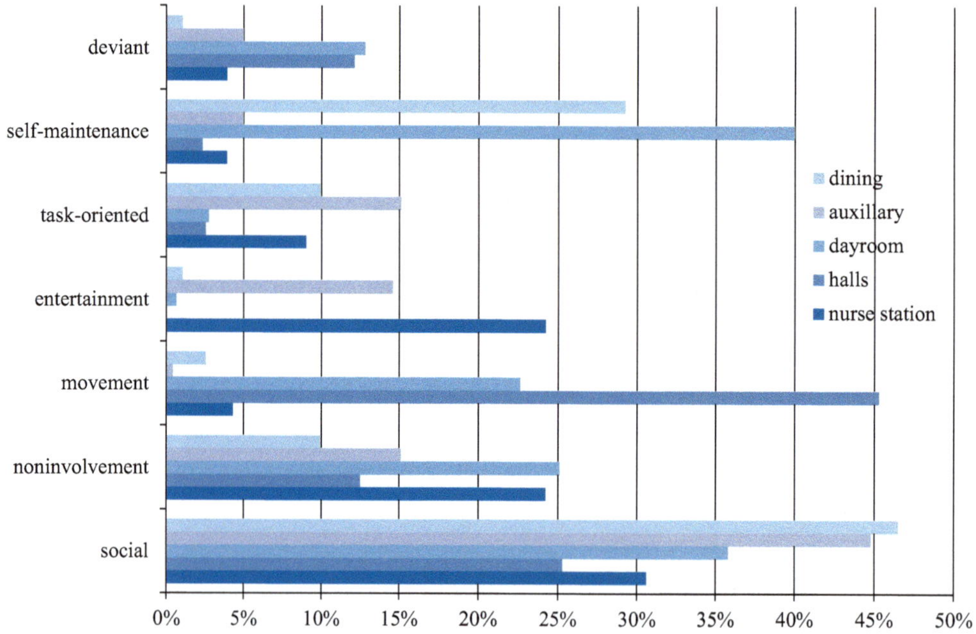

Figure 6.11: *Behavior activities, types of behavior by location (Data source: Fairbanks et al., 1977)*

therapy, group therapy, community meetings, being alone, with a patient, with a nurse, and at lunch. They were asked to rate the settings in terms of dichotomous descriptors: attentive-inattentive, friendly-hostile, outgoing-shy, sure-unsure, trusting-suspicious, and relaxed-tense. Their study showed that different ward settings can elicit different reactions from staff members. In their study, staff felt more secure, trusting, extroverted, and sociable in individual therapy than in group therapy. They also found that among different staff members, senior staff felt more secure, trusting, extroverted, and sociable in any therapy session. They concluded that different staff members function best in different ward settings depending on their expertise, seniority, and personality.

Whitehead, Polsky, Crookshank, and Fik (1984) conducted a pre- and post-occupancy evaluation of four inpatient mental health units in a federal hospital using behavioral observation and surveys. The redesign of the psychiatric unit was patient-centered and employed a "psychoenvironmental" model premised on an interaction between the psychotherapeutic environment and the physical milieu (Whitehead et al., 1984). Also, "social organizer" was the driving concept behind architectural solutions that motivated social interaction in the ward environment (Whitehead et al., 1984). The researchers developed four hypotheses to evaluate the impact of the psychiatric unit redesign:

1. There is a correlation between architectural modifications and alterations in social behavior. The findings of the study showed that the socially related interactions shifted from hallways to spaces such as the cafeteria, the dayroom, and the visiting room in the redesigned facility. No significant net difference in social behaviors was found on the ward; however, there was a substantial change in the location of the social interactions.

2. There is a correlation between architectural modifications and "altered spatial distribution of behavior." Findings showed a significant increase in utilization of dayroom by staff. Patients spent significantly more time in the redesigned cafeteria and less in the visiting room and hallways, which supports the function of cafeteria as a "social organizer." A significant decrease in hallway visits was evident for the visitor population. They used the visiting room significantly more frequently after redesign.
3. There is a correlation between architectural modifications and reduction in psychopathology. For the overall redesigned environment, findings showed a small decrease in observed psychopathology; however, a significant reduction was observed on the psychopathology rates relative to the dayroom in the redesigned unit. Opening up the spaces and supporting patient-staff interaction were psychoenvironmental strategies utilized in the redesign of the dayroom.
4. "Social organizers" – such as an open nursing station, a ward cafeteria, and a dayroom – can be utilized as spaces for which effective socializing and therapeutic design modifications may occur. The findings of the study supported "the concept of the cafeteria as a social organizer": it supported more social interactions and was utilized more frequently by the patients after redesign.

Regarding the configuration of the nursing station in the redesigned environment, researchers observed that the openness of the nurse station encouraged staff to leave the space and interact more frequently with patients. This feature facilitated staff observation of the dayroom and spaces used by patients from the nursing station. However, very few patients spent time close to the open nurse station. Nurses were often concerned about patients' abuse of the opportunity of easy interaction with staff, although the findings of the research contradicted this.

Objective and subjective outcomes of the study illustrated differences in opinion of patients and staff regarding the impact of the overall new environment. On a scale of 0–7, patients believed that the renovated facility made them feel better (5.6), but staff perceived the physical environment as less impactful (4.8). (See Figure 6.12.)

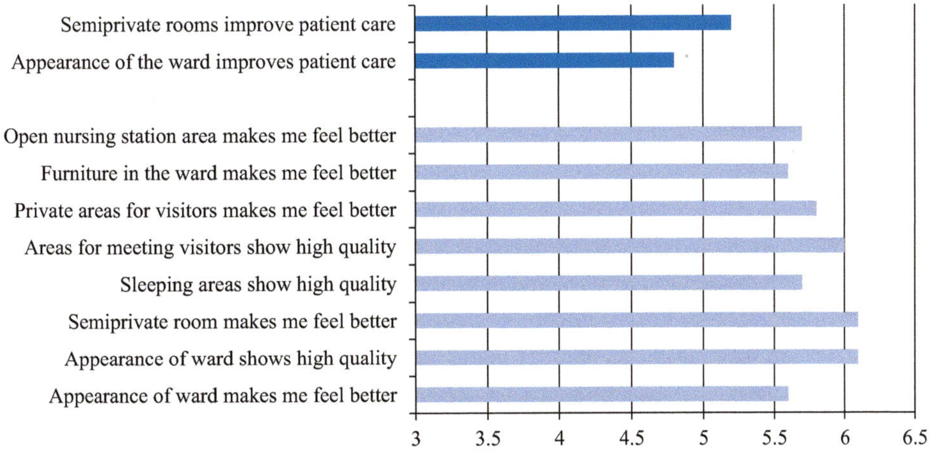

Figure 6.12: *Evaluation of new inpatient unit (light blue lines indicate staff evaluation, light blue indicates patient evaluation) (Data source: Whitehead, Polsky, Crookshank, & Fik 1984)*

6.4 Design goals for facilities for war veterans

6.4.1 *Inpatient environments*

Karlin and Zeiss (2006), from Psychology Service, Veterans Affairs, Palo Alto, recommend multiple goals in support of patient-centered care. (See Figure 6.13.)

The *Mental Health Facilities Design Guide* (2010) published by Department of Veterans Affairs states that the typical location of inpatient psychiatric units in VA medical centers should be in close proximity to the emergency department, which allows for convenient treatment of comorbid medical problems, as well as providing easy access for patients, families, and staff (Department of Veterans Affairs, 2009). Key goals for designing inpatient psychiatric units have been identified as:

- Attention should be given to architectural and interior design details that contribute to a home-like and noninstitutional environment.

Figure 6.13: *Karlin and Zeiss' environmental goals for patient-centered care (Karlin & Zeiss, 2006)*

Intervention	*Description*
Ambient features	Lighting should be soft, indirect, and full spectrum; spotlight lighting should be used in limited areas; natural daylight, good air quality; neutral colors
Architectural features	Single or non-dormitory rooms; private visiting areas; multiple large, low windows; views of nature; outdoor gardens; avoid long corridors; flexible dividers for large areas; seclusion rooms acoustically separated from nurse stations; staff respite spaces; support for technology; support for families
Interior design features	Clearly identifiable reception area; reflection of symbolic meaning
Furnishings	Reduced institutional feel
Familiarity	Upholstered furniture; interchangeable pieces; resistance to damage; soothing artwork; carpeting where appropriate
Color	Avoid monochromatic or trendy schemes; warm blue colors; avoid blue-green colors; seclusion rooms should not be white or gray
Other	Should accommodate patients who need stimulation but not overstimulate patients who are agitated; use color, light, and finishes to designate areas; plants; shatterproof windows; lockable cabinets; avoid blind corners; avoid highly polished floors
Social features	Spaces where patients can retreat, form social relationships; avoid overcrowding; provide privacy; open and flexible dayrooms; small group circular seating
Specific issues	
Nursing stations	Open nursing stations recommended
Older patients	Moderate environmental stimulation; familiar images; appropriate lighting; shorter corridors; more visual cues

- A bright and open design should be employed in the layout and color scheme of the building.
- Long corridors should be avoided to achieve a "pod-like" unit configuration that promotes social interaction among patients and staff, and creates a less institutional environment.
- Blind corners should be avoided in designing layouts. The office suites and spaces that require constant supervision by staff should be designed to be blocked off after hours to reduce extra monitoring.
- Physical and visual access to natural environments that support healing should be incorporated in layout design. Access to secure and attractive outdoor spaces should be provided directly outside the unit. Healing gardens should also be considered in addition to courtyard spaces. Access to ample natural daylight and views should be incorporated in the design of indoor spaces for patient activity areas besides providing suitable acoustic control.
- Choose furnishings, fixtures, and equipment with the minimum potential to be utilized as an anchor for hanging or as a weapon.
- Design clusters of multiple patient rooms within the unit should be provided to acknowledge separation of various patient subgroups.
- Nurse stations should have direct visual access to all patient activity areas and promote informal social interaction with patients while securing the confidentiality of patient records.
- Provide a recognizable reception and lobby space for greeting visitors, patients, and their families immediately outside the unit. Sufficient signage should be employed for easy wayfinding and direction to this area.

Figure 6.14 is based on an adjacency diagram provided in the *Mental Health Facilities Design Guide* and illustrates relationships in an inpatient mental health unit.

Positive distractions such as art and nature have been studied in outpatient settings for war veterans. Regarding art, Nanda, Gaydos, Hathorn, and Watkins (2010) conducted a literature review and case study analysis to determine recommendations for artwork for veterans with post-traumatic stress disorder. Their suggestions for content are as follows:

1. Waterscapes that are calm and nonturbulent
2. Landscapes with depth or open foreground, savannah landscapes, trees with extensive canopies, and dense vegetation
3. Culturally positive artifacts such as old houses and barns
4. Healthy, fresh, easily identifiable flowers
5. Diverse, emotionally positive figurative faces

Visual and physical access to nature have been found to be beneficial in general healthcare settings. Wagenfeld, Roy-Fisher, and Mitchell (2013) found no peer-reviewed publications that connected

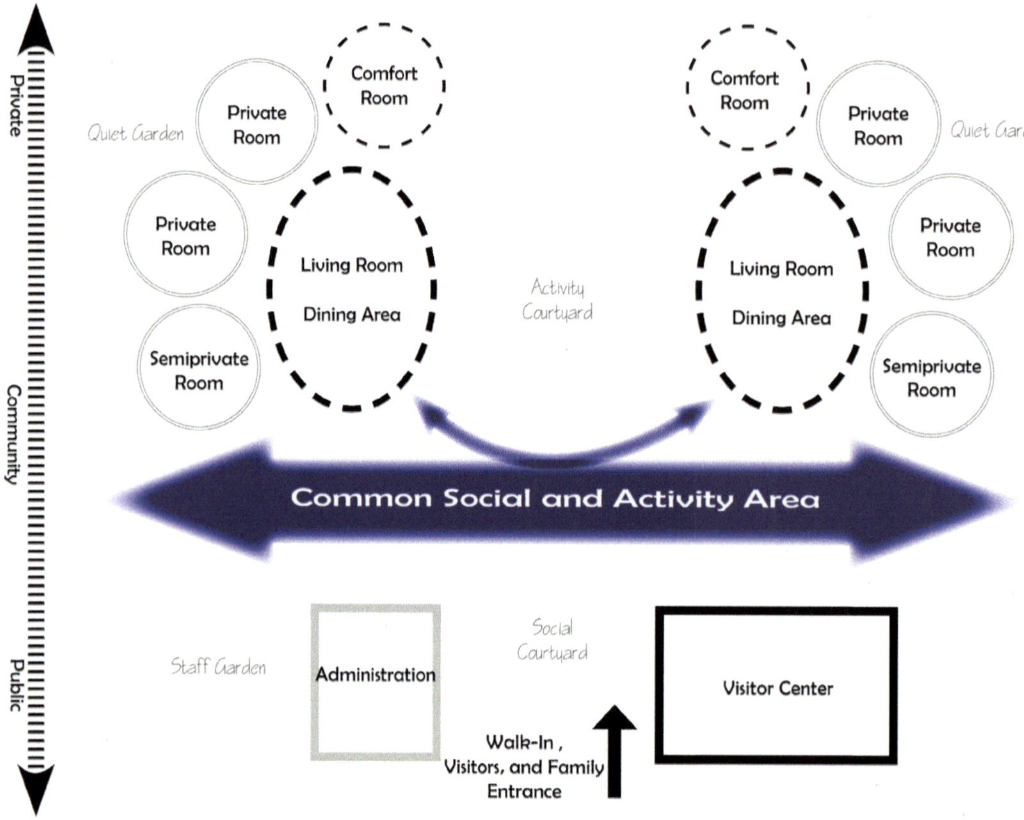

Figure 6.14: *Adjacency diagram for residential mental health facility (Based on:* Mental Health Facilities Design Guide, *2010)*

positive health outcomes in veterans with PTSD to access to healing nature. However, they used their literature review on healthcare environments to conceptualize a model to suggest benefits of access to nature for this unique population. (See Figure 6.15.)

6.4.2 *Outpatient environments*

The *Mental Health Facilities Design Guide* (2010), published by the Department of Veterans Affairs, identifies four main components of outpatient mental health facilities in the VA mental healthcare system as:

- Mental health clinic
- Substance abuse clinic
- Psychosocial rehabilitation recovery center (PRRC)
- Psychological services

Figure 6.15: *PTSD criteria, treatment concepts, and supportive outdoor design features (Wagenfeld, Roy-Fisher, & Mitchell, 2013)*

PTSD criterion	*Treatment concept*	*Design features*
Stressor	Adaptation level and sense of control	Public space that "affords" options for degrees of social interaction
Recollection	Nature and positive distraction	Water, flora, and fauna
Avoidant	"Soft" fascination	Distant views of "soft" landscape
Hyper-arousal	Social interaction	Picnic areas, barbecue pits, basketball courts, and smoking areas
Duration	Managed graded stressors	Physical courses with increasing levels of challenge
Functional significance	Meaningful activities	Naturalistic settings supporting service dog training, sustainable farming, physical/ psychological rehab

The authors note that outpatient mental health services might be provided as a functional addition to a primary care clinic or as an addition to an inpatient mental health center, or as part of a VA medical center (Department of Veterans Affairs, 2009). PRRCs are ideally located independently from other psychiatric facilities (Department of Veterans Affairs, 2009).

Mental health clinics provide outpatient general and special mental health evaluation, diagnosis, and treatment for veterans. Key goals for designing mental health clinics have been identified as follows:

- Patient dignity and privacy for a diverse population of veterans should be maintained throughout the planning and design of the clinic. Therapeutic and attractive environments should be provided for patients.
- Corridors and circulation paths in the clinic should be wheelchair-accessible (minimum of 6 feet clear for passage of two wheelchairs) and open, with direct visual access from the reception desk. Clear and ample signage as well as appropriate lighting should be incorporated throughout the space and hallways for convenient navigation.
- An identifiable reception area in close proximity to a comfortable waiting area should be included for greeting family members and patients. The waiting area should afford for some privacy as well.
- Suitable acoustic control should be provided for therapy rooms.
- Access to outdoor spaces should be provided to facilitate social interactions among patients when possible.

A diagram based on the *Mental Health Facilities Design Guide* illustrating the relationships in an outpatient mental health unit is replicated in Figure 6.16.

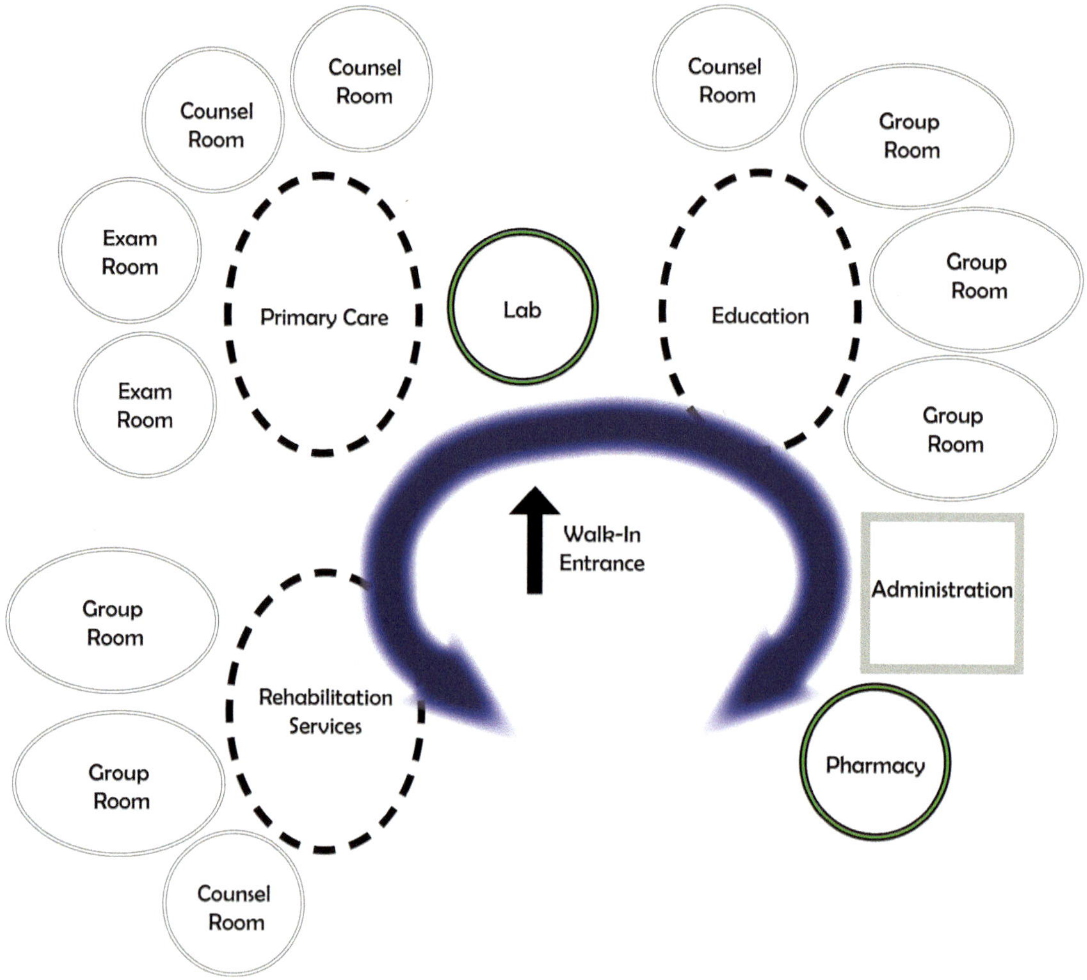

Figure 6.16: *Adjacency diagram for an outpatient mental health facility (Based on:* Mental Health Facilities Design Guide, *2010)*

6.5 Case study

6.5.1 *Acute Inpatient Psychiatric Replacement Facility Palo Alto, Veterans Affairs*

Location: Palo Alto, CA
Designer/Architect: The Design Partnership and Keller Mitchell & Co.
Client: U.S. Department of Veterans Affairs
Completion: June 2012
Area: 91,000 square feet

Awards: Award of Merit in the health-care category of ENR California's annual "Best Projects" competition; American Society of Landscape Architects Honor Award

Client, service users, and services

The facility is intended to represent the new standard for VA facilities by providing better care for veterans with mental health disorders. The project served as the basis for the Veterans Administration's recent "Design Guide for Mental Health Facilities."

Mission and goals

Creating a noninstitutional patient-centered facility has been the main goal in designing the facility. The care is focused on recovery in a setting with residential qualities where patient safety and engagement are emphasized. The facility intends to increase patient engagement by removing barriers to patient and staff interaction and includes large dayrooms and spacious semi-open nurse stations to achieve this objective. Patient respect and dignity was encouraged by supplanting conventional dorm-style rooms with private and semiprivate patient rooms.

Site

The complex is located near a residential suburban neighborhood less than 10 miles away from the Palo Alto city center. It was constructed to replace an existing facility built in 1960, which was seismically and functionally inadequate. The facility is accessible from an expressway along which several other commercial campuses are located.

Program

The program consists of four 20-bed psychiatric acute inpatient care units, with outdoor enclosed gardens for the patients. Swing beds between each pair of 20-bed units permit census to range from 18 to 22. Thirty percent of the beds are private, and the rest are double occupancy. Each unit has access to two open space gardens. A large recreation courtyard includes a combination of passive and active places, which are geared toward meditation and social activities, respectively. Activities include playing sports, horticultural therapy, and walking. The single-story bed units have direct access to gardens, and each unit, based on the population and acuity level, are adjacent to specific gardens. For example, quiet view gardens are adjacent to units dedicated to older patients.

Other clinical programs available on the hospital campus include an emergency department, imaging, laboratory, the Bone and Joint Center, and the Spinal Cord Injury service. A separate administrative pavilion includes functions such as ambulatory care center, research spaces, a conference center, and staff recruitment and training services. Offices are modular and all have windows, simplifying assignment of offices. The consolidation of an acute care center with ambulatory care services in one complex has been instrumental in facilitating accessibility and supporting responsive care management and recovery strategies.

Configuration and construction

The complex is composed of buildings connected by a covered walkway that wraps around the central garden courtyard, linking program functions through easy wayfinding for visitors, staff, and patients. A single-story building that includes the patient beds is constructed of slab-on-grade with a timber platform framing and plywood shear walls. The two-story administrative facility uses braced steel framing. Both structures are finished by cement plaster and brick veneer to match the campus palette. Arched roof elements use standing-seam metal, and flat roofs use single-ply membrane coverage. The building incorporates many sustainable design elements including use of high-efficiency water and heating systems and recycled and low-emission material that can be maintained using local resources. Ninety-five percent of interior occupied spaces are naturally lit.

Case study bibliography

The Design Partnership. (2015). Project information and other in-house publication materials.

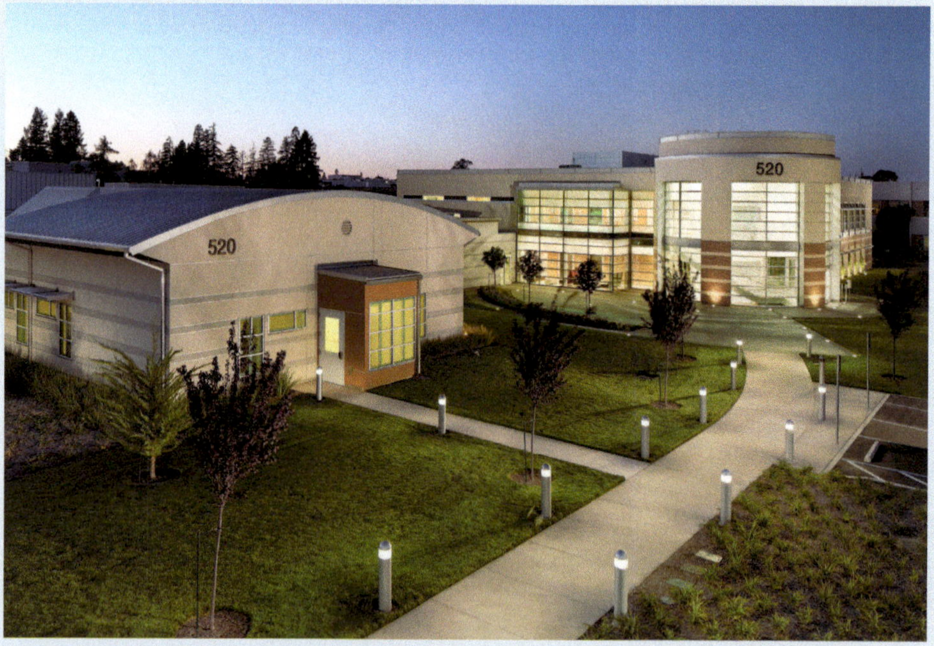

Figure 6.17: *VA Palo Alto Mental Health – exterior night (Architects: The Design Partnership; Photo credit: Will Lee)*

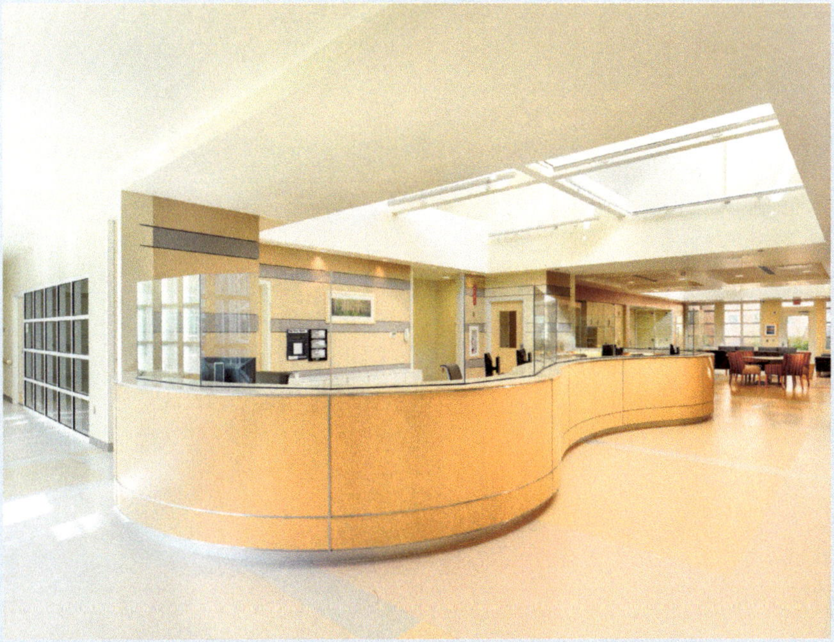

Figure 6.18: *VA Palo Alto Mental Health – nurses' station (Architects: The Design Partnership; Photo credit: Rien van Rijthoven)*

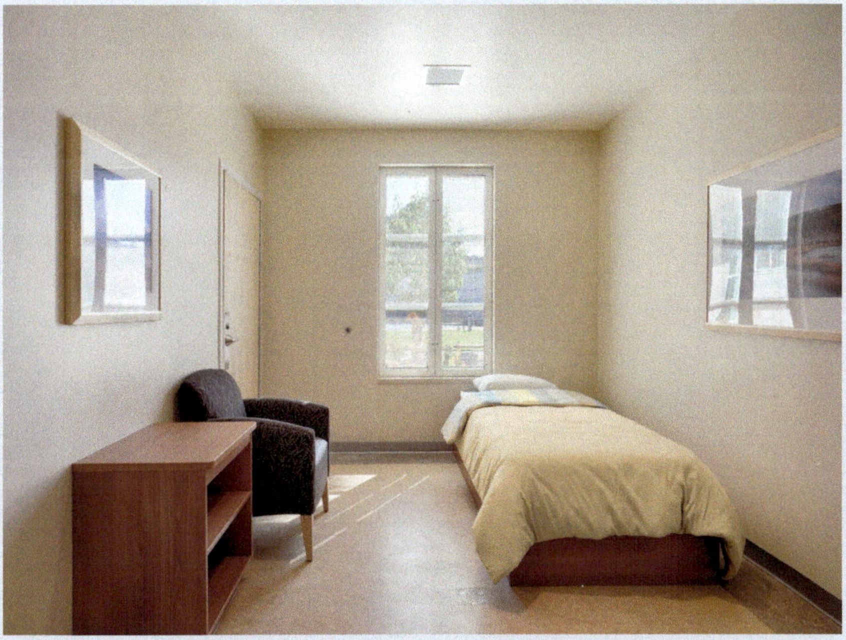

Figure 6.19: *VA Palo Alto Mental Health – private patient room (Architects: The Design Partnership; Photo credit: Rien van Rijthoven)*

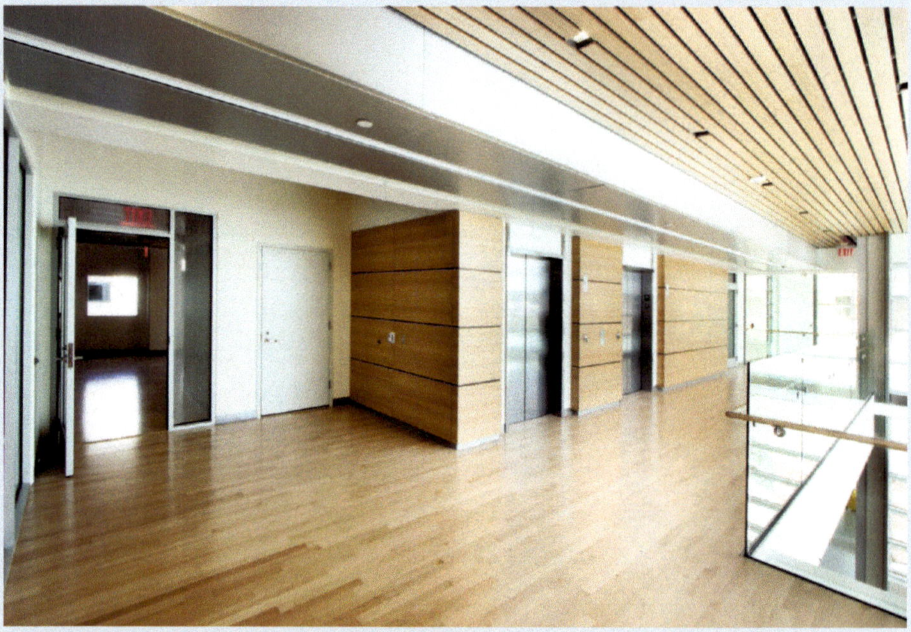

Figure 6.20: *VA Palo Alto Mental Health – elevator lobby (Architects: The Design Partnership; Photo credit: Chelsea Olsen)*

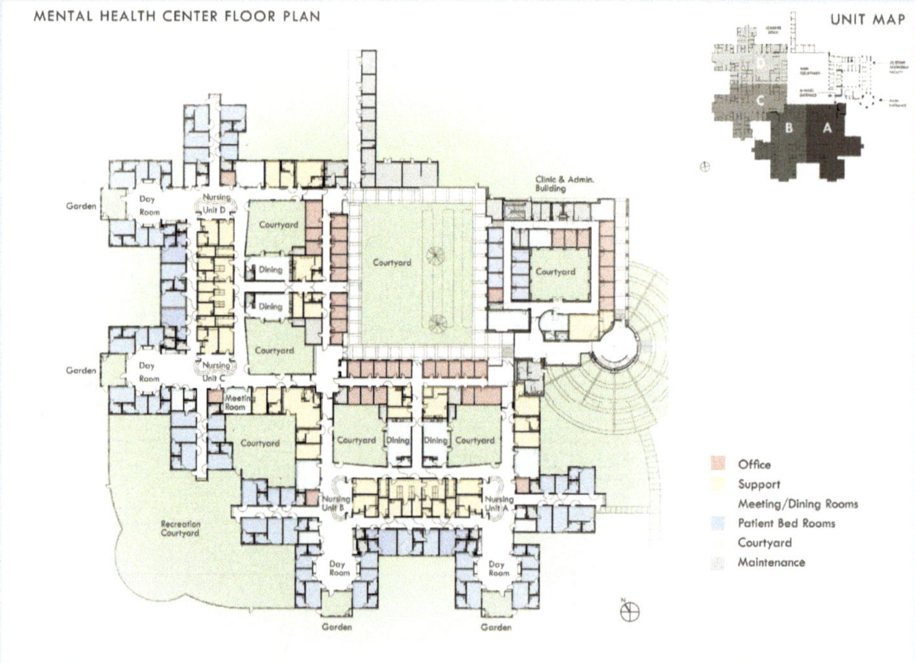

Figure 6.21: *VA Palo Alto Mental Health – floor plan (Source: Veterans Affairs, Acute Inpatient Psychiatric Replacement Facility Palo Alto, CA. Plan courtesy of The Design Partnership)*

References

Bowersox, N. W., Szymanski, B. J., & McCarthy, J. F. (2013). Associations between psychiatric inpatient bed supply and the prevalence of serious mental illness in veterans affairs nursing homes. *American Journal of Public Health*, *103*(7), 1325–1331.

Bryan, C. J., Rudd, M. D., & Wertenberger, E. (2013). Reasons for suicide attempts in a clinical sample of active duty soldiers. *Journal of Affective Disorders*, *144*(2023), 148–152.

Butterfield, M. I., Forneris, C. A., Feldman, M. E., & Beckham, J. C. (2000). Hostility and functional health status in women veterans with and without posttraumatic stress disorder: A preliminary study. *Journal of Traumatic Stress*, *13*(4), 735–741.

Cook, J. M., Dinnen, S., O'Donnell, C., Bernardy, N., Rosenheck, R., & Hoff, R. (2013). Iraq and Afghanistan veterans: National findings from VA residential treatment programs. *Psychiatry*, *76*(1), 18–31.

Department of Veterans Affairs. (2009). *Review of veterans health administration residential mental health care facilities*. Retrieved from www.va.gov/oig/54/reports/VAOIG-08-00038-152.pdf

Department of Veterans Affairs. (2015). *History – Department of Veterans Affairs (VA)*. Retrieved from www.va.gov/

Epidemiology Program Post-Deployment Health Group, Office of Public Health, Veterans Health Administration, Department of Veterans Affairs. (2015). *Analysis of VA health care utilization among Operation Enduring Freedom, Operation Iraqi Freedom, and Operation New Dawn veterans, from 1st Qtr. FY 2002 through 2nd Qtr. FY 2015*. Washington, DC: U.S. Department of Veteran's Affairs. Retrieved from www.publichealth.va.gov/epidemiology

Fairbanks, L., McGuire, M., Cole, S., Shordone, R., Silers, F., & Richards, M. (1977). The ethological study of four psychiatric wards: patient, staff and system behaviors. *Journal of Psychiatric Research*, *13*, 193–209.

Fontana, A. F., & Rosenheck, R. A. (2008). Treatment-seeking veterans of Iraq and Afghanistan: Comparison with veterans of previous wars. *Journal of Nervous and Mental Disease*, *196*, 513–521.

Karlin, B. E., & Zeiss, R. A. (2006). Environmental and therapeutic issues in psychiatric hospital design: Toward best practices. *Psychiatric Services*, *57*(10), 1376–1378.

Klett, S. L., Berger, D. G., Sewall, L. G., & Rice, C. E. (1963). Patient evaluation of the psychiatric ward. *Journal of Clinical Psychology*, *19*(3), 347–351.

McGuire, M. T., Fairbanks, L. A., Cole, S. R., Sbordone, R., Silvers, F. M., Richards, M., & Akers, J. (1977). The ethological study of four psychiatric wards: Behavior changes associated with new staff and new patients. *Journal of Psychiatric Research*, *13*(4), 211–224.

Mental health facilities design guide. (2010) (1st ed.). Retrieved from www.cfm.va.gov

Mills, P. D., King, L. A., Watts, B. V., & Hemphill, R. R. (2013). Inpatient suicide on mental health units in Veterans Affairs (VA) hospitals: Avoiding environmental hazards. *General hospital psychiatry*, *35*(5), 528–536.

Moos, R., & Daniels, D. (1967). Differential effects of ward settings on psychiatric staff. *Archives of General Psychiatry*, *17*(1), 75–82.

Nanda, U., Gaydos, H. L. B., Hathorn, K., & Watkins, N. (2010). Art and posttraumatic stress: A review of the empirical literature on the therapeutic implications of artwork for war veterans with posttraumatic stress disorder. *Environment and Behavior*, *42*(3), 376–390.

National Center for Veterans Analysis and Statistics – Veteran population. (2015). Retrieved from www.va.gov/vetdata/veteran_population.asp

Rice, C. E., Berger, D. G., Klett, S. L., Sewall, L. G., & Lemkau, P. V. (1963). The ward evaluation scale. *Journal of Clinical Psychology*, *19*(2), 251–258.

Rice, C. E., Berger, D. G., Klett, S. L., Sewall, L. G., & Point, P. (1966). Measuring psychiatric hospital staff opinions about patient care. *Archives of General Psychiatry*, *14*(4), 428–434.

Seal, K. H., Bertenthal, D., Miner, C. R., Sen, S., & Marmar, C. (2007). Bringing the war back home: Mental health disorders among 103,788 US veterans returning from Iraq and Afghanistan seen at Department of Veterans Affairs Facilities. *Archives of Internal Medicine*, *167*(5), 476–482.

Seal, K. H., Maguen, S., & Cohen, B. E. (2015). Mental health problems and treatment utilization of Iraq and Afghanistan veterans enrolled in department of veterans affairs health care. In M. Safir, H. Wallach, & A. Rizzo (Eds.), *Future directions in post-traumatic stress disorder* (pp. 329–345). New York: Springer.

Street, A. E., Vogt, D., & Dutra, L. (2009). A new generation of women veterans: Stressors faced by women deployed to Iraq and Afghanistan. *Clinical Psychology Review*, *29*(8), 685–694.

Wagenfeld, A., Roy-Fisher, C., & Mitchell, C. (2013). Collaborative design: Outdoor environments for veterans with PTSD. *Facilities*, *31*(9/10), 391–406.

Watts, B. V., Young-Xu, Y., Mills, P., DeRosier, P., Kemp, J., Shiner, B., & Duncan, W. (2012). Examination of the effectiveness of the mental health environment of care checklist in reducing suicide on inpatient mental health units. *Archives of General Psychiatry*, *69*(6), 588–592.

Whitehead, C., Polsky, R., Crookshank, C., & Fik, E. (1984). Objective and subjective evaluation of psychiatric ward design. *American Journal of Psychiatry*, *82*, 454–462.

Child and adolescent psychiatric care 7

7.1 Introduction

7.1.1 History of child and adolescent care in the United States

The history of child and adolescent mental and behavioral care in the United States is loosely linked to the evolution of professional psychiatric organizations. The American Academy of Child Psychiatry was founded in the mid-1950s. It followed the creation of the American Psychiatric Association and the American Medical Association by more than 100 years (Houston & Martini, 2013). Various political interventions have also played a role in the development and objectives of the profession; in recent years the provision of mental health services has been impacted by Medicare, Medicaid, the Community Mental Health Act, managed care, and HMOs (Houston & Martini, 2013).

Child psychiatry originated with pediatric guidance clinics in the 1920s in response to juvenile delinquency (Houston & Martini, 2013). These ambulatory settings served as a training ground for child psychiatrists working with interdisciplinary teams of social workers and pediatricians. At the same time, the field of psychoanalysis and the individual treatment of children in intensive therapy gained momentum (Houston & Martini, 2013).

Three factors – the Health Maintenance Act of 1973, over-hospitalization for adolescents in the 1980s, and managed care in the 1990s – resulted in overutilization of psychopharmacology and the diminishment of the value of diagnostics, therapy, and consultation (Houston & Martini, 2013). In spite of the potentially transformative evolution, children and adolescents are still underserved. According to Houston and Martini, we are currently facing a fragmented system that leaves 80% of pediatric patients without treatment.

According to the National Research Council and Institute of Medicine report (2009), an estimated 13%–20% of children living in the United States suffer from a diagnosable mental disorder in a given year, and an estimated $247 billion is spent annually on mental disorders of persons under 24. According to Soni (2009), treating mental disorders in children was among the highest reported healthcare expenditures in 2006. Children's mental disorders are a critical public health issue impacting children, families, and communities in the United States. The American Academy of Pediatrics (2009) Task Force on Mental Health asserts that no other illnesses impact children so significantly. At the same time, they recognize that early identification and treatment have the potential to reduce the impact of mental illness and its multiple outcomes.

7.1.2 Data regarding the pediatric psychiatric population

A review of the data associated with pediatric mental and behavioral health patients is useful in the development of needs assessments for this population and the related facility requirements. Although more current data would be desirable, the most recent studies are based on data gathered prior to 2011.

Merikangas et al. (2010a) describe the 12-month prevalence estimates for behavior and mental disorders among U.S. children utilizing data from the National Health and Nutrition Examination Survey, a collaboration between the National Institute for Mental Health and the National Center for Health Statistics. The data, which is based on 3,042 children 8–15 years of age, represents a probability sample of noninstitutionalized children. In this group 8.6% were diagnosed with attention deficit/hyperactivity disorder (ADHD), 3.7% with mood disorders, 2.1% with conduct disorder, 0.7% with panic or anxiety disorder, and 0.1% with eating disorders. Unfortunately, only half had accessed treatment with a mental health professional during that period. The distribution of disorders is summarized in Figure 7.1.

Regarding teenagers, 49.5% of 13- to 18-year-olds have or have had a psychiatric disorder, and 21.4% have or have had a severe disorder (Merikangas et al., 2010b). Among the most common are anxiety disorders (31.9%), conduct disorders (19.2%), and mood disorders (14.3%) (Merikangas et al., 2010b). (See Figure 7.2.)

The data in Figures 7.1 and 7.2 invite a comparison. Regarding children between 8 and 15, ADHD, mood, and conduct disorders are the most prevalent diagnoses, in that order. Among children between 13 and 18, anxiety, conduct, and mood disorders are the most common. Interestingly, ADHD, which is a significant issue for the younger children (16.4%), is greatly reduced in their adolescent years. Panic disorders, on the other hand, increase. Also notable is that adolescents represent 49% of the children with disorders, as opposed to 24% of younger children. (See Figure 7.3.) In both cases, severe disorders present in about 40% of the total population. In spite of the significant discussion in public forums regarding eating disorders, they represented a marginal portion of the pediatric population, despite the fact that there is an increase in late adolescence. Regarding facility implications, data like these suggest that older children are more likely to be the primary patients in mental health settings.

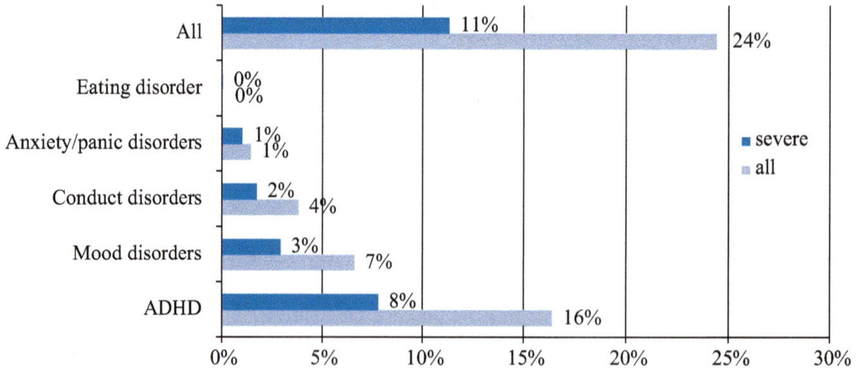

Figure 7.1: *Type of disorder for children 8–15, (rounded %) (Data source: Merikangas et al., 2010a)*

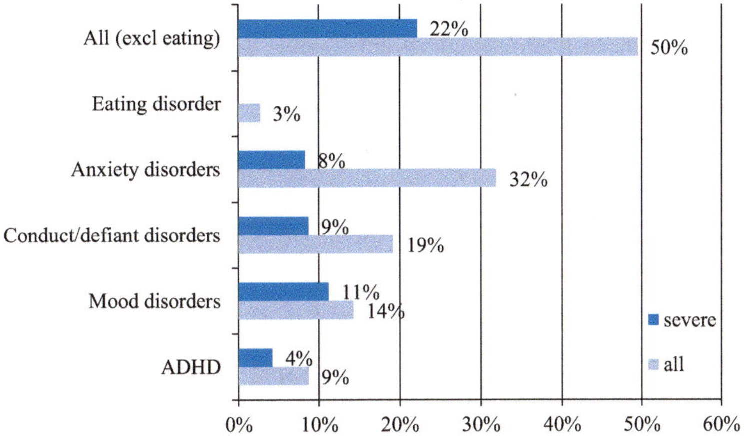

Figure 7.2: *Type of disorder for children 13–18, (rounded %) (Data source: Merikangas et al., 2010b)*

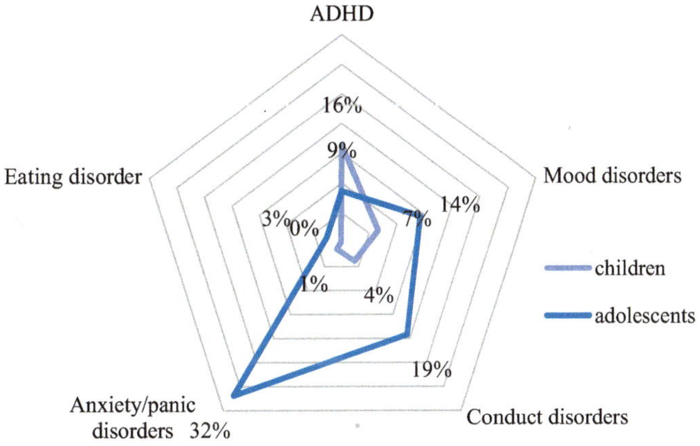

Figure 7.3: *A comparison of Merikangas et al.'s 2010 data on children and adolescents*

The relationship of the trajectory of these data as compared to that of adults is of interest. Olfson, Blanco, Wang, Laje, and Correll's (2014) assessment of U.S. national trends regarding 446,543 outpatient children, adolescents, and adults, utilizing data from the *National Ambulatory Medical Care Survey*, indicates that between 1995–1998 and 2007–2010, visits by teenagers resulting in psychiatric disorder diagnoses per 100 persons increased significantly, from 7.78 to 15.30. By contrast, adults with psychiatric disorder diagnoses only increased from 23.23 to 28.48 visits per 100 persons. A similar growth pattern for adolescents was associated with psychotherapy and psychotropic medication. This suggests that the difference between older children and younger may be increasing and that the early years may be critical to later mental health.

What are the potential factors contributing to this increase in mental health issues in children? In 1993 Wells and Whittington provided a snapshot of a 111-patient adolescent residential treatment facility population. These children tended to come from impoverished backgrounds with frequent family breakdowns. The median income was half that of all U.S. families, and only 14% had both biological parents in their homes. The youths had diverse symptoms and compromised social competencies and were difficult to diagnose as having a single illness. Additionally, the children in the study had utilized a variety of services over their lifetime and been in crisis for the year prior. Eighty-three percent had behavioral problems prior to adolescence, 93% had used out-of-home placement, and 86% used outpatient therapy. Their families tended to be less cohesive; 59% did not want their child to "live at home now" and 56% reported that there was abuse in their family. From the perspective of facility design, designers should thoroughly contemplate the components of a "homelike" environment, focusing on concepts such as safety rather than a particular aesthetic.

7.1.3 Characteristics and needs of children

Our intuitive understanding of children as well as a vast body of literature tells us that their healthcare needs, both physical and psychological, are very different from the needs of adults. However, clinicians and designers may not discriminate. De Andres-Trelles (2015) notes that psychopharmaceuticals are frequently studied and used by adults and the inclination is to extrapolate this to children. However, there is little evidence to support this approach. Within the pediatric population, stages of development, diagnoses, and needs vary. Additionally, children vary widely in terms of their developmental status.

Piaget's (1952) writings on pediatric development are among the classic resources for understanding the developmental process. His theories have been updated (and sometimes challenged), but the foundation provides a useful perspective. Piaget modeled children's development on the notion of "increasingly powerful logicomathematical structures," while a more contemporary approach addresses "conceptual knowledge structures" and may be linked to their social environmental circumstances (Case, 1991). The gist of most developmental theories is that children interact with their social and physical environment at increasingly complex levels as they age. This does not just refer to preferences, but is intricately linked to a child's or adolescent's ability to respond to and process experiences. A 6-year-old has radically different responses to his or her social and physical environment from those of a 12-year-old or a 17-year-old.

The relationship between child development and the physical environment is discussed at length by Gary Evans and others, including the impact on children of behavioral toxicology, noise, crowding, housing and neighborhood quality, schools, and day care environments. With particular reference to crowding, Evans (2006) notes the difficulty that children experience in dense social conditions that might manifest itself in resistance to cooperation, increased aggression, and neuroticism. Developmental differences have been found relative to art preferences (Eisen, Ulrich, Shepley, Varni, & Sherman, 2008), color preferences (Read & Upington, 2009), need for privacy (Laufer & Wolfe, 1977), access to nature (Wells & Evans, 2003), and spatial processing (Ishikawa & Montello, 2006).

7.2 Characteristics of residential pediatric mental healthcare facilities

Three important factors contribute to the description of a residential healthcare setting: average length of stay, average daily census, and number of beds. Length of stay is important because amenities and the complexity of the space may be different depending upon the duration of exposure to the environment. Daily census and number of beds dictate the density and distribution of patient clusters.

7.2.1 Length of stay

Regarding the length of stay (LOS) in pediatric facilities, Meagher, Rajan, Wyshak and Goldstein (2013) found a significant decrease between 1991 and 2008. (See Figure 7.4.) In less than 20% of facilities, children stayed for longer than a year on average. Data analyzed by Ireys, Achman, and Takyi (2006) demonstrated that longer length of stay was more prevalent in facilities with three to 16 residents, compared to the facilities with an average of 17 or more residents. This is an appropriate environmental response, as long-term patients are more likely to need a more personal care experience.

More current data suggest that the LOS has leveled off. Torio, Encinosa, Berdahl, McCormick, and Simpson (2015), in an investigation of national trends (2006–2011) in hospital utilization noted that expenditures and costs for patients aged 1 to 17 reported no significant increase in LOS for hospitalized pediatric patients with mental health illnesses. The mean LOS in 2006 was 7 days and in 2011 was 7.2 days. Torio et al. (2015) attributed this apparent stability in length of stay to the stabilization in the effects of managed care and utilization of management policies.

While it is difficult to compare hospitalization with group-home treatment, some gender differences may be seen. In an investigation of gender differences among adolescents in group-home residential treatment, Handwerk, Clopton, Huefner, Smith, Hoff, and Lucas (2006) found that the mean LOS for boys and girls was 17.6 months. Boys had a mean LOS of 16.9 months and girls had a mean of 18.8 months.

Age at entry into the system and the severity of symptoms appear to predict LOS (Hussey & Guo, 2005). Hussey and Guo (2005) noted a 30% increase in the rate of discharge for every year of increase in age at admission to the residential facility. At the end of the study period, the slowest rate of discharge (80% remaining in care) was noticed for children who entered the residential facility at the age of 5; only 18% of 13-year-olds remained in the facility.

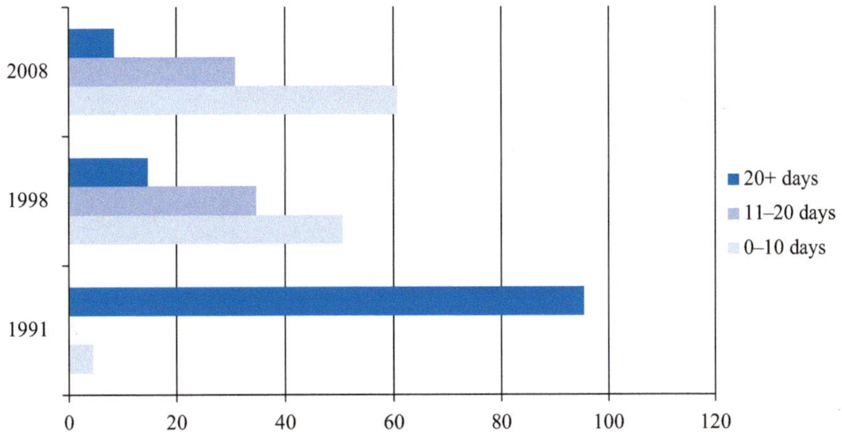

Figure 7.4: *Length of stay, 1991 versus 2003 (Data source: Ireys, Achman, & Takyi, 2006; Witkin, 1974)*

7.2.2 *Average daily census*

In 2002, in a study of 21 states, North Carolina and California were recorded as having the highest average daily census (ADC) for children in state-operated facilities (Ireys et al., 2006). This hierarchy reminds us that state population may not be related to census. The National Association of State Mental Health Program Directors (NASMHPD) data only include information for the residential care organizations owned or operated by state mental health agencies. According to NASMHPD, residential beds are defined as providing either: (1) 24-hour mental healthcare besides psychiatric services in any setting other than a hospital, or (2) 24-hour mental healthcare along with supervised living and support services in any setting other than a hospital (Ireys et al., 2006). Good data are hard to come by. Few states track the number of children in state-operated facilities receiving mental health treatment (Pear, 2003). (See Figure 7.5.)

7.2.3 *Number of beds and facilities*

The number of beds per capita for children by state also varies broadly and, as with the ADC, is not necessarily related to total state population. One of the larger states, California, has the fewest number of beds and fewest number of community treatment facilities, possibly due to inadequate funding for access to home and community-based settings (Stortz, 2003). (See Figure 7.6.)

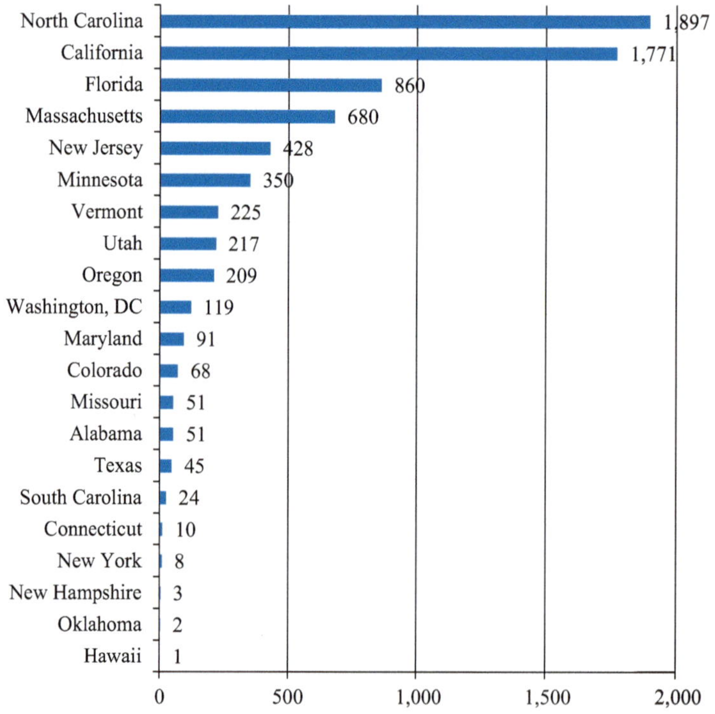

Figure 7.5: *Average daily census of children under 21 years in 24-hour residential care operated by state mental health agencies in 21 states, 2002 (Data source: Ireys, Achman, & Takyi, 2006)*

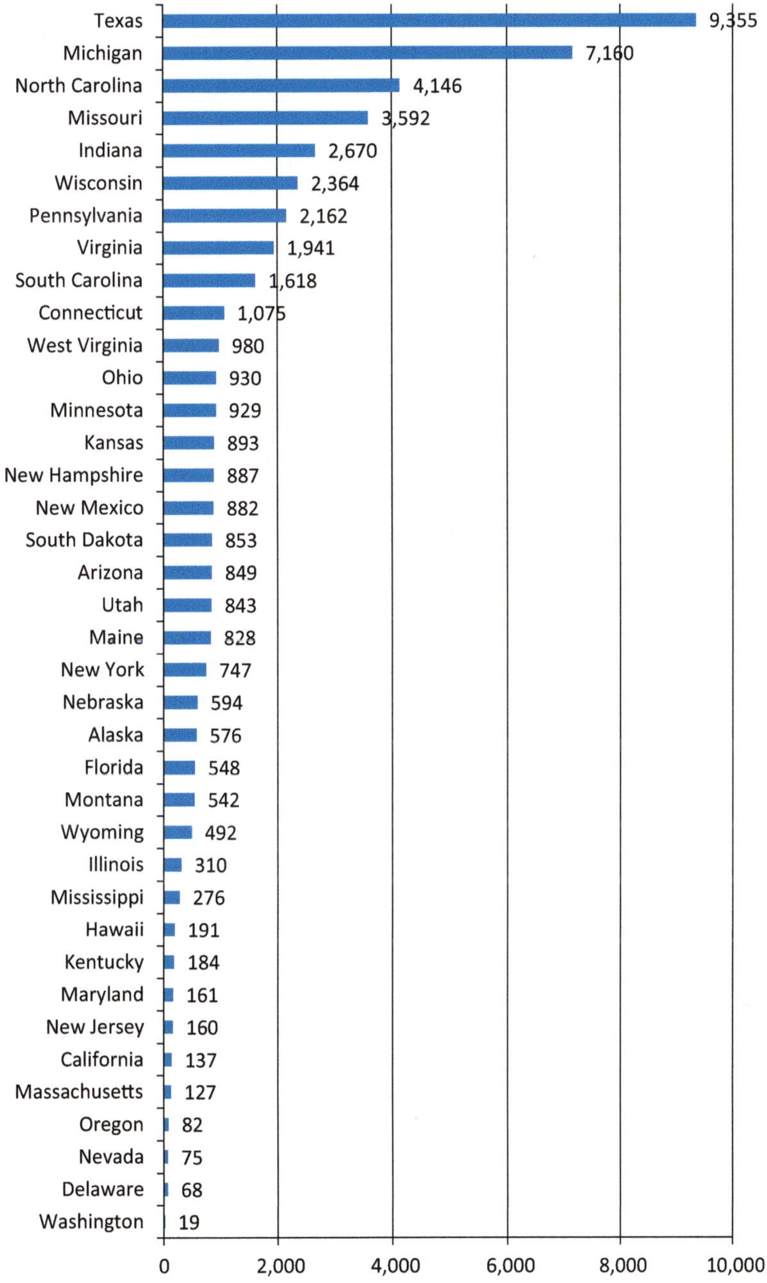

Figure 7.6: *Number of beds for children with mental illness by state (38 states), 2003 (Data source: Ireys, Achman, & Takyi, 2006)*

U.S. national data on beds and facilities indicates that 63% of beds are in 28% of the facilities – those in which the facility capacity is 17 or more. (See Figure 7.7.)

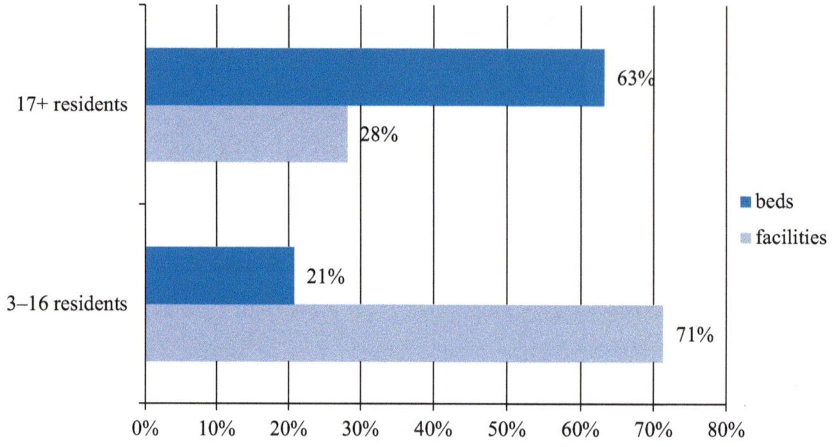

Figure 7.7: *Residential facilities of children with mental illness and associated facilities and beds, by average number of residents, 2003 (Data source: Ireys, Achman, & Takyi, 2006)*

7.3 Characteristics of outpatient and emergency room pediatric mental healthcare facilities

7.3.1 Pediatric outpatient data

Olfson, Blanco, Wang, Laje, and Correll (2014) analyzed data from nationally representative surveys of outpatient visits to physicians comparing children (0–13 years) and adolescents (14–20 years). Disruptive behavior disorders accounted for most of the child mental disorder visits (Olfson et al., 2014). According to Hoagwood, Burns, Kiser, Ringeisen, and Schoenwald (2001), the present evidence and the ongoing study of therapies in clinical practice settings suggest that symptoms associated with pediatric mental disorders could be successfully reduced by psychosocial interventions for children when administered in research-based outpatient settings. Moreover, to meet the challenge, Olfson et al. (2014) identified a pressing need for suitably trained mental healthcare specialists as well as the development and implementation of effective models of collaboration among pediatricians and other nonpsychiatric physicians who treat children and adolescents.

Regarding race/ethnicity of office visits resulting in a mental health disorder diagnosis, in a study conducted between 2007 and 2010, 71.77% were non-Hispanic White, 12.86% were non-Hispanic Black, and 15.3% were Hispanic. Children and adults represented a similar percentage of mental health disorder visits relative to ethnicity, although the data suggest that non-Hispanic White adults are more likely to account for adult visits and Hispanic and non-Hispanic Black children are more likely to account for pediatric visits. (See Figure 7.8.)

Interesting outcomes are noted regarding gender in outpatient settings. Males are more likely to be participating in visits when they are younger and women are likely when they are older (Olfson et al., 2014). (See Figure 7.9.)

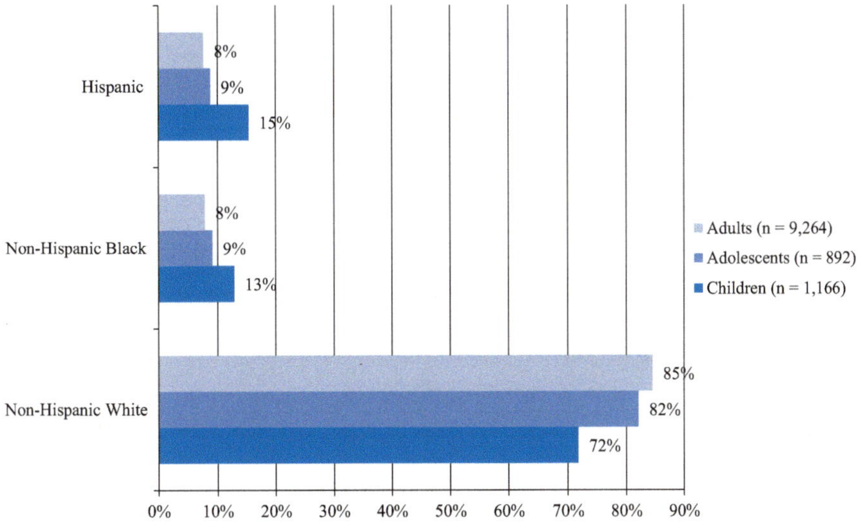

Figure 7.8: *Percentage of visits resulting in mental disorder diagnosis of children, adolescents, and adults who made office-based physician visits by race/ethnicity, 2007–2010 (Data source: Olfson, Blanco, Wang, Laje, & Correll, 2014)*

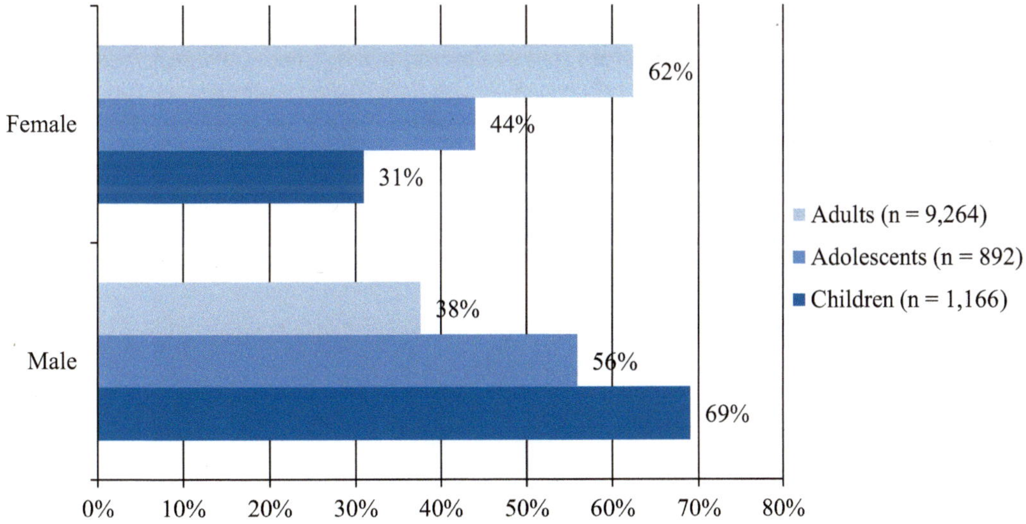

Figure 7.9: *Percentage of visits resulting in mental disorder diagnosis of children, adolescents, and adults who made office-based physician visits by gender, 2007–2010 (Data source: Olfson, Blanco, Wang, Laje, & Correll, 2014)*

In terms of visit diagnosis, the data (see Figure 7.10) indicate that children are more likely to be diagnosed with disruptive behaviors. All other diagnoses, except comorbid disorders, were more common among adults.

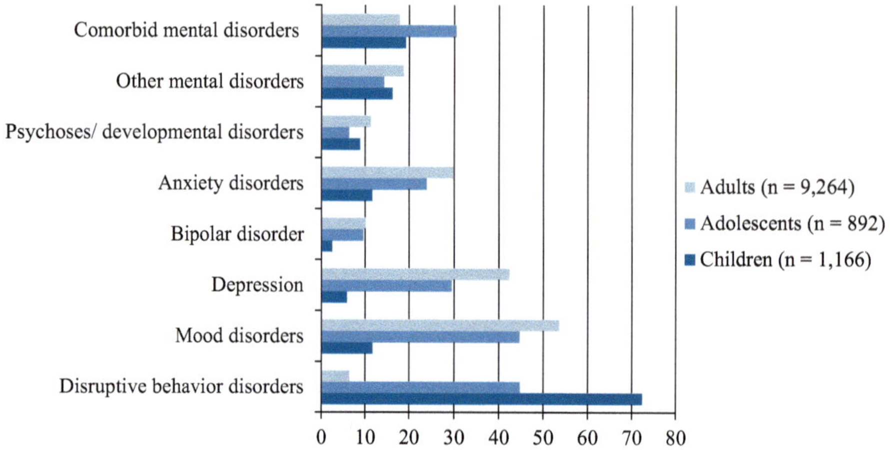

Figure 7.10: *Percentage of visits resulting in mental disorder diagnosis of children, adolescents, and adults who made office-based physician visits by mental disorder, 2007–2010 (Data source: Olfson, Blanco, Wang, Laje, & Correll, 2014)*

7.3.2 *Pediatric emergency department data*

Data from North America suggest a reduction in inpatient days, increasing non-urgent ED visits, and a shortage of child psychiatrists (Carlisle, Mamdani, Schachar, & To, 2012). Pediatric mental health visits to emergency departments were more likely than non-mental health visits to arrive by ambulance and be admitted or triaged for rapid evaluation (Case, Case, Olfson, Linakis, & Laska, 2011). The median LOS was longer for behavioral health patients, 169 minutes as opposed to 108 minutes, thereby placing significant demands on emergency departments. More detail on outpatient and emergency room pediatric mental healthcare is provided in Chapters 3 and 4.

7.4 Pediatric inpatient, outpatient and emergency room design goals

7.4.1 *Pediatric inpatient environments*

7.4.1.1 Research on pediatric inpatient design

Regarding behavioral health facilities for children and adolescents, four research projects in the early 1990s provide a good spectrum of the type of research that was being conducted at that time: Potthoff's 1991 and 1995 explorations on adolescent rehabilitation facilities (discussed in Chapter 5), Wilson, Soth, and Robak's 1992 study on group size in an adolescent psychiatric facility, Shepley's 1995 pre- and post-occupancy study on spatial design and negative behavior in a children's facility, and Glod et al.'s 1994 examination of the impact of color in quiet rooms (timeout rooms) in children's facilities. Additional research projects are described in Chapter 9.

Wilson, Soth, and Robak (1992) used interviews to examine the impact of dividing a group of 40 adolescents into physical environments that supported four groups of 10. As a result of the smaller clusters, there were reductions in vandalism, theft, and acting out on the part of patients and an increased feeling of belonging, competence, and satisfaction on the part of staff. Shortcomings included patient restlessness in an enclosed space and resistance on the part of patients to interact in the larger hospital environment.

Shepley (1995) conducted a pre- and post-occupancy evaluation of a new children's psychiatric facility using questionnaires, interviews, drawings, and incidents of disruptive behavior data. The old facility had dormitory-style sleeping accommodations off a double-loaded corridor, while the new facility incorporated private and semiprivate rooms, eliminated corridors, and created visual access to the outdoors throughout. The researchers found that the number of incidents reduced significantly during the period immediately after the building completion. Also of note was that more negative behaviors occurred in the new semiprivate rooms than the old dormitories, although the behaviors were less harmful.

Glod et al. (1994) explored whether the introduction of rose-colored walls, carpeting, and a nature mural would calm children in a psychiatric facility quiet room. Quiet rooms, sometimes referred to as timeout or seclusion rooms, are where patients are placed when their behavior becomes threatening to themselves or others. The researchers found that overall aggression ratings were 45% lower in the remodeled quiet room.

Huffcut (2010), in a series of interviews of adolescents in a residential facility, identified several desirable features: private "calm down" spaces with positive distractions, blue and purple color schemes, good daylight, seating options, and the desire to connect to peers.

7.4.1.2 Pediatric inpatient design recommendations and features

Cotton and Geraty (1984) made clear recommendations regarding the design of children's psychiatric facilities. Cotton and Geraty (1984) supported the idea that treatment goals are articulated through design details, and the physical environment can support or hinder environmental factors used for carrying out treatment goals. Physical characteristics that demonstrate behavioral cues to the patients could be identified as siting and size of building, layouts of floor plans, corridors, windows, and interior design elements such as lighting fixtures, air quality, color textures, and furniture (Cotton & Geraty, 1984). Cotton and Geraty (1984) address five treatment goals:

- Goal 1: To provide a friendly, warm, adaptive setting for pediatric patients and their families that will convey an eagerness for tolerating psychological difficulties without despair, judgment, or avoidance. To fulfill this goal, the institutional quality of the building and monotony must be minimized. Spaces should be kept in simple, small and manageable sizes. A unit kitchen might be included for a weekly community supper and evening snacks prepared by staff and children. Wall decorations should be minimal; appropriate proportions of the walls should be covered with blank bulletin boards to promote spontaneity and allow for the posting of children's artwork. Movable, attractive and simple furniture should be arranged in both sociopetal and sociofugal groupings in the living room. Paint colors can convey a positive message. Colors with institutional connotations such as muddy grays, greens, and browns and washed-out pastels should be avoided.
- Goal 2: To provide spaces that support a continuum of external controls and can be adjusted to the requirements of different patients and groups of patients as their capacities to use internal controls fluctuates. The tension between "freedom and protection" in open-door and

closed-door environments is also reflected in the design of the psychiatric units. The design throughout the facility should "afford" the treatment philosophy: to close down when activities become unmanageable and open up when patients regain composure. Quiet rooms could be designed for the treatment of intensely disturbed pediatric patients and as a replacement for dependence on psychotropic medication in transitory behavioral crises. Quiet rooms should also serve multiple purposes such as reading, peer play, napping, tutoring, or therapy. Another high-security area in the design of pediatric psychiatric facilities is the bathroom, since children are allowed to be alone in this particular space. No plumbing or wiring should be visible, and the material for tub and shower stalls should be simple and indestructible.

- Goal 3: To support the patient throughout all developmental levels. Cotton and Geraty (1984) referred to the adaptability of spaces in response to the level of functioning. Overwhelmed patients respond better to a more consistent, organized, and controlled environment. Over time, as patients begin to heal, more sophisticated and enriched spaces are desirable; namely, incorporation of "private nooks" and breaking up the corridors with "play spaces" where children can interact in small groups.
- Goal 4: To provide opportunities for private times and constructive peer relations. The architectural design goal of promoting social interaction among children should be realized in the design of the floor plans, furniture groupings, and room arrangements. Separations should be provided by low-height dividers and nooks rather than doors and walls. Furniture could be arranged to promote interaction and encourage spontaneous conversations. Cotton and Geraty (1984) pointed out the unconventional utilization of architectural elements by children as furniture: built-in toy boxes on walls could be climbed by children so as to sit and look out the windows.
- Goal 5: To redirect and substitute pathological, maladaptive behavior for more adaptive behavior. Redirection and substitution are two processes that are crucial for successful treatment of "ego-deficit" children. The overarching design strategy should anticipate destructiveness and respond by selecting durable furniture, vandal-proof lighting fixtures, and floor coverings which are hard to rip, stain, or puncture, and concealing pipes and wiring behind walls. Assaultive behavior could be minimized by designing short and interrupted corridors.

In her ethnographic study of two children's residential psychiatric facilities, Tapak (2012) offered the following considerations for facility design: (1) involve children in the design development process, (2) enhance the residential quality of the space, (3) support patient safety, (4) provide privacy, (5) exhibit sensitive treatment to the design of patient bedrooms, (6) choose appropriate decoration, and (7) provide exercise areas. In reviewing the websites of multiple children's psychiatric facilities – Fairmont Behavioral Health System (2013), University of Minnesota Amplatz Children's Hospital (2013), Meriter UnityPoint Health (2015), and Seattle Children's Hospital (2014) – we found that the inpatient psychiatric facility settings included all or some of the following components:

- private rooms;
- semiprivate beds;
- private intensive treatment rooms;
- family reception areas;
- living rooms;

- dining and social areas;
- group therapy rooms;
- academic classroom(s);
- gym;
- therapy pool;
- outdoor recreational areas;
- calming/comfort rooms;
- sensory and music therapy rooms;
- game rooms;
- overnight rooms for parents furnished with pullout couches, showers, and TVs;
- sibling units; and
- adolescent chemical dependency/dual diagnosis units.

Potential relationships among these amenities in a pediatric residential facility are described in Figure 7.11.

As Bailey summarized in his 2002 literature review, the physical environment supports interactions between children and their caretakers. A poor environment, on the other hand, might create iatrogenic illnesses, that is, illnesses resulting from the treatment itself. He identified eight design factors as being critical to an appropriate environment: control, symbolism, crowding, privacy, interior design, the development of specific domestic areas, the outdoors, and healing culture. Control is critical to achieve confidence and efficacy, which are important for development and therapeutic processes (Bartlett, 1997).

Bailey notes that an aesthetic environment, including art, sculpture, stained glass, and landscaping, carries a symbolic message in and of itself. Regarding symbolism,

> some youth may perceive a treatment facility as a "prison" where they must "do time" and thus adopt a "prisoner mentality" during their stay there. More generally, however, youth can perceive the facility in which they stay as a place for "bad kids" and then embody that belief about themselves.
>
> (Bailey, 2002, p. 17)

Regarding the effects of crowding, Maxwell (1996) suggests that home and day care facility crowding communicates a lack of personal power and status, which in turn results in undesirable behaviors such as aggression, hyperactivity, impulsiveness, competitiveness, and withdrawal. Evans, Lepore, and Schroeder (1996) recommend spatial depth as a way of dealing with overcrowding and the subsequent infringement upon privacy. He defines depth as the number of spaces transited to arrive at a destination. Bailey recommends a series of open shelves or half-height walls to support simultaneous supervision, daylight, and windows. Also recommended are noise-absorbing materials, and comfortable and homelike furniture.

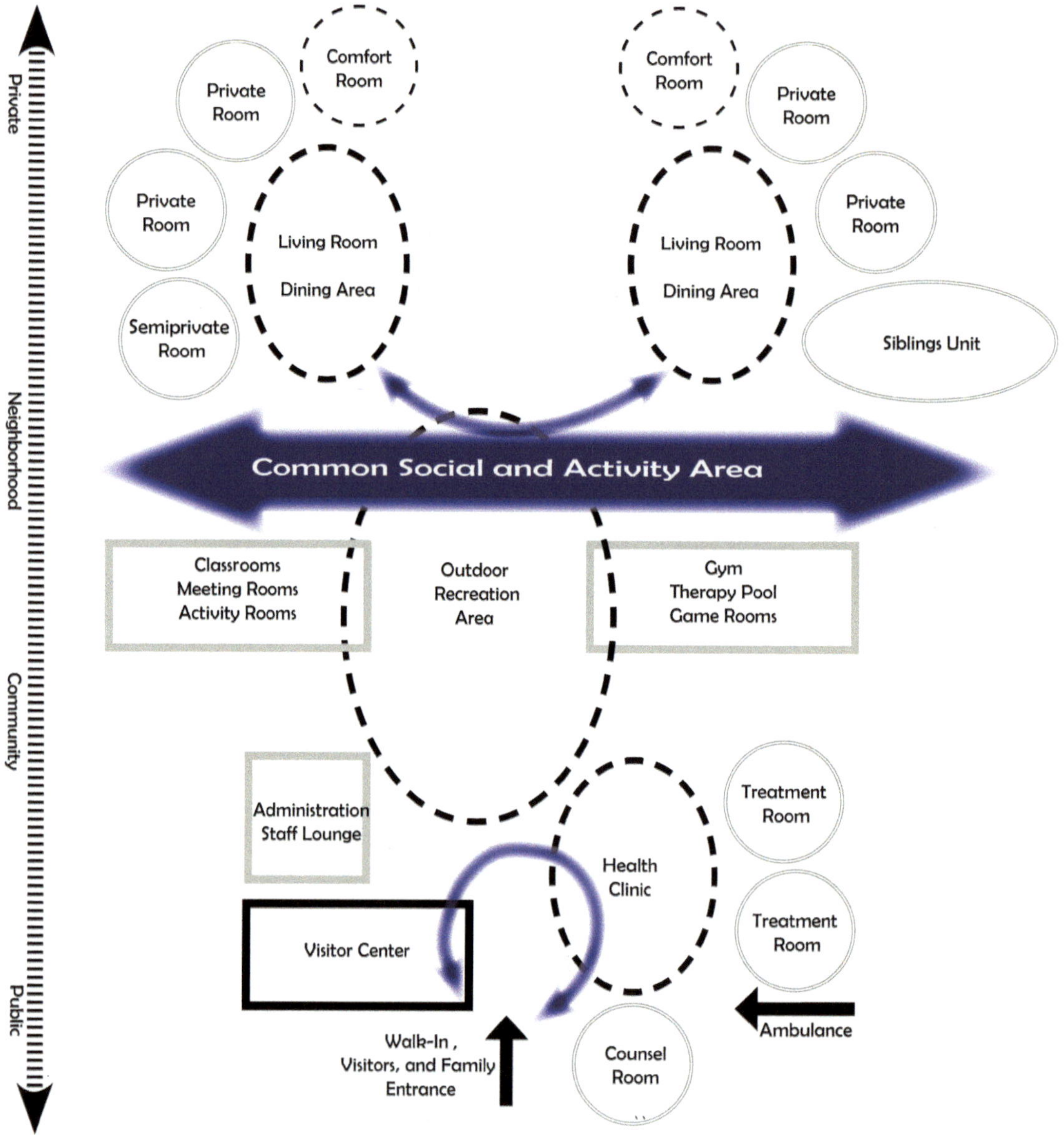

Figure 7.11: *Adjacency diagram for a pediatric inpatient facility*

Lastly, privacy is a critical contributor to the development of personal autonomy (Csikszentmihalyi & Rochberg-Halton, 1981), a characteristic recommended by experts. Patients, particularly adolescents, are concerned that the private details of their lives are shared with strangers, and therefore, they may continually feel exposed (Bailey, 2002).

Bailey provides guidelines for the design of kitchens and bathrooms. Citing prior research, Bailey recommends a spatial configuration that allows patients to watch the preparation of food and provides round-the-clock accessibility to snacks. The bathroom should "be a place of safety and privacy for the child to come to terms with his or her body, find acceptance for its care and function, and learn to live more comfortably in it" (Bailey, 2002, p. 23).

Access to outdoor recreational activities is needed for appropriate physical, psychological, and cognitive development. This is particularly true for adolescents who may not have had the chance to engage in developmentally appropriate play as younger children. Erikson (1963) hypothesized that difficult childhood issues might be resolved through play. Outdoor play areas such as sandboxes and water features can be used as therapeutic tools. Rose (2004) notes that adolescents, due to their energy level and educational needs, require very sturdy furniture and the support of additional educational and social activities.

7.4.2 Pediatric outpatient environments

Research on pediatric outpatient design is summarized in Chapters 3 and 9. Regarding outpatient design goals, Garland et al. (2013) pointed out the alarming levels of fragmentation and ineffectiveness of community-based outpatient mental health clinics in the treatment of children. They highlight the urgent need for the improvement of community-based and specialty outpatient mental health settings for children and families through delivery of evidence-based practices, access and engagement with services, and outcome accountability.

In reviewing the websites of several behavioral outpatient centers for children and adolescents (e.g., *New Behavioral Healthcare Center for Children, Youth & Families on Lake Burien*, n.d.), we found that the typical outpatient psychiatric facility design includes the following components:

- primary medical care clinic for preventive and regular medical care;
- treatment spaces for individual, group, and family psychotherapy;
- drug and alcohol assessment and treatment spaces; and
- spaces for behavioral support of youth with developmental disabilities.

A discussion of general outpatient facilities is provided in Chapter 3.

7.4.3 Pediatric emergency department environments

Pediatric emergency room design research is summarized in Chapters 4 and 9. Regarding design goals, recommendations cover all scales (from community planning to furnishings) of the design.

The issues begin at the community level where more facilities are required. Cooper and Masi (2007) point to the negative consequences of limited access to community-based mental health services, which could be associated with increased emergency use rates for mental health-related ED visits by children and youth. Well-trained pediatric emergency department providers are more likely to be successful in the identification and reporting of child abuse and the treatment of pediatric patients with intensive needs (Cooper & Masi, 2007).

Another design issue is related to the accommodation of families. Cooper and Masi (2007) note the movement toward family engagement in emergency healthcare visits. The evidence regarding family-centered practices in emergency departments is still growing, and the results are mixed in practices that advocate inclusion of family members in emergency healthcare (Cooper & Masi, 2007). It appears, however, that families need to be accommodated in the waiting and treatment room spaces. Accommodations for siblings are also recommended (Cooper & Masi, 2007).

Grover and Lee (2013) recommend the use of Lean Six Sigma to guide room design, equipment placement, and patient movement. Elements promoted in their research included camera-monitored patient rooms with recessed lighting, hospital beds with removable chairs, door hinges that allow doors to swing both ways, televisions protected by shatterproof glass, mobile equipment to avoid ligature, sinks and patient bathrooms with an automatic flush, and an alert button rather than a cord.

Security is critical in pediatric emergency departments, as with adult facilities, to ensure children's safety and protection (Vickery, 2011). Secured and visually open vestibules, clear and easy wayfinding between check-in, triage, and treatment rooms, and well-situated signage and registration desks are all important factors in children's security (Vickery, 2011). Treatment rooms are required to accommodate patients, caregivers, and family members/guardians (Vickery, 2011).

7.5 Case studies

7.5.1 *Mary Graham Children's Shelter*

Location:	French Camp, CA
Designer/Architect:	The Design Partnership
Client:	San Joaquin Co. Capital Projects
Completion:	August 2003
Area:	33,000 square feet

Client, service users, and services

The Mary Graham Children's Foundation is a private nonprofit 501(c)(3) organization founded in 2001 that supports local youth who have been subject to neglect, abuse, or abandonment. The Mary Graham Children's Center provides temporary shelter for children. The facility has the capacity for housing up to 60 children. After an average length of stay of two to three weeks, children are placed in foster homes, satellite homes, or treatment programs. The Mary Graham Children's Foundation also raised funds to establish an advocacy center located in the shelter complex. The advocacy center, as a vital part of the shelter program, provides medical and dental care and sexual abuse evaluations. Mary Graham Children's Shelter is operated under the direction of the San Joaquin County Human Services Agency.

Mission and goals

The Mary Graham Children's Center supports children who need temporary shelter in a comfortable and protective environment. The mission, according to the foundation website, is to "provide support that rebuilds hope and strengthens our youth's skills and education to successfully move from the foster care system to life on their own." The foundation raises funds to supplement county funds for the education and enrichment programs, trade school and college scholarship opportunities, as well as equipment and capital improvements that directly benefit the children at the shelter. Acknowledging the void in the continuum of care for foster children, especially when they reach adulthood, the foundation also contributes to subsidized housing, special needs stipends, tutoring services, and a mentoring program.

Site

The campus is located in French Camp, California, in a Central Valley farming community. French Camp is the oldest settlement in San Joaquin County. The historical precedents of nearby buildings through scale, planning, and materials were influential in site planning and design of the facility. The eight-acre campus complex replaced an old county facility. Nine buildings encompass a commons lawn offering a range of outdoor activities for children of different ages.

Program

The center hosts a variety of functions, including accommodation and educational, administrative, and clinical roles. The reception and intake building is part of the administrative program through which children are welcomed and assessed. This building includes interview and therapy rooms and staff offices. Several of the children who arrive at this building do not use the center's accommodations as they are immediately placed in foster or group homes in the community. The Child Advocacy Center is located in a smaller building that hosts clinical functions of the program. Forensic interviews take place in this building. The separation of this function from the residential, administrative, and educational sections of the program was intentional to ensure confidentiality as well as reducing the effects of negative association.

Parental visits, under supervision, take place in the visitor center. Children who have left the shelter may still come back to this building for their planned visitations with their parents. Similar to the clinical program, this part of the program was intentionally separated from the rest for confidentiality and children's safety. Two duplex cottages and four living units of 12 beds make up a total of 60 beds. Each cottage includes living and dining space and a full kitchen. To accommodate population fluctuations, six swing beds are designated between each pair of living units.

Educational programs provided to children during their stay are coordinated with the Office of Education. The education program is placed in three separate structures on the site and includes four classrooms, a library, a teacher's center, and a multipurpose building. A separate building is used as a storage and arts building.

Configuration and construction

The shelter adheres to the model of a boarding school campus, where the program is fitted in a number of smaller structures, which encloses an outdoor activity area, thereby taking advantage of the mild climate. The placement of functions in separate buildings responds to confidentiality and safety considerations, and addresses different design needs in each of the program functions. The facility was constructed to withstand excessive abuse. Through experimentation and cost research, the designers determined that two layers of 5/8" gypsum wallboard were equally effective and less costly than one layer of gypsum wallboard with one layer of plywood backing. Accordingly, this material was used to build most of the interior walls. The facility has been designed to exceed Title 24 Energy Efficiency standards. Indigenous plant species have been used for landscaping to reduce irrigation needs.

Case study bibliography

Mary Graham organization website at http://marygrahamfoundation.org/
The Design Partnership. (2015). Project information and other in-house publication materials.

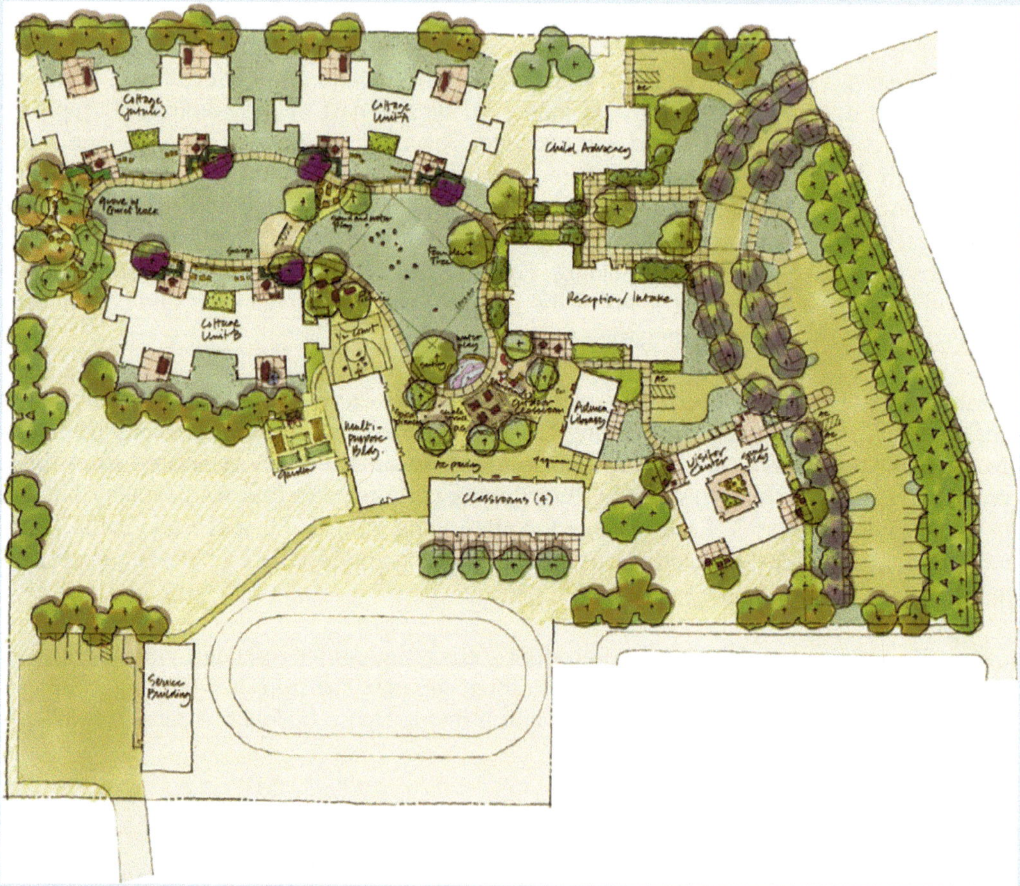

Figure 7.12: *Mary Graham – landscape site plan (Architects: The Design Partnership; Photo credit: Frank Domin)*

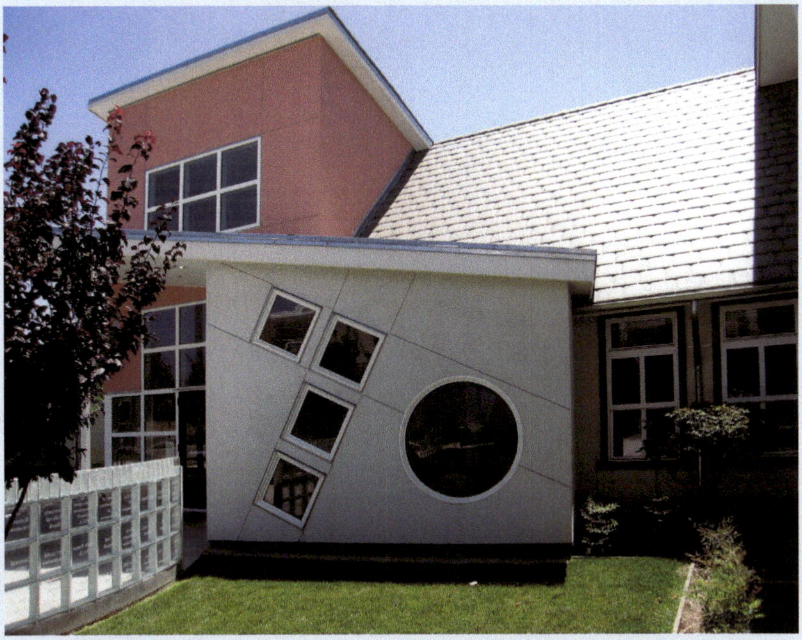

Figure 7.13: *Mary Graham – reception-intake entry detail (Architects: The Design Partnership; Photo credit: Frank Domin)*

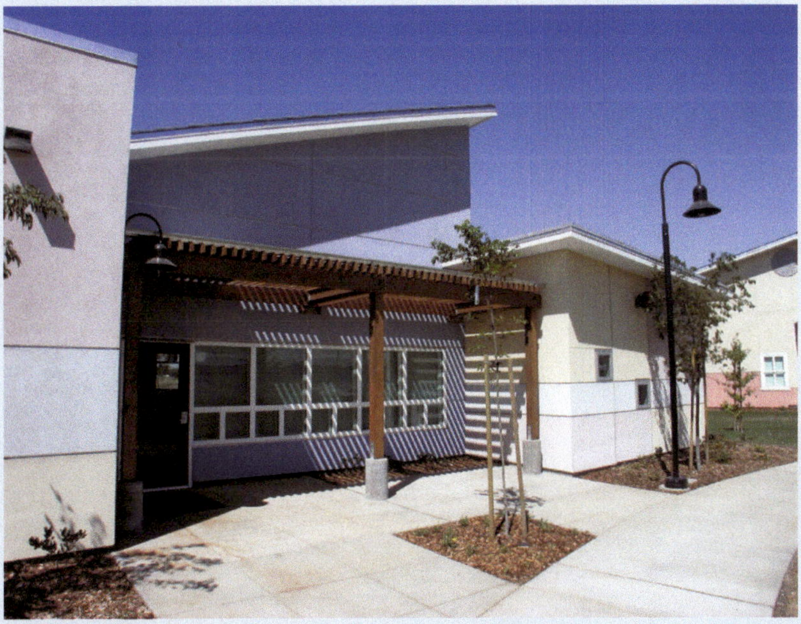

Figure 7.14: *Mary Graham – residential unit entry (Architects: The Design Partnership; Photo credit: Frank Domin)*

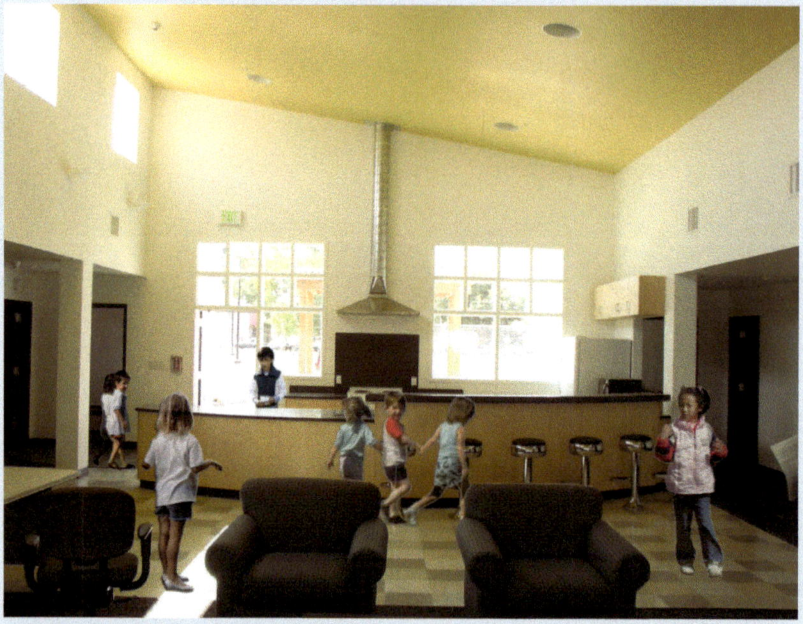

Figure 7.15: *Mary Graham – residential unit with children (Architects: The Design Partnership; Photo credit: Frank Domin)*

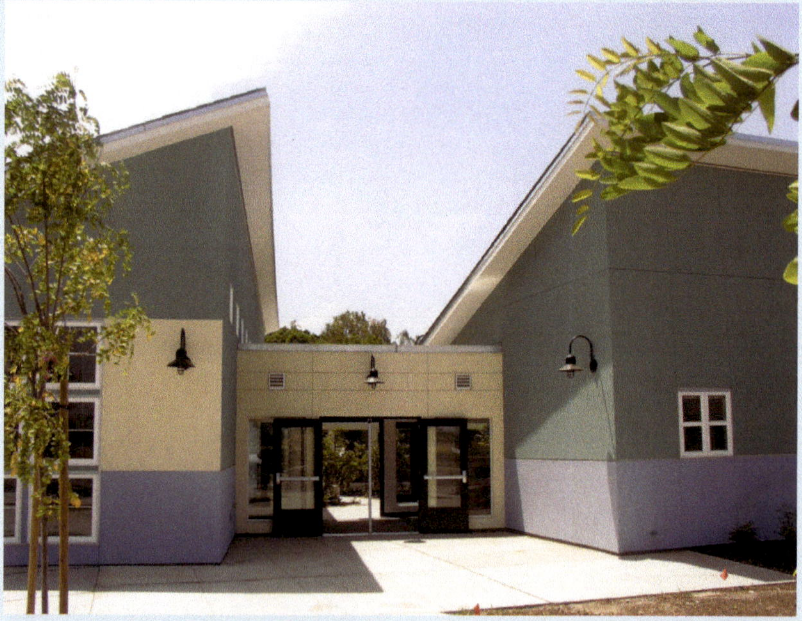

Figure 7.16: *Mary Graham – visitor center entry (Architects: The Design Partnership; Photo credit: Frank Domin)*

7.5.2 Placer County Children's Emergency Shelter

Location:	Auburn, CA
Designer/Architect:	The Design Partnership and the HLA Group
Client:	Placer County Facility Services
Completion:	2007
Area:	20,000 square feet

Client, service users, and services

Placer County Children's Shelter provides short-term housing for children aged 6 to 18 who have been removed from their families. Having experienced domestic problems or mental health issues, these children usually suffer from low self-esteem. Children typically use the shelter as a safe, temporary home until they can be returned to their families or until another permanent solution has become available.

Mission and goals

The main goal of this project is to provide a healing and homelike environment for children in crisis. Teaching the children how to prepare simple meals or complete their own daily tasks is a mission of the shelter to help children feel confident and independent. Cultivating a sense of family and strengthening the children's ability to reconnect to the larger community is another goal that the shelter aims to achieve.

Site

The shelter is located in a rural area adjacent to the new County Center in Auburn, California. Located in the Sierra foothills, the seasonal climate can range from hot dry summers to snow in the winter. The site originally housed a water treatment facility and a retention pond. Over a 30-year period leading up to the shelter project, the pond was reclaimed as a natural fresh water pond with several large native oak trees. The pond and trees were preserved during construction of the shelter and accommodated by the design plan. A new bridge over the pond was constructed to provide access to the shelter from the main road.

Program

The shelter has the capacity to house up to 30 children. Five separate units host teen boys, teen girls, preteens, siblings who want to stay together, and children who exhibit behavioral issues. Each unit includes two to four double occupancy rooms, two shared bathrooms, a living room, and a storage space. All of these units open into the main living room, which is open, spacious, and provides daylight and nature views through a floor-to-ceiling window wall. The admitting unit, dining room, and kitchen also have direct access to the main living room. The admitting unit is composed of a lobby, office, break room, storage space, and toilets and lockers for children. The administration and clinical cottage is connected to these units through a trellis and includes the entrance lobby, staff offices, an interview room, an observation room, an examination room, and a visiting room. In addition to living and clinical spaces, several outdoor and indoor recreational spaces and a 5,000-square-foot school building are the other components of this program.

Configuration and construction

The buildings were planned in a way that *preserved* existing nature amenities. A simple campus plan was adopted for the program, which incorporated design elements of the local rural setting. Four separate buildings on this campus include the main shelter building, a school, a gymnasium, and an administration/staff building. These buildings are intended to be identified as "home," "school," and "play" by children. The support buildings are arranged to surround the central main shelter, creating a sense of privacy and protection. The administrative building serves as the front door, while the school and gymnasium are located closer to the children's living area for easier daily access.

Case study bibliography

The Design Partnership. (2015). Project information and other in-house publication materials.

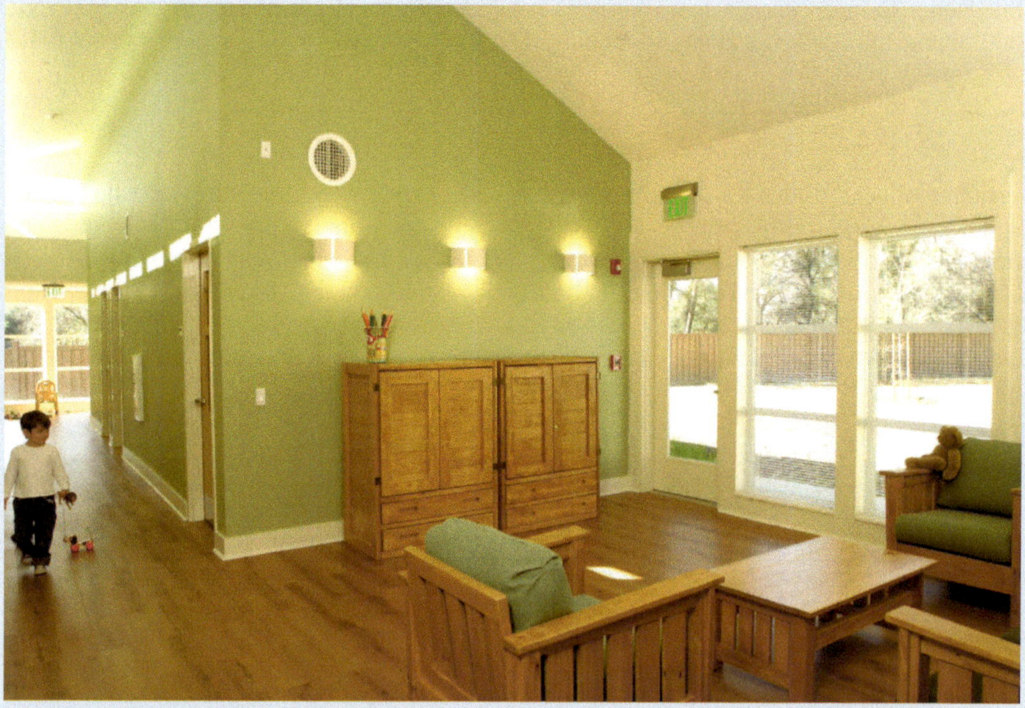

Figure 7.17: *Placer County Children's Emergency Shelter – unit living room (Architects: The Design Partnership; Photo credit: Bernard Andre)*

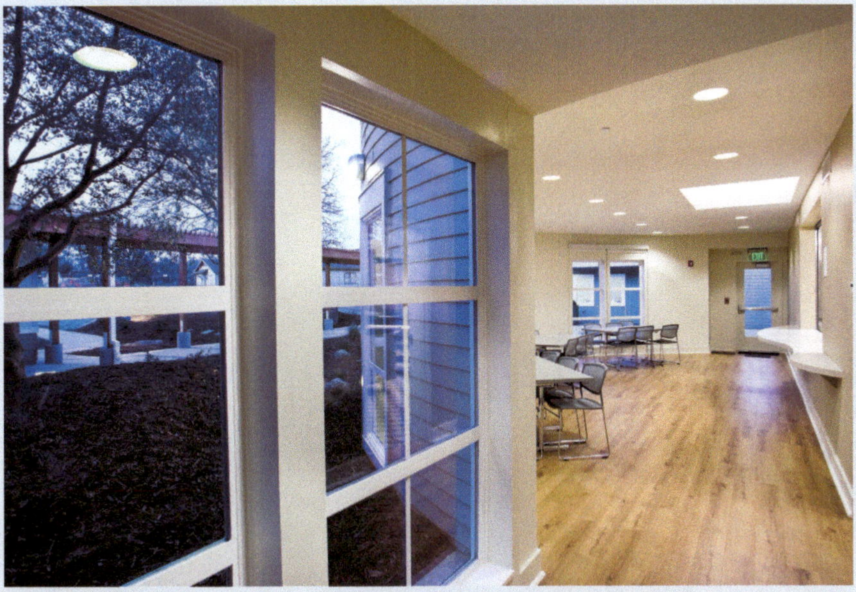

Figure 7.18: *Placer County Children's Emergency Shelter – dining room interior (Architects: The Design Partnership; Photo credit: Bernard Andre)*

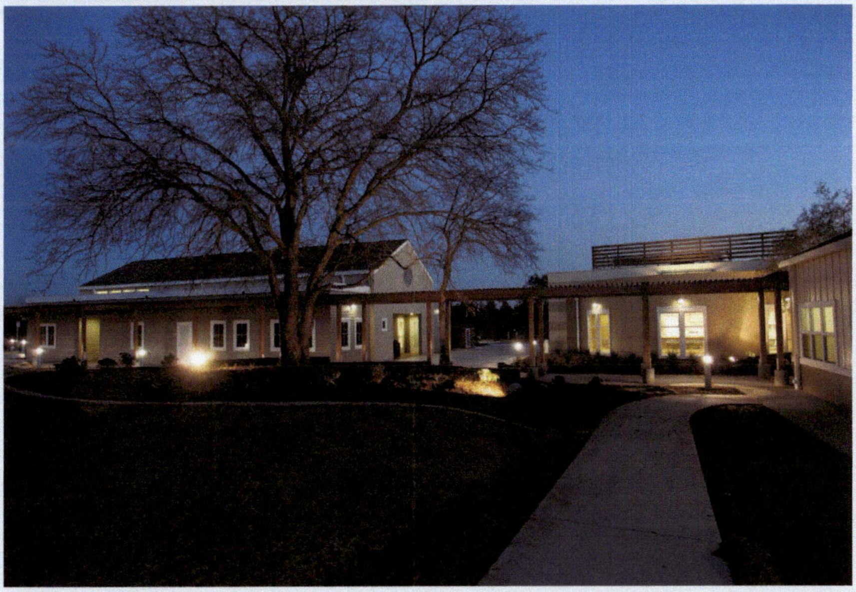

Figure 7.19: *Placer County Children's Emergency Shelter – evening administration trellis, administration (Architects: The Design Partnership; Photo credit: Bernard Andre)*

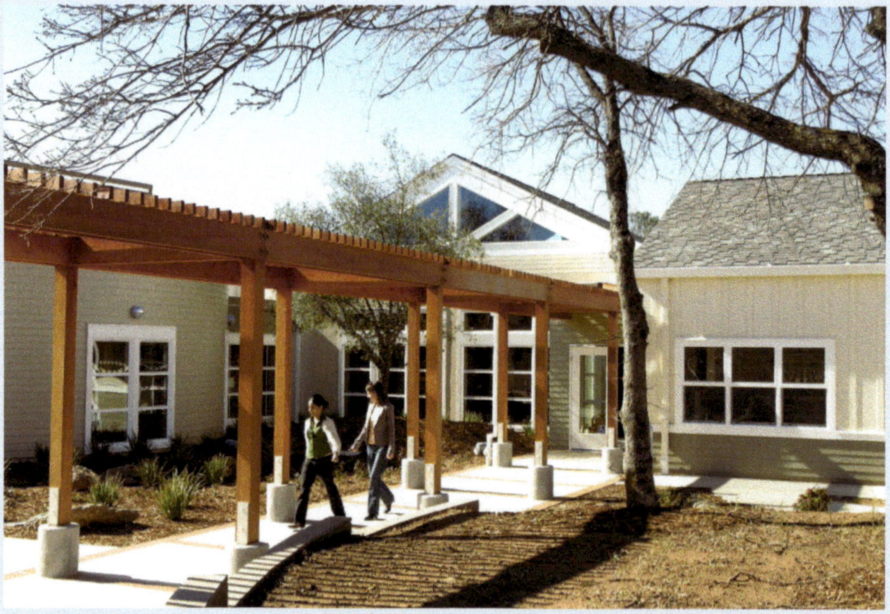

Figure 7.20: *Placer County Children's Emergency Shelter – trellis, main living room, admitting unit (Architects: The Design Partnership; Photo credit: Bernard Andre)*

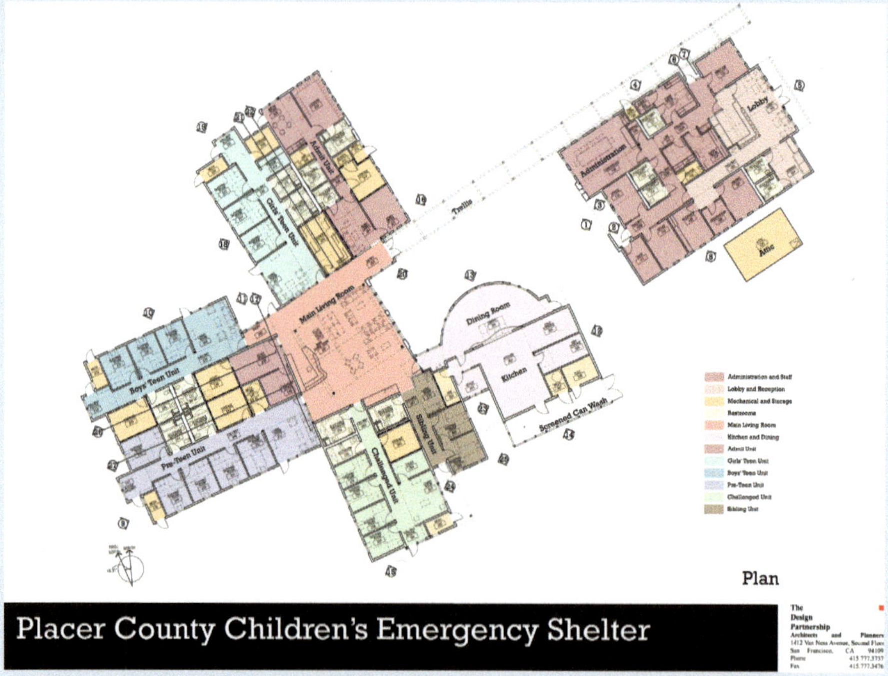

Figure 7.21: *Placer County Children's Emergency Shelter – floor plan (Architects: The Design Partnership; Photo credit: Bernard Andre)*

References

American Academy of Pediatrics. (2009). Improving mental health services in primary care: Reducing administrative and financial barriers to access and collaboration. *Pediatrics, 123*(4), 1248–1251.

Bailey, K. A. (2002). The role of the physical environment for children in residential care. *Residential Treatment for Children & Youth, 20*(1), 15–27.

Bartlett, S. N. (1997). Housing as a factor in the socialization of children: A critical review of the literature. *Merrill-Palmer Quarterly, 43*, 169–198.

Carlisle, C. E., Mamdani, M., Schachar, R., & To, T. (2012). Aftercare, emergency department visits, and readmission in adolescents. *Journal of the American Academy of Child & Adolescent Psychiatry, 51*(3), 283–293.

Case, R. (1991). Stages in the development of the young child's first sense of self. *Developmental Review, 11*(3), 210–230.

Case, S. D., Case, B. G., Olfson, M., Linakis, J. G., & Laska, E. M. (2011). Length of stay of pediatric mental health emergency department visits in the United States. *Journal of the American Academy of Child & Adolescent Psychiatry, 50*(11), 1110–1119.

Cooper, J. L., & Masi, R. (2007). *Child and youth emergency mental health care: A national problem*. New York: National Center for Children in Poverty, Columbia University.

Cotton, N. S., & Geraty, R. G. (1984). Therapeutic space design: Planning an inpatient children's unit. *American Journal of Orthopsychiatry, 54*(4), 624–636.

Csikszentmihalyi, M., & Rochberg-Halton, E. (1981). *The meaning of things: Domestic symbols and the self*. New York: Cambridge University Press.

De Andres-Trelles, F. (2015). Psychiatric diseases moving towards adolescents and children: How much room is there for extrapolation. *European Neuropsychopharmacology, 25*, 1039–1044.

Eisen, S. L., Ulrich, R. S., Shepley, M. M., Varni, J. W., & Sherman, S. (2008). The stress-reducing effects of art in pediatric health care: Art preferences of healthy children and hospitalized children. *Journal of Child Health Care, 12*(3), 173–190.

Erikson, E. (1963). *Childhood and society*. New York: Norton.

Evans, G. W. (2006). Child development and the physical environment. *Annual Review of Psychology, 57*, 423–451.

Evans, G. W., Lepore, S. J., & Schroeder, A. (1996). The role of interior design elements in human responses to crowding. *Journal of Personality and Social Psychology, 70*, 41–46.

Fairmont Behavioral Health System. (2013). *Child and adolescent inpatient services*. Retrieved from http://fairmontbhs.com/program-services/child-and-adolescent-inpatient.

Garland, A. F., Haine-Schlagel, R., Brookman-Frazee, L., Baker-Ericzen, M., Trask, E., & Fawley-King, K. (2013). Improving community-based mental health care for children: Translating knowledge into action. *Administration and Policy in Mental Health and Mental Health Services Research, 40*(1), 6–22.

Glod, C. A., Teicher, M. H., Butler, M., Savino, M., Harper, D., Magnus, E., & Pahlavan, K. (1994). Modifying quiet room design enhances calming of children and adolescents. *Journal of the American Academy of Child & Adolescent Psychiatry, 33*(4), 558–566.

Grover, P., & Lee, T. (2013). Dedicated pediatric behavioral health unit: serving the unique and individual needs of children in behavioral health crisis. *Pediatric Emergency Care, 29*(2), 200–202.

Handwerk, M., Clopton, K., Huefner, J., Smith, G., Hoff, K., & Lucas, C. (2006). Gender differences in adolescents in residential treatment. *American Journal of Orthopsychiatry, 76*(3), 312–324.

Hoagwood, K., Burns, B. J., Kiser, L., Ringeisen, H., & Schoenwald, S. K. (2001). Evidence-based practice in child and adolescent mental health services. *Psychiatric Services, 52*(9), 1179–1189.

Houston, J. M., & Martini, D. R. (2013). The delivery of mental health care: where are we and where are we going? *Journal of the American Academy of Child & Adolescent Psychiatry*, *52*(11), 1128–1130.

Huffcut, J. (2010). Can design promote healing? Evidence-based design can make a difference for adolescent patients. *Healthcare Design*, *10*(2), 33–35.

Hussey, D. L., & Guo, S. (2005, Fall). Forecasting length of stay in child residential treatment. *Child Psychiatry and Human Development*, *36*(1), 95–111.

Ireys, H., Achman, L., & Takyi, A. (2006). *State regulation of residential facilities for children with mental illness*. Rockville, MD: U.S. Department of Health & Human Services, Substance Abuse and Mental Health Services Administration.

Ishikawa, T., & Montello, D. R. (2006). Spatial knowledge acquisition from direct experience in the environment: Individual differences in the development of metric knowledge and the integration of separately learned places. *Cognitive Psychology*, *52*(2), 93–129.

Laufer, R. S., & Wolfe, M. (1977). Privacy as a concept and a social issue: A multidimensional developmental theory. *Journal of Social Issues*, *33*(3), 22–42.

Maxwell, L. E. (1996). Multiple effects of home and day care crowding. *Environment and Behavior*, *28*, 494–511.

Meagher, S.M., Rajan, A., Wyshak, G., & Goldstein, J. (2013). Changing trends in inpatient care for psychiatrically hospitalized youth: 1991–2008. *Psychiatric Quarterly*, *84*(2), 159–168.

Merikangas, K. R., He, J. P., Brody, D., Fisher, P. W., Bourdon, K., & Koretz, D. S. (2010a). Prevalence and treatment of mental disorders among US children in the 2001–2004 NHANES. *Pediatrics*, *125*(1), 75–81.

Merikangas, K. R., He, J. P., Burstein, M., Swanson, S., Avenevoli, S., Cui, L., Benjet, C., Georgiades, K., & Swendsen, J. (2010b). Lifetime prevalence of mental disorders in U.S. adolescents: Results from the National Comorbidity Survey Replication – Adolescent Supplement [NCS-A]. *Journal of the American Academy and Child Adolescence Psychiatry*, *49*, 980–989.

Meriter UnityPoint Health. (2015). *Child & adolescent psychiatry*. Retrieved from www.Meriter.com/services/psychiatry-program/child-adolescent-psychiatry

National Research Council and Institute of Medicine. (2009). *Preventing mental, emotional, and behavioral disorders among young people: Progress and possibilities*. Washington, DC: The National Academic Press.

New behavioral healthcare center for children, youth & families on Lake Burien. (n.d.). Retrieved from www.navos.org/behavioral-healthcare-center

Olfson, M., Blanco, C., Wang, S., Laje, G., & Correll, C. U. (2014). National trends in the mental health care of children, adolescents, and adults by office-based physicians. *JAMA Psychiatry*, *71*(1), 81–90.

Pear, R. (2003). *Mental care poor for some children in state custody*. Retrieved from www.nytimes.com/2003/09/01/us/mental-care-poor-for-some-children-in-state-custody.html.

Piaget, J. (1952). *The origins of intelligence in children*. New York: International Universities Press.

Potthoff, J. (1991). Young adult male satisfaction with drug and alcohol rehabilitation facilities: Interior design implications. *Journal of Alcohol and Drug Education*, *37*(1), 38–45.

Potthoff, J. (1995). Adolescent satisfaction with drug/alcohol treatment facilities: Design implications. *Journal of Alcohol and Drug Education*, *41*, 62–73.

Read, M. A., & Upington, D. (2009). Young children's color preferences in the interior environment. *Early Childhood Education Journal*, *36*(6), 491–496.

Rose, J. (2004). The residential care and treatment of adolescents. In P. Caming (Ed.), *From toxic institutions to therapeutic environments: Residential settings in mental health services* (pp. 219–132). London, UK: The Royal Society of Psychiatrists.

Seattle Children's Hospital. (2014). *Seattle children's hospital unveils new inpatient psychiatry unit*. Retrieved from: www.seattlechildrens.org/press-releases/2014/seattle-children-s-hospital-unveils-new-inpatient-psychiatry-unit/

Shepley, M. (1995). The location of behavioral incidents in a children's psychiatric facility. *Children's Environments, 12*(3), 352–361.

Soni, A. (2009). *The five most costly children's conditions, 2006: Estimates for the U.S. civilian noninstitutionalized children, ages 0–17*. Rockville, MD: Agency for Healthcare Research and Quality.

Stortz, M. (2003). *A tale of two settings: Institutional and community-based mental health services in California since realignment in 1991*. Retrieved from www.disabilityrightsca.org/pubs/540301.htm#_Toc103486125

Tapak, D. M. (2012). *"Don't speak about us without us:" Design considerations and recommendations for inpatient mental health environments for children and adolescents*. (Unpublished master's thesis). Winnipeg, Canada: University of Manitoba.

Torio, C. M., Encinosa, W., Berdahl, T., McCormick, M. C., & Simpson, L. A. (2015). Annual report on health care for children and youth in the United States: national estimates of cost, utilization and expenditures for children with mental health conditions. *Academic pediatrics, 15*(1), 19–35.

University of Minnesota Amplatz Children's Hospital. (2013). *Creating a safe haven for behavioral healthcare*. Retrieved from www.healthcaredesignmagazine.com/article/creating-safe-haven-behavioral-healthcare

Vickery, C. (2011). *Design choices in pediatric emergency departments*. Retrieved from www.healthcaredesignmagazine.com/blogs/cgvickery/design-choices-pediatric-emergency-departments

Wells, K., & Whittington, D. (1993). Characteristics of youths referred to residential treatment: Implications for program design. *Children and Youth Services Review, 15*(3), 195–217.

Wells, N. M., & Evans, G. W. (2003). Nearby nature: A buffer of life stress among rural children. *Environment and Behavior, 35*(3), 311–330.

Wilson, M. R., Soth, N., & Robak, R. (1992). Managing disturbed behavior by architectural changes: making spaces fit the program. *Residential Treatment for Children & Youth, 10*(2), 63–74.

Witkin, M. J. (1974). *Residential psychiatric facilities for children and adolescents*. Rockville, MD: Alcohol, Drug Abuse and Mental Health Administration.

Mental and behavioral health community residential settings

8

8.1 Introduction

8.1.1 History of residential facilities in the United States

On October 31, 1963, the Community Mental Health Act was signed into law that provided grants to states for establishment of community mental health centers that moved people with mental illnesses back into communities (Public Law 88–164). Implementation of this act was made feasible with new psychotropic medications and psychotherapy approaches, and was motivated by former psychiatric patients who shared their experiences of hospitalization (Caplan, 1969). The initial plan for community care was developed by the National Institute of Mental Health and consisted of case managers who would manage all of the services needed for people with severe and persistent mental disorders, thus allowing them to continue living in the community (Turner & TenHoor, 1978). By that time a growing body of evidence had shown success and cost-effectiveness of care in community settings compared to traditional psychiatric hospitals. Since then, the organizations providing community care services have evolved to provide more diverse and comprehensive services (National Council for Behavioral Health, 2015).

Doyle, Lanoil, and Dudek (2013) report that in 1948, prior to the inception of the concept of community mental health centers and community residential facilities, patients discharged from a New York psychiatric hospital gathered to discuss alternate programs to treat persons with behavioral health challenges. Their goal was to start an alternative support system they referred to as a clubhouse. Since then, many clubhouses have formed around the world, many of them named Fountain House after the original model in New York (Doyle et al., 2013). The initial concept that led to the creation of Fountain House was that engaging in work on a routine daily schedule can bring normalcy into the lives of persons with mental illnesses, which could help remove the stigma associated with mental illnesses (Doyle et al., 2013). For such a concept to be realized, members joining a clubhouse are recognized as persons capable of making contributions rather than patients in need of repair. In this capacity, members join forces with staff to help deliver the social services they will also use (Doyle et al., 2013, pp. 60–61). While Fountain House is not typically a residential setting, the model can be applied to residential care.

During this time frame, especially in France and the United Kingdom, many functions of care, other than acute care, were transferred from the hospital to the community. These community services spanned aftercare, accommodations, rehabilitation, and occupational therapy (Chrysikou, 2014).

The social awareness and medical advances that originated the concept of community care centers in the United States were also the driving forces behind normalization theory (Chrysikou, 2014).

This theory is the underlying care concept for promoting the use of domestic settings that allow mental and behavioral health patients to live and engage with the community. A primary goal is supporting patterns of everyday life and regular circumstances of living for all people with disabilities. Regular circumstances include housing, schooling, employment, exercise, recreation, and freedom of choice while following the regular rhythm of life (Nirje, 1982). Because normalization is sometimes erroneously associated with imposing a "normal life" on people with disabilities, in 1983, Wolfensberger formulated the term social role valorization (SRV) (Wolfensberger & Thomas, 1983). In its latest definition, SRV calls for the application of empirical knowledge to enhance a person's or group's competencies and image (Wolfensberger & Thomas, 2005).

Development of community-based mental health centers in the 1960s in the United States was initiated by the deinstitutionalization movement and has evolved since its initial inception (Stroman, 2003). However, many early recommendations, such as financial aid to families, foster care services, leisure and recreation, and employment opportunities, still hold (Bank-Mikkelsen, 1969; Smith & Brown, 1992). Chrysikou (2014) notes that, although the new community care model was opposed to institutional practices, these practices continue to be present in community care settings.

The Community Mental Health Act has had mixed success in the United States. Since enactment of the law, a high percentage of beds for psychiatric patients have been cut at state hospitals (Smith, 2013), resulting in a population drop from over 500,000 to less than 150,000 in large public mental hospitals (Dixon & Goldman, 2003). However, many communities did not have sufficient facilities to replace the reduction in beds (Koran & Meinhardt, 1981). This led to an increase in the number of homeless persons with mental illnesses (Hynes, 1987).

To offset shortcomings of the community care model, the concept of balanced care has been investigated by the World Health Organization (WHO). *Balanced care* consists of community-based services that are incorporated within local settings (HEN, 2003). Balanced care aims to provide individualized treatments that address both disabilities and symptoms, and it incorporates a combination of modern hospitals for acute cases, long-term residential facilities, as well as mobile services that can reach out to patients at home or in rural areas (HEN, 2003).

8.1.2 Data regarding residential facility population

Community involvement is the main driver in shaping the concept of community residential facilities. The community can be both the immediate community or group or the broader community in which the facility is nested. Residents are responsible for performing daily chores and helping to clean and cook (Fitzpatrick, 2007). Residents who are more independent may acquire jobs and create stronger bonds with the community (Fitzpatrick, 2007). The general idea is to help residents reach their potential in independent living. Community residential facilities should empower patients in all areas of their life, including housing, accountability, medication, and employment. However, many patients who enter the residential care setting after being discharged from the hospital have not learned to cope with their illness; homelessness and readmission to hospitals creates a vicious cycle that entangles many of the patients who leave the community residential setting prematurely (Burt, 2006).

A study by Forchuk, Ward-Griffin, Csiernik, and Turner (2006) of 90 individuals with mental health disabilities in both urban and rural regions of Ontario noted three steps toward achieving stability in the lives of persons with serious mental health diagnoses.

1. Losing ground: Limited control over housing conditions
2. Struggling: Trying to survive with the support of community services
3. Stability: Securing personal space through rebuilding relationships

Perkins, Born, Raines, and Galka (2005), among others, have emphasized the importance of a supported housing approach to prevent homelessness for people living with mental disabilities.

8.2 Characteristics of residential facilities

8.2.1 Types of programs and settings

According to the National Alliance on Mental Illness (NAMI, 2016), the three types of housing available to people with mental disabilities can be broken down into the following categories, which loosely show the transition from a custodial model toward a supportive housing model:

- Supervised group housing: Trained staff would be present in-house to assist for medication, treatment management, daily living tasks, meals, and transportation.
- Partially supervised group housing: Residents perform their daily tasks and may hold a part-time job and can call for help if needed.
- Supportive housing: The residents live almost independently; however, resources would be available to them if they need help.

Research shows that patients who preferred to live either alone or with a significant other or a friend, rather than with other mental health patients, need consistent access to staff who do not live in with them (e.g., Schutt, Goldfinger, & Penk, 1997). This model is more accessible through supported housing programs that enable more independent living arrangements for persons with mental health diagnoses (NAMI, 2016).

Supported housing is based on the concept that persons with mental disabilities "choose, get, and keep" the housing options. The U.S. Housing and Urban Development department has dedicated funds for establishing supported housing for very low- and extremely low-income adults with disabilities. Properties using these funds are known as Section 811 housing and must have subsidized rent to provide affordable housing (HUD, 2016a). Section 8 housing is a program for public housing tenants who have been forced to move because of rehabilitation or demolition of their public housing unit (HUD, 2016b). Supported housing may be based on rental or homeownership models:

- Rental housing: Residents are considered completely independent and may have a job or have custody of children. Rent can be paid by the resident or a third party such as the government or a nonprofit agency.

- Homeownership: Although homeowners may still get some assistance from various resources, they are highly independent in paying their bills, managing their treatment and medication, and involvement with the surrounding community.

Each housing approach may seem appropriate for different consumer populations; however, research shows that they may not have the same level of success and effectiveness. For example, Segal and Kotler (1993) found that custodial care could increase dependence and assisted social functioning. Patients who are recently discharged from hospitals and join a community residential program would still need help for managing day-to-day tasks before they can live independently. While this presence is needed and can be provided by either live-in or visiting staff, less restrictive regimes have been shown to be more successful (Dickey, 2000). Subsequently, recent literature reviews suggest that supportive care can be more effective compared to custodial care (e.g., Leff et al., 2009). These studies found the programs to be successful in providing choice and control, satisfaction, reduced hospitalization, and reduced substance use (Cheng, Lin, Kasprow, & Roosenheck, 2007).

Success and failure of community residential programs is also dependent on the community and its resources functioning as a system. For example, differences in rural settings versus urban settings and circumstances and resources of each community can create different outcomes. Bruce (2003) noted that limitations in smaller towns and rural areas, including small and low-quality housing markets, aging population, poverty, and lack of mental healthcare services, make implementation of community care services in rural areas less successful.

Improvements and changes are needed in most communities to make them supportive hosts for community mental health services. Such changes can be categorized as first-order versus second-order change (Watzlaic, Weakland, & Fish 1974) or ameliorative versus transformative change (Nelson & Prilleltensky, 2010). First-order (ameliorative) change focuses on improving existing infrastructure, while second-order (transformative) change emphasizes revisiting the system values and operations. With this background, Nelson (2010) identified custodial and supportive housing as types of first-order or ameliorative change, while supported care was considered a second-order or transformative change.

8.2.2 Number of facilities and participation rates

The primary impediment to gathering information about persons with mental illnesses is that national surveys do not sample populations such as homeless people, people residing in hospitals or residential care facilities, or people incarcerated in prisons or jails (SAMHSA, 2012). A percentage of these populations need services but are less likely to receive treatment that meets professionally recommended guidelines.

According to the WHO (2011) *Mental Health Atlas*, for every 100,000 persons in the United States, there are community residential facility beds available for 22 persons. These rates drop to 15 beds per 100,000 for children. A comparison of the number of beds in mental and general hospital psychiatric wards demonstrates that community mental health facilities treat approximately one-third of the population with mental illnesses (Figure 8.1). Community residential facilities include individuals residing in supervised settings, such as group homes, halfway houses, and residential institutions, and minors residing with parents, guardians, or in foster care. The majority of facilities that offer residential services are in the private sector. (See Figure 8.2.)

On average for each month in 2012, 4.2% of the U.S. population received housing benefits, almost 50% of which involved continued participation between 37 and 48 months. The U.S.

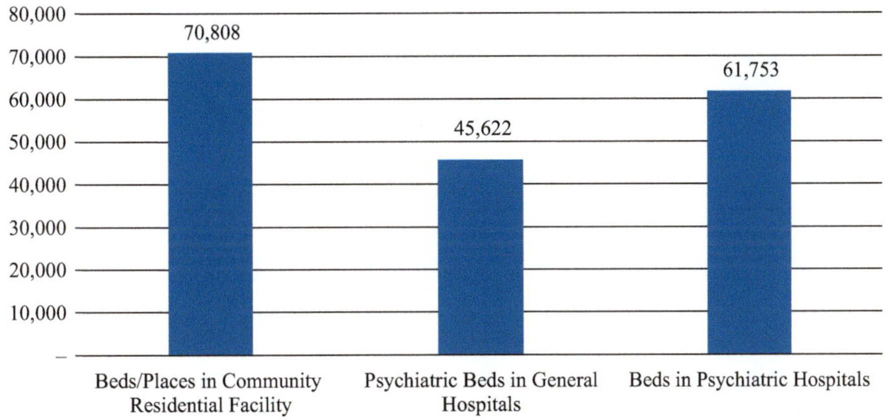

Figure 8.1: *Available beds for persons with psychiatric diagnosis in the United States (Source: WHO* Mental Health Atlas, *2011)*

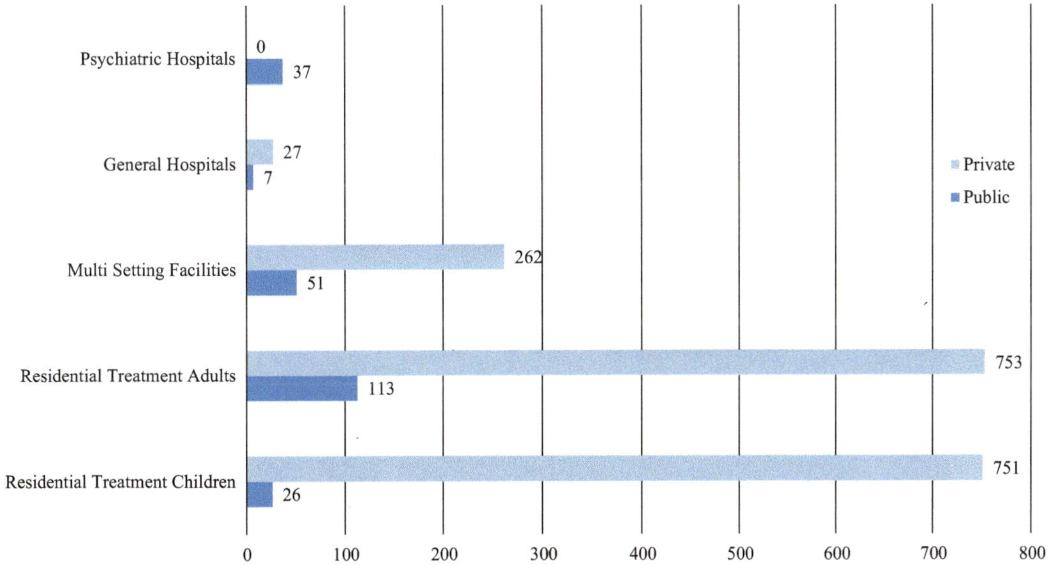

Figure 8.2: *Number of mental health facilities that provide residential services, United States, 2010 (SAMHSA, 2012)*

Northeast region has the highest participation rates, and the South and Midwest regions had the lowest participation rates (Figure 8.3).

Among U.S. homeless adults who stay in shelters, approximately 26% live with a serious mental illness, and an estimated 46% live with severe mental illness and/or substance use disorders (HUD, 2015). According to HUD (2015), over 50% of the homeless population in the United States were in five states: California (21%), New York (16%), Florida (6%), Texas (4%), and Massachusetts (4%). California, Oregon, Montana, and Hawaii had unsheltered homeless rates exceeding 50%. (See Figure 8.4.)

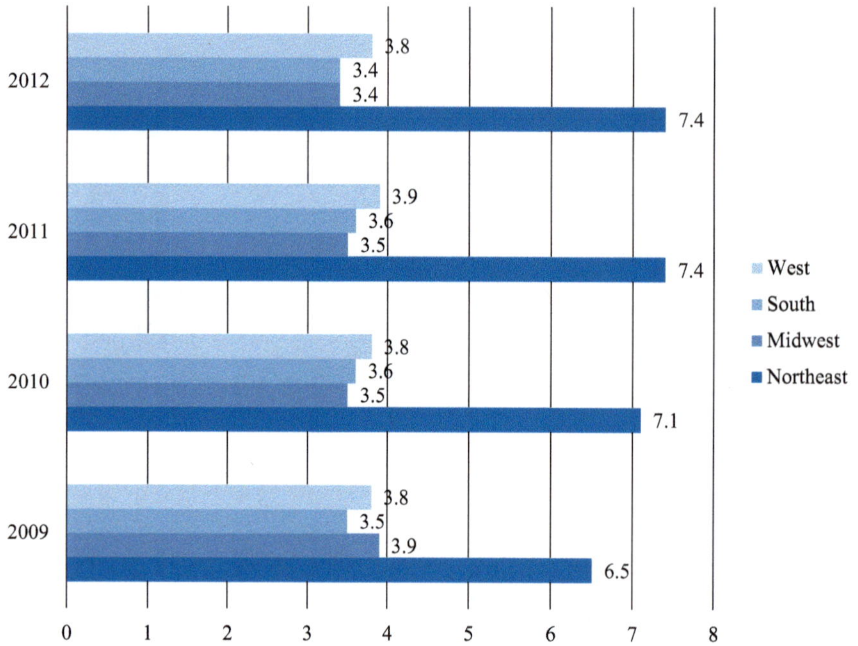

Figure 8.3: *Average monthly participation rates for housing assistance by region (by percentage), U.S. Census data (Irving & Loveless, 2015)*

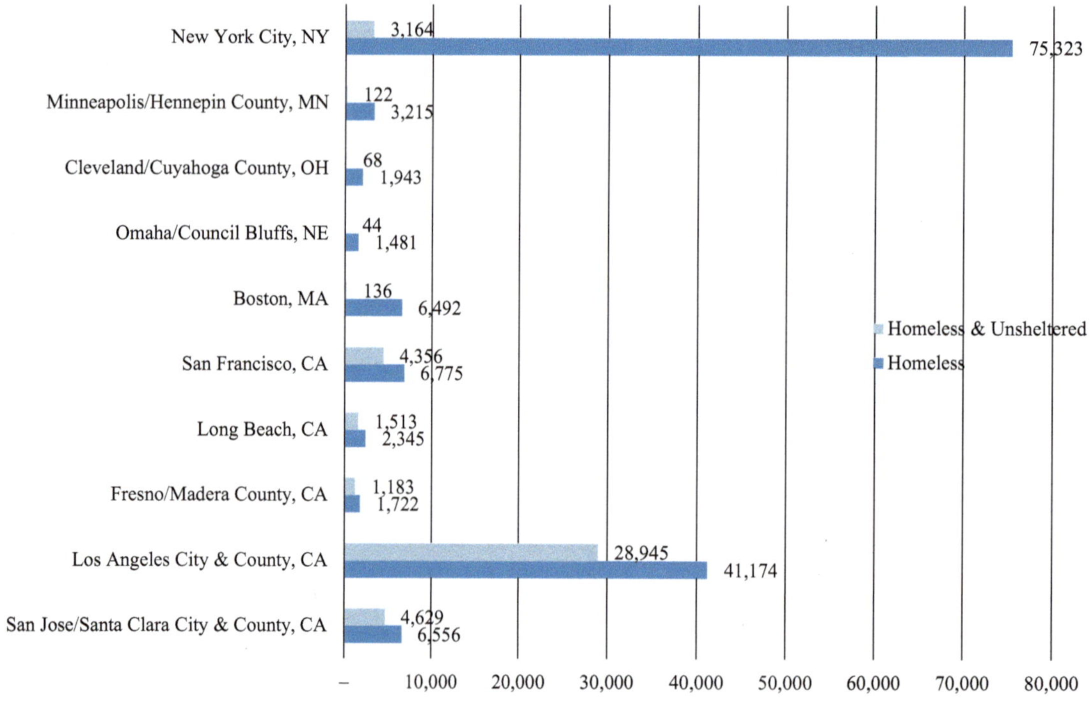

Figure 8.4: *Major U.S. cities with highest and lowest ratio of unsheltered homeless (HUD, 2015)*

Overall homelessness declined by 2% (or 11,742 people) between 2014 and 2015 and by 11% (or 82,550) since 2007; however, the high numbers are still concerning. According to HUD (2015), in January 2015, on average 564,708 people were homeless on a given night; one-quarter of them were children under the age of 18.

8.3 Mental and behavioral health design goals

Discussions about the need for flexibility and integration with the community started around the mid-1960s (e.g., Dorsett & Brown, 1965) and continues today. A 1998 article argues that an architect's attempt to build a relationship with the surrounding community can help with the success of the future community-based mental health facility. The article framed flexibility in design in terms of program requirements, technological infrastructure, treatment methods, and relationships with the health system (Inland Architect, 1998).

In their 1965 article, Dorsett and Brown listed desirable CMHC services as diagnostic services, rehabilitation, community-based pre-care and aftercare, training of professionals, and research and evaluation. It is noteworthy that at that time the concept of community mental health services was not fully implemented, and, as other researchers argue, the community mental health centers were planned and managed by a continuation of the institutionalization mindset that created psychiatric hospitals. Rather than a more "normalized" environment, these facilities were characterized by custodial care in low-quality buildings for an extended period of time.

More recent research shows that quality housing facilities in supportive communities can help patients recover by enhancing feelings of acceptance and reducing feelings of loneliness (Browne & Courtney, 2004) as well as perceiving a higher quality of life (Horan, Muller, Winocur, & Barling, 2001). Browne and Courtney (2004) noticed that lower-quality housing situations predicted higher hospital readmission rates.

PASS (Demaine, Silverstein, & Mayeda, 1980; Flynn & Heal, 1981; Wolfensberger & Glenn, 1975 and PASSING (Flynn, LaPointe, Wolfensberger, & Thomas, 1991) are two rating systems that evaluate services based on implementation of normalization goals. Demaine et al. (1980) tested the validity of PASS 3 and conducted a factor analysis of the tool using data from 98 residential facilities in Southern California dedicated to developmentally disabled persons. They identified six factors, including: (1) the application of normalization principles, (2) policies, (3) integration of services with the surrounding community, (4) administrative structure, (5) location and proximity of service, and finally, (6) comfort and appearance. The factors structure provides a concise explanation of variables that PASS 3 aims to evaluate. Of these factors, 5 and 6 are the only factors for which environmental design items have a strong presence. Factor 5 includes access, local proximity, physical resources, and regional proximity. Factor 6 includes environmental beauty, physical comfort, internal design and appointments, and "deviant staff juxtaposition."

More recently, Cardoso et al. (2016) reported the use of another standardized tool, the Quality Indicator for Rehabilitative Care (QuIRC). The QuIRC tests for reliability and validity (Killaspy et al., 2013) and consists of seven domains of care, including: (1) living environment, (2) therapeutic environment, (3) treatments and interventions, (4) self-management and autonomy, (5) recovery-based practice, (6) social inclusion, and (7) human rights. They found a correlation between better quality of care and service users' autonomy and their ratings of the therapeutic milieu consisting of recovery-based practices such as collaborative care planning and promotion of independent living skills.

8.3.1 Recommendations by designers

An international set of design recommendations are revealed via the case studies on four projects, one in Johannesburg, one in Ontario, one in New York, and one in London. A short description of a halfway house in Johannesburg appeared in a 1995 issue of *Architectural Review*. Slessor (1995) described the new block addition to what was previously an old hotel. This building was created as a halfway home, for individuals with psychiatric diagnoses mostly discharged from hospitals, that would provide psychosocial skills needed for living in society. Large windows that brought in daylight and allowed views of the outside was the major therapeutic design attribute discussed in the article.

Fitzpatrick (2007) proposes a supportive housing facility formed around a courtyard in urban Waterloo, Ontario. The urban location can provide both a sense of privacy as well as connectivity to the community. She proposes a public face for the building with amenities such as a café, library, pharmacy, and grocer that can be accessed by the public and residents. The receptionist located at the entrance lobby of the facility serves to monitor possible public infiltration into private patient spaces. The facility program, in addition to patient living units and staff spaces, includes indoor and outdoor dining areas, laundry, crafts installation space, various indoor and outdoor exercise spaces (aerobics, cardio, weights), rooftop garden, greenhouse, playground, occupational therapy kitchen, quiet lounge, activity lounge, computer lab, chapel, guest suite, and several meeting rooms and lobbies. The spaces are arranged into two wings, with group, individual, and family therapy spaces located in the public wing of the facility.

Regarding design goals, Fitzpatrick recommends:

- natural and incandescent lighting;
- landscaped areas;
- natural ventilation;
- natural, textured, light-colored, and sound absorbent finishes that create a sense of relaxation, security, stability, and openness;
- corridors that are wide enough to put patients at ease while passing by people;
- circular routes and secondary access to spaces to help put paranoid minds at ease; and
- screening in lobbies and lounges to aid residents in seeing people who are about to join them in the space.

Fountain House has a small residential program, the physical environment for which follows similar patterns to their clubhouse. The physical environment is organized to foster collegiality, voluntarism, and choice. The character of the space follows the "person in environment" approach that provides places designed to reduce feelings of exclusion (Doyle et al., 2013).

Curtis, Gesler, Priebe, and Francis (2009) conducted unstructured discussions with a group of administrative staff and psychiatrists in a custodial community care facility in London. The psychiatrists

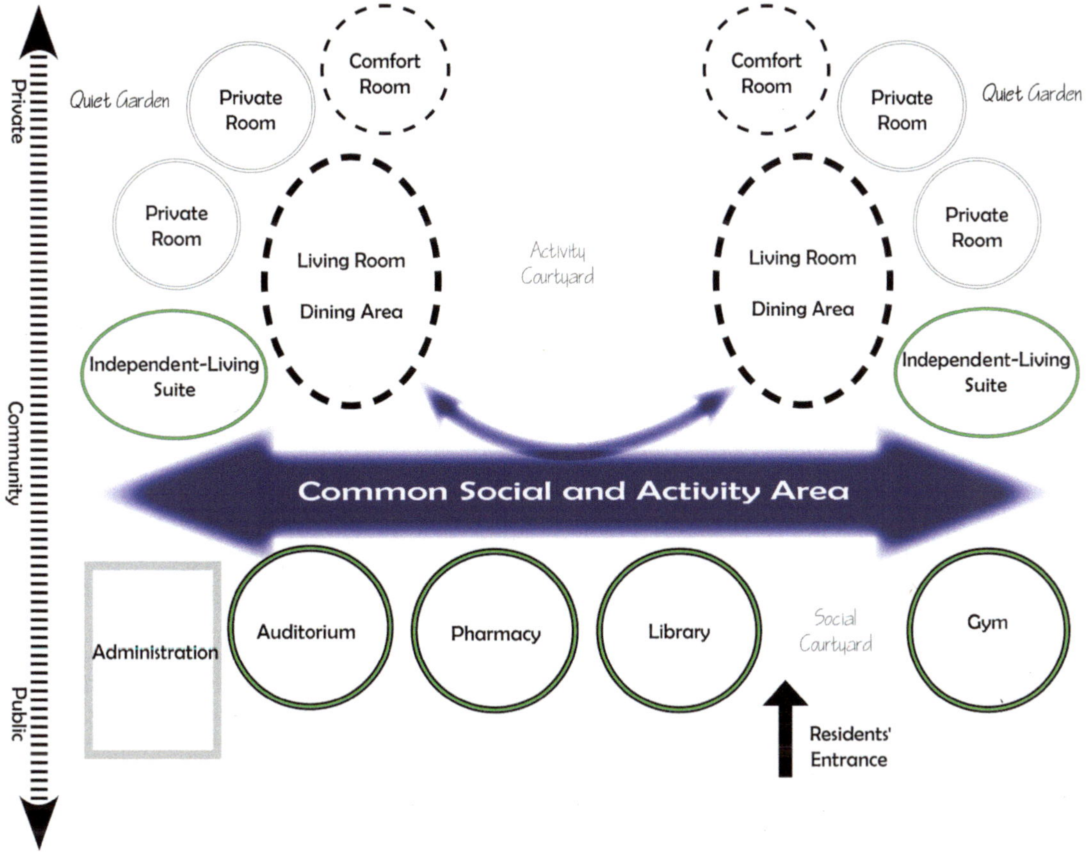

Figure 8.5: *Adjacency diagram for a community residential facility*

recruited seven people with psychiatric diagnoses who were in a healthy state during the course of study. The main focus of the study was to investigate specific features of the facility, including physical layout and activities, that were either beneficial or harmful to the well-being of the staff and patients. Due to the small and self-selective group of participants, the findings of the study might not be generalizable; however, they provide insight into some counterintuitive aspects of design and therapy, and are described in the next section.

Based on the concepts discussed in this chapter, Figure 8.5 provides a recommendation for a community residential facility.

8.3.2 *Psychological factors influencing the effectiveness of community facilities*

One of the psychological features raised in the literature on community residential facilities is the concept of attachment. In the Curtis study (2009), patients moved from an older facility to a new one with considerably better design and presence of therapeutic elements. However, these patients mentioned a sense of longing for the older place and the people they had come to know.

This finding was in alignment with prior research that demonstrates people who have spent a long time in mental care institutions are more likely to come back to visit the grounds, even if the institution were closed (Parr, Philo, & Burns, 2003). This attachment can be beneficial to residents in helping them develop a sense of community. However, it can also prevent residents from moving on to live as independent individuals in the society if they become too dependent on the social support they receive in the facility (Segal & Kotler, 1993).

The facility as a space of refuge, where patients can step outside of the building and engage in various activities while still on the facility's grounds and feel protected, was appealing to patients (Curtis et al., 2009). Managing a permeable interface for the facility where the community infiltrates into the facility and patients use surrounding community services as part of their care was discussed by Curtis. Greater permeability was desired; however, the need for refuge and staying away from stresses of the daily life was deemed essential.

The state of transition, which is the core focus of community care for people who need to be ready to engage with the community, also seemed confusing to the staff. It was challenging to make the environment more homelike and keep patients engaged while encouraging transition. A user discussed the experience as a sense of "abandonment." The limited aftercare the patient had received during the transition period compared to when he was a psychiatric inpatient made him skeptical about the advantages of a facility (Curtis et al., 2009).

The clinical care provided during the inpatient care, however, could be perceived in two different ways. As mentioned, a patient described it as more protective and felt abandoned after the care was changed in the transition period. However, it was suggested by others that the formal part of the care in the transition period felt like a clinical regimen and as a result had created a sense of disengagement and apathy toward the treatment. Curtis et al. (2009) suggested moving as much of the care regimen as possible to the informal spaces of the facility to soften the regimen-like aspects of the care.

8.4 Case studies

8.4.1 The Next Door

Location:	Nashville, TN
Designer/Architect:	ESa Architects
Completion:	2014
Area:	42,600 square feet

Awards: 2015 ULI Nashville Excellence in Development; Award of Excellence for the ABC (Associated Builders and Contractors) of Greater Tennessee

Client, service users, and services

The Next Door, an 82-bed residential facility, was built for The Next Door, Inc., a nonprofit organization, the mission of which is to support women in crisis and provide temporary residential and recovery support services for individuals transitioning from rehabilitation centers, domestic violence shelters, or correctional facilities.

The facility is described as providing a spectrum of care including:

- six-month reentry program with case management, work force development, counseling, and addiction relapse services;
- medical detoxification;
- residential treatment;
- outpatient treatment;
- aftercare to support prior clients of all programs with educational and community activities;
- recovery, life skills, and counseling programs for women currently residing at the Tennessee Prison for Women; and
- link to the adjacent Freedom Recovery Community, an independent housing complex for women and children.

Mission and goals

The mission of The Next Door is to "provide a continuum of evidence-based care for women and their families impacted by addiction, mental illness, trauma, and/or incarceration." A faith-based organization, The Next Door is open to all women. The organization requested a "human-centered design" that conveyed a sense of community and well-being. The exterior was intended to resemble an apartment to enhance contextualization with the local urban fabric; the facility provides views of the adjacent community. In keeping with the social mission, the design team provided their services pro bono, with subspecialties offering reduced rates.

Site

The site is adjacent to related facilities, including an independent housing complex (the Freedom Recovery Center) for individuals "graduating" from The Next Step. The Next Steps is, an integrated support and engagement program assisting individuals with self-management skills, while focusing on their self-identified area of concern. The Freedom facility is visually accessible to residents in The Next Step as an incentive for recovery. Located on a 1.05-acre site, nearby are the American Red Cross and the American Cancer Society, as well as commercial and residential land uses. This facility was designed to replace the previous 12,000-square-foot facility, which was razed to make room for a new hotel desired to support increased visitors to the Music City Convention Center. The new location allows for 100% expansion in adjacent areas as the program grows. Potential expansion might serve up to 250 women in medically monitored detox and residential beds, 175 individuals in outpatient services, and 175 in aftercare services.

Program

The program includes bedrooms, classrooms, a fitness room, laundry, and staff support. The chapel, clinic (supported in association with Vanderbilt School of Nursing), clothing boutique, computer lab, children's space, administrative offices, and dining and food services for 100+ persons are on the ground floor. The second floor accommodates six medically monitored detox beds and 36 residential treatment beds and provides a dedicated kitchenette, dining room, classrooms, and rehabilitation services. The third floor is dedicated to halfway house accommodations (40 beds) and related amenities. Bedrooms are semiprivate except in the "social detox" area on the second floor, which is an open plan with staff space at the core. Regarding access to nature, features include large windows to enhance natural light and a landscaped courtyard.

Configuration and construction

The L-shaped floor plan configuration is characterized by support services in the core (bathroom, laundry, etc.), and resident rooms, offices, dining rooms, and lounges around the perimeter. The "L" wraps a courtyard on the north side. Exterior materials include brick, Hardi-Plank siding, EIFS (exterior insulation finishing system), and curtain walls. The engineers and contractor were reported to have been engaged early in the design process in order to control and monitor construction costs. Sustainability features were considered, although the principles did not conform to a specific system.

Case study bibliography

Chandler, D. (2014). "Holistic, whole-person care" at The Next Door. *Worship Today, 1*(3)4–5.
ESa. (2015). Community experience and other in-house publication materials.
The Next Door. (Winter 2014). The Next Door Nashville's grand opening marks a successful milestone for women and the community. *The Next Door Newsletter*.

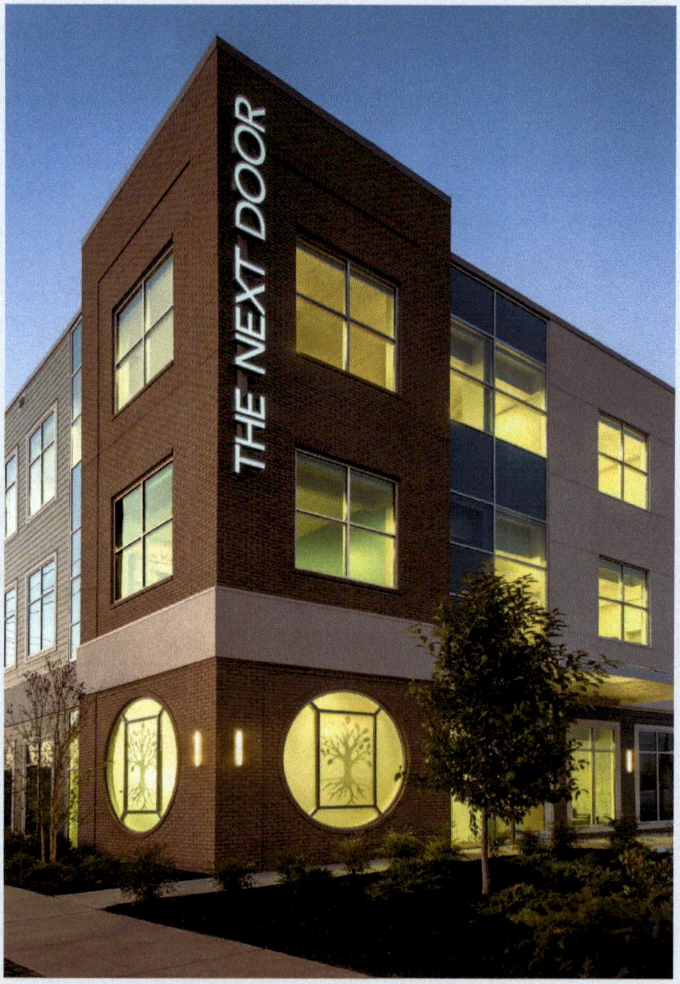

Figure 8.6: *The Next Door – exterior view (Architects: ESa Architects)*

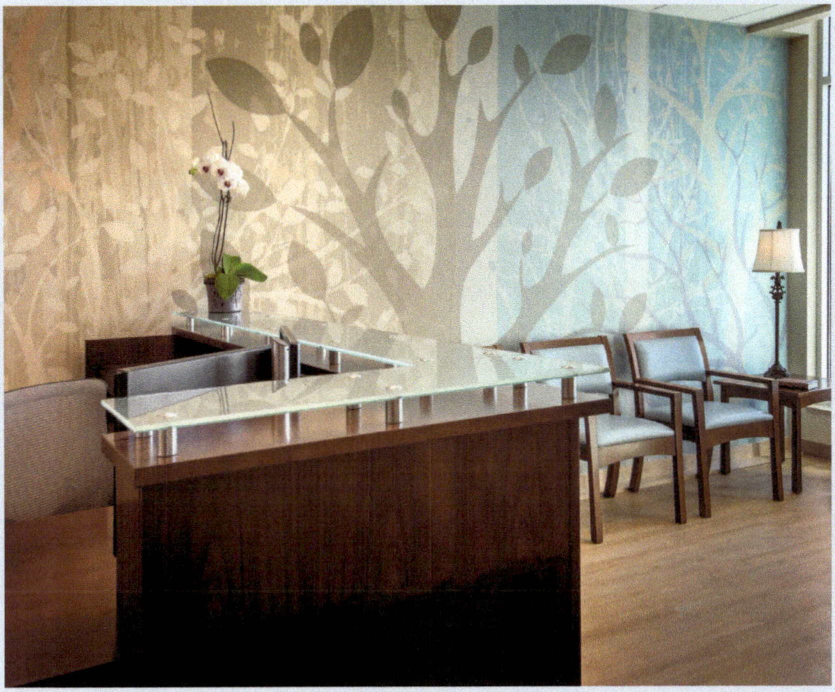

Figure 8.7: *The Next Door – lobby (Architects: ESa Architects)*

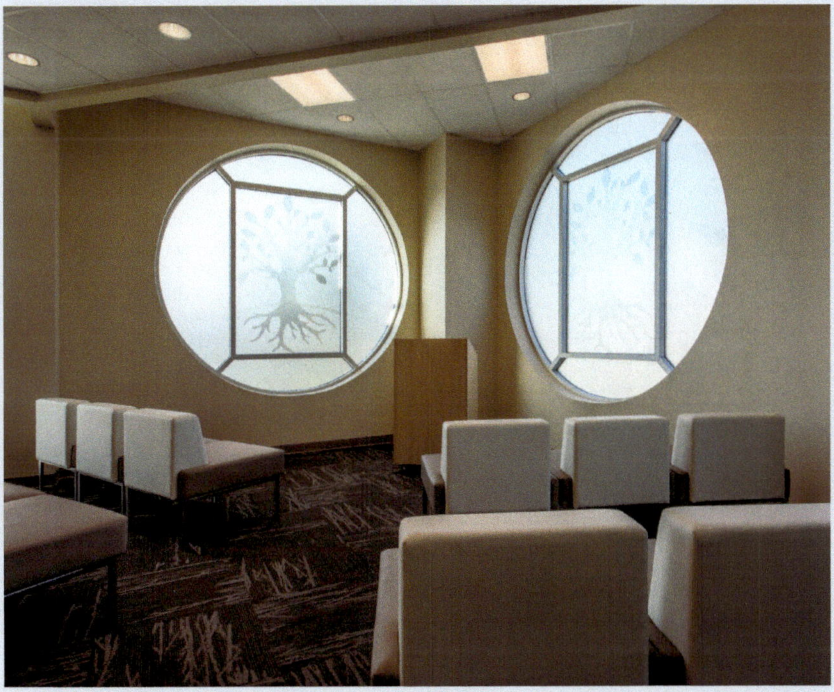

Figure 8.8: *The Next Door – chapel (Architects: ESa Architects)*

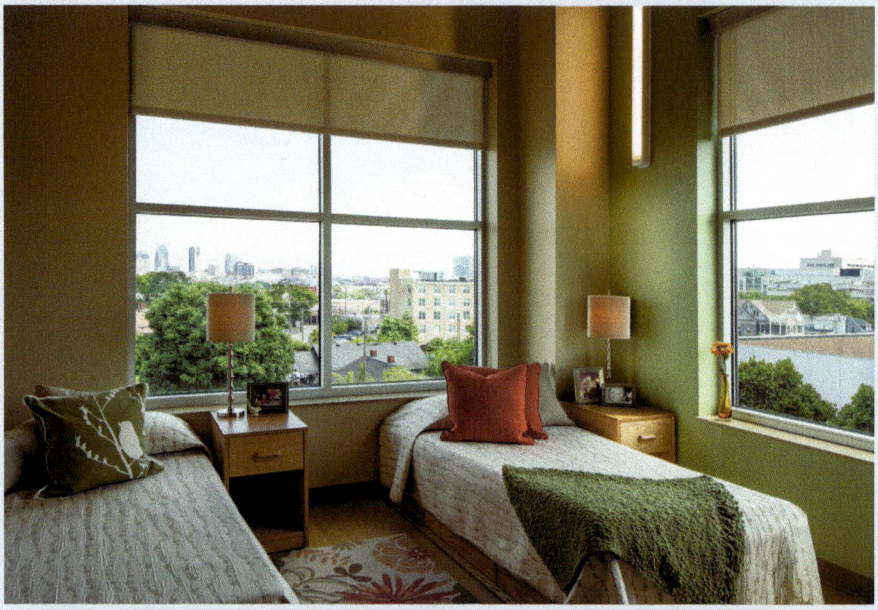

Figure 8.9: *The Next Door – resident bedroom (Architects: ESa Architects)*

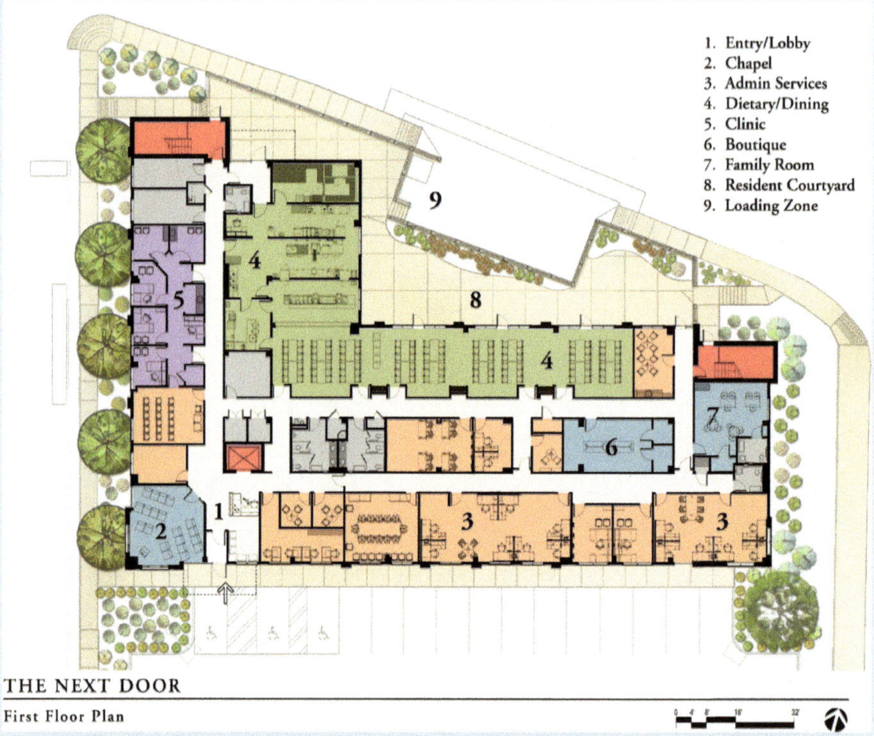

Figure 8.10: *The Next Door – first floor (Architects: ESa Architects)*

8.4.2 *Tiny Homes at the Farm at Penny Lane*

Location:	Chatham County, North Carolina
Designer/Architect:	Habitat for Humanity and Bold Construction
Client:	XDS Inc/UNC Center for Excellence in Community Mental Health
Completion:	2016 (first home)
Area:	336 square feet per house; 10 total houses planned

Client, service users, and services

The homes are intended to serve clients of the UNC Center for Excellence in Community Mental Health. The program is specifically intended to provide affordable housing to those living on Supplemental Security Income or other federal benefits and for those individuals with disabilities.

Mission and goals

The Farm at Penny Lane is intended to provide permanent supportive housing, employment, and meaningful learning opportunities for individuals living with major mental illnesses. The major goals of the farm are to:

1. Maximize social, cognitive, physical, and psychological functioning of participants.
2. Enhance the general health and wellness of individuals.
3. Facilitate entrepreneurship for program participants.
4. Break down barriers in the community and reduce the stigma associated with mental illness.

Lastly, this tiny house program is directed at addressing the low-income housing shortage and giving people, who might not ordinarily have the funds for their own home, "a place to call their own."

Site

The property is located between Chapel Hill and Pittsboro, North Carolina, on 40 acres in a rural forested track of land. An Assertive Community Treatment team has offices on-site. The ACT team is a group of clinicians including nurses, doctors, and people who serve individuals with severe mental illness in the community. One home has been completed and will eventually be joined by nine others. Other structures on the site include a variety of greenhouses and agricultural buildings. An effort is being made to locate a bus stop nearby.

Program

The farm will provide opportunities for physical activity and generating food with the intention of making it self-sufficient. The land is currently being developed agriculturally and has a facility for training dogs that can serve as emotional support for veterans and others with post-traumatic stress disorder and other mental health conditions. The Tiny Home project is currently being evaluated via a research project, the first phase of which is feedback via staff and client focus groups. Stage two will involve clients taking turns living in the home for a short period and obtaining their feedback.

Configuration and construction

The tiny house is a 12' by 28' one-story wood structure, consisting of a living room/kitchen (11' 4" × 14' 5"), a bathroom (7' 10" × 5' 0"), and a bedroom (11' 4" × 7' 3").

Case study bibliography

Bail, B. (2015, August 19). In Chatham County, a nonprofit will build tiny homes for the homeless. *Indy Week*.

Bonner, L. (2016, February 14). Building a community: Houses for NC people with mental illness. *The News & Observer*.

Cohen, T. (2015, August 7). Tiny homes to shelter the homeless. *Triangle Business Journal*.

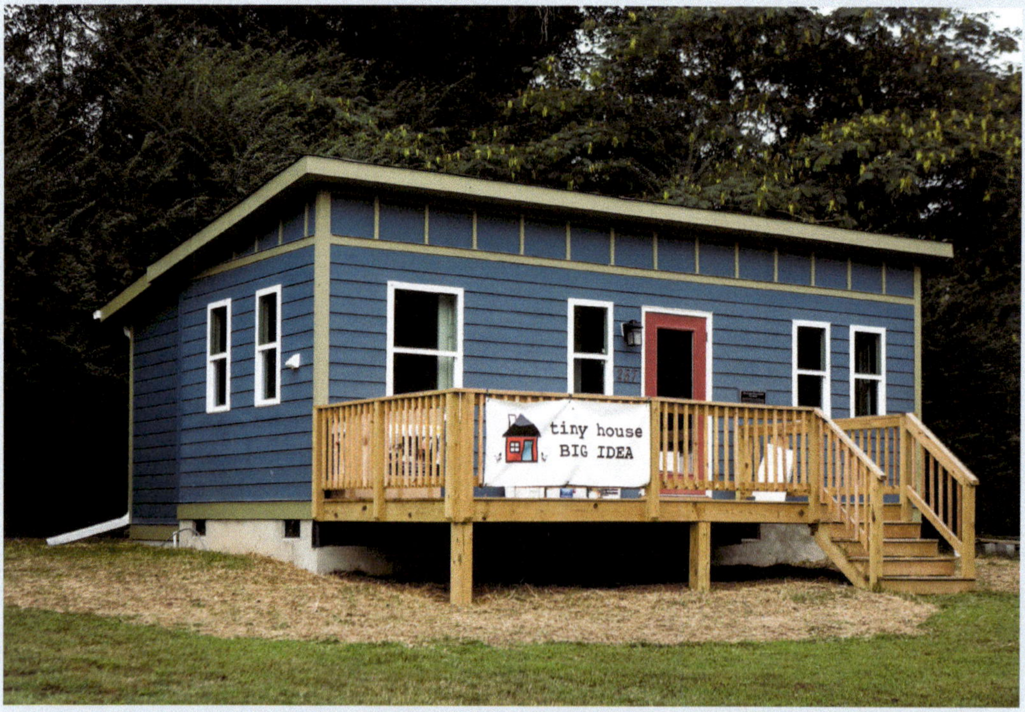

Figure 8.11: *Penny Lane – exterior (Architects: Habitat for Humanity and Bold Construction)*

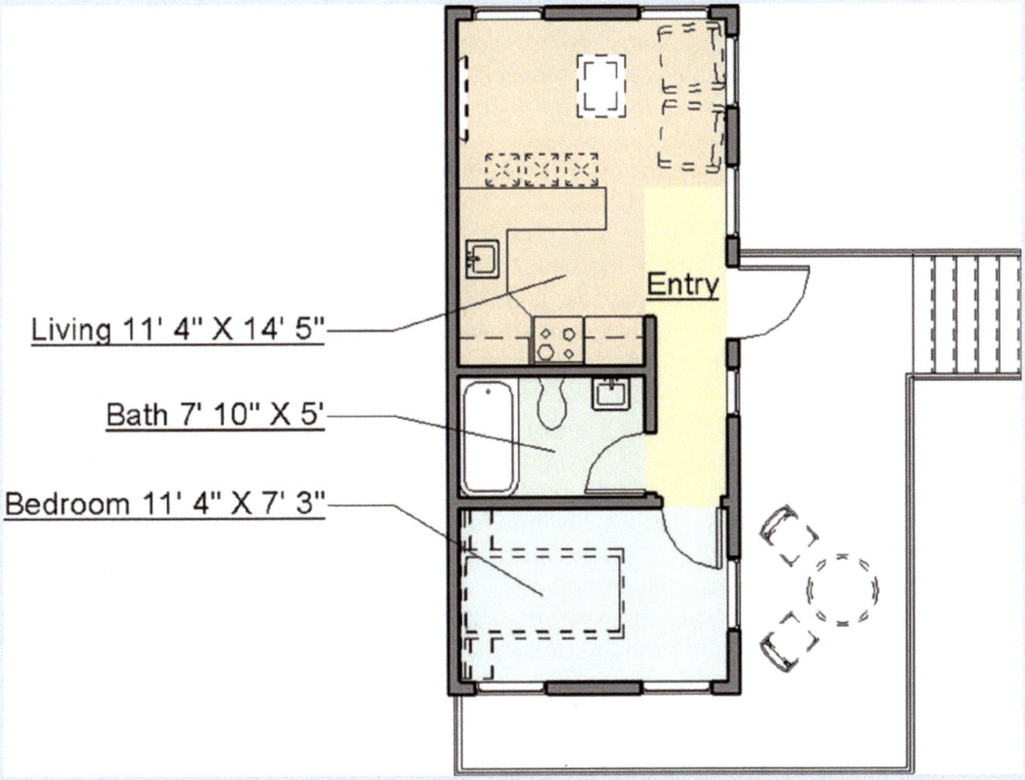

Figure 8.12: *Penny Lane – floor plan (Architects: Habitat for Humanity and Bold Construction)*

References

Bank-Mikkelsen, N. (1969). Part VI, Ch. 10: A metropolitan area in Denmark, Copenhagen. In R. B. Kugel & W. Wolfensberger (Eds.), *Changing patterns of residential services for the mentally retarded*. Washington, DC: President's Committee on Mental Retardation. 227–224.

Browne, G., & Courtney, M. (2004). Measuring the impact of housing on people with schizophrenia. *Nursing Health Sciences*, *6*(1), 37–44.

Bruce, D. (2003). Housing needs of low-income people living in rural areas. *Canadian Mortgage and Housing Corporation*, 1–6. Retrieved from www.cmhc-schl.gc.ca/publications/en/rh-pr/socio/socio03-012-e.pdf

Burt, M. (2006). *Characteristics of transitional housing for homeless families*. Washington, DC: Urban Institute. Retrieved from www.urban.org/sites/default/files/alfresco/publication-pdfs/411369-Characteristics-of-Transitional-Housing-for-Homeless-Families.PDF

Caplan, R. B. (1969). *Psychiatry and the community in nineteenth century America*. New York: Basic Books.

Cardoso, G., Papoila, A., Tome, G., Killaspy, H., King, M., & Caldas, J. (2016). Living conditions and quality of care in residential units for people with long term mental illness in Portugal – a cross sectional study. *BMC Psychiatry*, *16*(34). doi:10.1186/s12888-016-0743-7

Cheng, A. L., Lin, H., Kasprow, W., & Roosenheck, R. (2007). Impact of supported housing on clinical outcomes: Analysis of a randomized trial using multiple imputation technique. *Journal of Nervous and Mental Disease*, *195*, 83–88.

Chrysikou, E. (2014). *Architecture for psychiatric environments and therapeutic spaces*. Amsterdam: IOS Press.

Curtis, S., Gesler, W., Priebe, S., & Francis, S. (2009). New spaces of inpatient care for people with mental illness: A complex rebirth of the clinic? *Health and Places*, *15*(1), 340–348.

Demaine, G. C., Silverstein, A. B., & Mayeda, T. (1980). Validation of PASS 3: A first step in service evaluation through environmental assessments. *Mental Retardation*, *18*, 131–134.

Dickey, B. (2000). Review of programs for persons who are homeless and mentally ill. *Harvard Review of Psychiatry*, *8*(5), 242–250.

Dixon, L., & Goldman, H. (2003). Forty years of progress in community mental health: The role of evidence-based practices. *Journal of Psychiatry*, *37*, 668–673.

Dorsett, C., & Brown, B. (1965). *Planning, programming, and design for the community mental health center*. Pittsburgh, PA: National Institute for Mental Health.

Doyle, A., Lanoil, J., & Dudek, K. (2013). *Fountain house: Creating community in mental health practice*. New York: Columbia University Press.

Fitzpatrick, H. (2007). *Supportive housing for mental health recovery: A bio-psycho-social approach* (Unpublished master's thesis). University of Waterloo, Ontario.

Flynn, R. J., & Heal, L. W. (1981). A short form of PASS 3: A study of its structure, interrater reliability, and validity for assessing normalization. *Evaluation Review*, *5*(3), 357–376.

Flynn, R. J., LaPointe, N., Wolfensberger, W., & Thomas, S. (1991). Quality of institutional and community human service programs in Canada and the United States. *Journal of Psychiatry and Neurosciences*, *16*(3), 146–153.

Forchuk, C., Ward-Griffin, C., Csiernik, R., & Turner, K. (2006). Surviving the tornado of mental illness: Psychiatric survivors' experiences of getting, losing, and keeping housing. *Psychiatric Services*, *57*(4), 558–562.

Health Evidence Network (HEN). (2003). *What are the arguments for community-based mental healthcare?* WHO Regional Office for Europe. Retrieved from www.euro.who.int/__data/assets/pdf_file/0019/74710/E82976.pdf

Horan, M. E., Muller, J. J., Winocur, S., & Barling, N. (2001). Quality of life in boarding houses and hostels: A residents' perspective. *Community Mental Health Journal*, *37*(4), 323–334.

HUD. (2015). *The 2015 annual homeless assessment report to congress*. Retrieved March 5, 2013, from www.hudexchange.info/resources/documents/2015-AHAR-Part-1.pdf

HUD. (2016a). *Section 811 supportive housing for persons with disabilities*. Retrieved from http://portal.hud.gov/hudportal/HUD?src=/program_offices/housing/mfh/progdesc/disab811

HUD. (2016b). *Section 8 assistance for public housing relocation/replacement*. Retrieved from http://portal.hud.gov/hudportal/HUD?src=/programdescription/phrr

Hynes, J. (1987). The California Mental Health Reform Act of 1985: A case study of policy reform in the post-welfare state. In L. J. Duhl & N. A. Cummings (Eds.), *The future of mental health services: Coping with crisis*. New York: Springer.

Inland Architect. (1998). The changing role of mental health facilities. *Inland Architect*, *115*(3), 63–66.

Irving, S., & Loveless, T. (2015). *Dynamics of economics wellbeing: Participation in Government programs 2009–2012: Who gets assistance?* Household Economic Studies. Washington, D.C.: US Census Bureau, US Department of Commerce.

Killaspy, H., Marston, L., Omar, R. Z., Green, N., Harrison, I., & Lean, M. (2013). Services quality and clinical outcomes: an example from mental health rehabilitation services in England. *British Journal of Psychiatry*, *202*, 28–34

Koran, L. M., & Meinhardt, K. (1981). Mental health expenditures in California counties. *American Journal of Psychiatry*, *138*(7), 936–940.

Leff, H. S., Chow, C. M., Peppin, R., Conley, J., Allen, I. E., & Seaman, C. A. (2009). Does one size fit all? What we can and can't learn from a meta-analysis of housing models for persons with mental illness. *Psychiatric Services*, *60*, 473–482.

NAMI. (2016). Securing stable housing. *National Alliance for Mental Illness*. Retrieved from www.nami.org/Find-Support/Living-with-a-Mental-Health-Condition/Securing-Stable-Housing

National Council for Behavioral Health. (2015). Community Mental Health Act. *The National Council*. Retrieved from www.thenationalcouncil.org/about/national-mental-health-association/overview/community-mental-health-act/

Nelson, G. (2010). Housing for people with serious mental illness: Approaches, evidence, and transformative change. *Journal of Sociology & Social Welfare*, *37*, 123–146

Nelson, G., & Prilleltensky, I. (2010). *Community psychology: In pursuit of liberation and wellbeing*. New York: Palgrave Macmillan.

Nirje, B. (1982). *The basis and logic of the normalization principle: Sixth International Congress of IASSMD*. Toronto, Canada: National Institute on Mental Retardation.

Parr, H., Philo, C., & Burns, N. (2003). "That awful place was home": Reflections on the contested meanings of Craig Dunain asylum. *Scottish Geographical Journal*, *119*(4), 341–360.

Perkins, D. V., Born, D. L., Raines, J. A., & Galka, S. W. (2005). Program evaluation from an ecological perspective: Supported employment services for persons with serious psychiatric disabilities. *Psychiatric Rehabilitation Journal*, *28*(3), 217–224.

Public Law 88–164. (1963). Mental Retardation Facilities and Community Health Centers Construction Act of 1963. *National Archives Catalog*. Retrieved on June 26, 2016, from https://research.archives.gov/id/299883

SAMHSA. (2012). *Behavioral health United States, 2012*. U.S. Department of Health and Human Services. Retrieved from www.samhsa.gov/data/sites/default/files/2012-BHUS.pdf

Schutt, R. K., Goldfinger, S. M., & Penk, W. E. (1997). Satisfaction with residence and with life: When homeless mentally ill persons are housed. *Evaluation and Program Planning*, *20*(2), 185–194.

Segal, S. P., & Kotler, P. L. (1993). Sheltered care residence: Ten year personal outcomes. *American Journal of Orthopsychiatry*, *63*, 80–91.

Slessor, C. (1995). Halfway house. *The Architectural Review*, *197*(1177), 60–63.

Smith, H., & Brown, H. (1992). Defending community care: Can normalization do the job? *British Journal of Social Work*, *22*(6), 685–693.

Smith, M. R. (2013, October 20). 50 years later, Kennedy's vision for mental health not realized. *The Associated Press*. Retrieved from www.seattletimes.com/nation-world/50-years-later-kennedy rsquos-vision-for-mental-health-not-realized/

Stroman, D. (2003). *The disability rights movement: From deinstitutionalization to self-determination*. Lanham, MD: University Press of America.

Turner, J., & TenHoor, W. (1978). The NIMH community support program: Pilot approach to a needed social reform. *Schizophrenia Bulletin*, *4*, 319–348.

Watzlawick, P., Weakland, J., & Fish, R. (1974). *Change: Principles of problem formation and problem solution*. New York: Norton.

Wolfensberger, W., & Glenn, L. (1975). *PASS 3: A method for quantitative evaluation of the human services field*. Toronto, Canada: National Institute on Mental Retardation.

Wolfensberger, W., & Thomas, S. (1983). *PASSING: Program analysis of service systems implementation of normalization goals*. Toronto, Canada: National Institute on Mental Retardation.

Wolfensberger, W., & Thomas, S. (2005). *Introductory social role valorization workshop training package*. Syracuse, NY: Training Institute for Human Service Planning, Leadership and Change Agency (Syracuse University).

World Health Organization. (2011). *Mental health Atlas 2011*. Department of Mental Health and Substance Abuse, World Health Organization. Retrieved from www.who.int/mental_health/evidence/atlas/profiles/usa_mh_profile.pdf

Part Three: The research

The role of the physical environment in mental and behavioral health research 9

9.1 History and status of research

Formally recognized design research on mental and behavioral health facilities dates back to the mid-twentieth century, (e.g., Griffin, Mauritzen, & Kasmar, 1969; Kasmar, Griffin, & Mauritzen, 1968). The topic experienced a surge in the 1970s in keeping with cultural and social values of the time. Studies waned during the 1980s and 1990s, but interest in this specialty has regained momentum since the turn of the century. Unfortunately, these more recent studies rarely manifested themselves in design guidelines or readily translatable findings.

The limited number of useful studies is evident when reviewing the literature on the impact of behavioral healthcare environments on patient outcomes, as demonstrated by the systematic reviews conducted by Devlin and Arneill (2003); Dijkstra, Piesterse, and Pruyn (2006); and Evans (2003). More recently, Connellan and colleagues (2013) conducted a broad review of health facility design research with a sub-focus on mental health. In this study, of the 165 articles, 25 were data driven and seven were literature reviews. The most frequent themes regarding mental health were light, workspace, homelike milieu, and gardens. More recently, a literature review by Richter and Hoffmann (2014) of 25 pre-post studies with control group conditions (no randomized controlled trials) suggested desirable impacts on psychopathology and aggression, but the body of research is limited.

While the examples of rigorous studies are few, a review of the research findings and clinical data of the past 50 years indicates that research-informed, patient-focused environmental interventions can positively impact the experience of patients and staff (Karlin & Zeiss, 2006; Richter & Hoffmann, 2014).

9.2 Methodology for literature review

The remainder of this chapter is a summary of research in the recent decades and the conclusions that can be drawn from them. It combines the literature review by Shepley & Pasha et al., (2013) and an in-depth subsequent exploration between 2013 and 2016. Approximately 800 articles were reviewed for possible incorporation, of which approximately 200 were deemed sufficiently substantive for mention in this chapter. The criteria for inclusion included (a) relevance to the topic of behavioral health facilities, (b) a demonstration of clear research methodology or practice/research supported guidelines, (c) post-1960 publication, and (d) publication in peer-reviewed journals. In a few cases, the publications occurred in non-peer-reviewed journals. In these cases, the structure of the data or the experience of the author(s) suggested that the research merited inclusion.

The authors accessed the following databases in pursuit of these research papers: EBSCO (academic and business), CAB Abstracts (Ovid), PubMed, MEDLINE, ERIC, PsycINFO (ProQuest), ScienceDirect (Elsevier), and Web of Science. Search terms included combinations of the following: psychiatric, behavioral, design, architecture, facility, health, environment, mental, and rehabilitation, as well as other synonyms for these terms. Within the typology of MBH facilities, the review does not include a summary of therapeutic environments for individuals with developmental disabilities, autism spectrum disorder, or dementia. Although the emphasis in the literature is placed on residential/inpatient facilities, the design principles also apply to outpatient environments.

9.3 Challenges to data collection involving patients

In addition to trying to address the wide range of settings and variety of diagnoses discussed in Chapter 1, researchers encounter other difficulties when trying to gather data from mental health patients and residents. First, the methods for gathering data must honor the privacy and preferences of subjects. Human subjects review boards are acutely aware of the vulnerability of this special population and impose restrictions on the type of information gathered and the identification of individual patients.

Second, the reliability and validity of subjects is critical to establishing credibility; particular concern has been expressed with regard to the capacity of mental health patients to respond clearly to evaluation surveys, as their responses might be influenced by "personalized and idiosyncratic responses which might be of questionable validity" (Rice, Berger, Klett, Sewall, & Lemkau, 1963, p. 251). Questions exist regarding the validity of responses considering patients' cognitive abilities, memory issues, and emotional stability. Additionally, as psychiatric patients are frequently evaluated for their personal characteristics, these evaluation tools might be perceived as a clandestine means of psychological state assessment and subjects might attempt to manipulate the results.

Avoiding interaction with patients by focusing on the perspectives of staff and family might not be appropriate. In studies of social or physical ward environments, staff evaluations of the physical and social environment have not always been found to accurately reflect patient evaluations. Brunt and Rask (2008) used the Ward Atmosphere Scale (WAS) to obtain psychiatric patient and staff perceptions of the ward atmosphere. They found that the two groups assess the ward social environment differently in terms of autonomy and involvement, program clarity and order, and organization. Main, McBride, and Austin (1991) surveyed psychiatric patients and staff using WAS and also concluded that staff and patients scored various categories of behaviors differently. For example, staff self-evaluations were higher than patient evaluations of staff regarding involvement, support, spontaneity, practical orientation, personal problem orientation, and program clarity. Meanwhile, patients rated staff higher than staff in categories perceived as negative (control). As another example of dissimilar responses, Marcheschi (2012) found that staff perception of the social climate was more positive than resident perception. Schjødt et al. (2003) also found differences in patient and staff ratings of the ward atmosphere, but concluded that such differences reflect "nuances in views rather than fundamental differences in opinion" (p. 215). To get the clearest understanding possible, Marcheschi (2012) recommends integrating users' and experts' environmental assessments to better understand the interaction between physical and social environment and related impacts on user well-being.

9.4 Behavioral health facility evaluation tools

Eleven MBH facility occupancy evaluation tools are described in this chapter. These tools are designed to evaluate the social or physical environment, and some of them cover the characteristics of the treatment plan as well. Most of the tools are focused on evaluating the psychiatric ward environment. However, a few can be used for all types of mental health facilities. Available tools also vary in terms of intended respondents; some of them are designed to be used by staff members, while others are designed to be used by both staff and patients to compare their perspectives on various characteristics of the social or physical environment. The tools are summarized in Figure 9.1.

The most recent of these tools is the Psychiatric Staff Environmental Design tool (Shepley et al., 2016). This pilot questionnaire, which was built on a literature review and 19 interviews with

Figure 9.1: *Tools for evaluating mental and behavioral health facilities (Based on: Shepley & Pasha et al., 2013 and Shepley et al., 2016)*

Abbreviation	*Name*	*Author*	*Setting*	*Focus*	*Outcomes*	*Respondents*
AEDET Evolution	Achieving Excellent Design Evaluation Toolkit	NHS Estates, 2013	Various	Social and physical environment	Functionality, impact, building performance	All stakeholder groups
ASPECT	A Staff and Patient Environment Calibration Toolkit	Department of Health, 2008	Various	Social and physical environment	Privacy, dignity, views, access to nature, comfort, control, legibility, interiors, facilities	Staff and patients
MHEOCC	Mental Health Environment of Care Checklist	Watts et al., 2012	VA Mental Health Hospital	Physical environment	Safety measures for physical features	Staff
PACI	Physical and Architectural Characteristics Inventory	Timko, 1996	Hospital and community psychiatric / substance abuse treatment	Social and physical environment	Community access, physical amenities, social/ recreational aids, prosthetics, safety, staff facility, space availability	Administrators
PFE	Practitioner-focused Facility Evaluation	Shepley, 2011	Healthcare	Physical environment	Pre- and post-occupancy evaluation tool	Design teams and building occupants
PSED	Psychiatric Staff Environmental Design tool	Shepley et al., 2016; Shepley et al., 2017	Various	Physical environment	Maintenance, access to nature, aesthetics, homelikeness, order	Staff

Abbreviation	*Name*	*Author*	*Setting*	*Focus*	*Outcomes*	*Respondents*
SATQ-98	Satisfaction AT Questionnaire	Müller, Schlosser, Kapp-Steen, Schanz, & Benkert, 2002	Various	Social environment and treatment plan	Satisfaction, doctor, medication, psychotherapy, care, nurses, social programs, food, equipment, visiting	Patients
SRAT	Safety Risk Assessment Tool	Center for Health Design, 2015	Six types including behavioral health	Physical environment	Safety measures for physical features	Multi-disciplinary project team
SRI	Setting-Response Inventory	Moos & Houts, 1968	Psychiatric Ward	Physical environment	Trust, extroversion, security, involvement, sociability	Staff
WAS	Ward Atmosphere Scale	Moos, 1989	Psychiatric Ward	Social environment	Relationship, personal development, system maintenance	Staff and patients
WES	Ward Evaluation Scale	Rice et al., 1963	Psychiatric Ward	Social and physical environment	Facilities, management of patients, services	Patients

experts, was tested on 134 nurses. The researchers sought to evaluate effectiveness and importance of environmental qualities and environmental features. The pertinent environmental qualities were: well-maintained, visual and physical access to the outdoors, attractive and aesthetically pleasing, deinstitutionalized and homelike, and orderly and organized.

Environmental features were:

- good staff safety and security mechanisms,
- good noise control,
- good daylighting,
- comfortable furniture,
- good electric lighting,
- damage-resistant furniture,
- spaces for staff respite, and
- attractive furniture.

9.5 Linking research to design

Via this book, the authors intended to link research and guidelines. Unfortunately, the number of rigorous studies is too limited to advance many EBD recommendations. However, recognizing that designers must create facilities regardless of whether the associated science is available, we propose that using the extant information is better than making uninformed decisions. In the best case, the research knowledge shared here will ultimately be supported by clusters of studies. In the worst case, designs based on the current level of knowledge summarized in this paper will serve as laboratories to examine the appropriateness of preliminary recommendations.

9.5.1 *Strong evidence and emerging evidence*

In order to formulate potential design guidelines, the authors sought a structure to use in order to categorize the implications of the literature content. Borrowing, in part, from the model generated by the *Active Design Guidelines* (ADG) (NYC, 2010) initiative, Shepley et al. (2013) developed strategies focusing on evidential support. In the ADG, *strong evidence* is defined as those strategies supported by evidence from at least two longitudinal or five cross-sectional studies, and *emerging evidence* is defined as strategies supported by a pattern of research.

There were an insufficient number of longitudinal or cross-sectional studies to create a category suggesting strong evidence. The highest category that the authors were able to substantiate was emerging evidence. Examples of emerging evidence are summarized in Figure 9.2. An additional category was added for the purposes of this exercise: studies requiring corroboration. This category refers to studies or pairs of studies that suggest potential conclusions but lack enough documentation to be considered evidence.

Figure 9.2: *Emerging evidence in behavioral health facility design (Based on: Shepley & Pasha et al., 2013)*

General	*Citation*
Provide a flexible and deinstitutionalized and homelike environment	Carr, 2011; Devlin, 1992; Grosenick & Hatmaker, 2000; McGonagle & Allan, 2002; Potthoff, 1995; Priebe & Broker, 1999; Shepley, Frohman, & Wilson, 1999; Shepley, et al., 2016; Shepley et al., 2017; Tapak, 2012; Ulrich, Bogren, & Lundin 2012; Whitehead, Polsky, Crookshank, & Fik, 1984; Wilson, Soth, & Robak, 1992
Support patient autonomy and spontaneity in the ward	Cleary, Hunt, & Walter, 2009; Donald, Duff, Lee, Kroschel, & Kulkarni, 2015; Middelboe, Schjødt, Byrsting, & Gjerris, 2001; Sorlie, Parniakov, Rezvy, & Ponomarev, 2010; Shepley et al., 2016; Shepley et al., 2017
Provide order and organization in the ward	Eklund & Hansson, 2001; Schjødt, Middelboe, Mortensen, & Gjerris, 2003; Shepley et al., 2016; Shepley et al., 2017
Provide high-quality maintenance, furniture, and landscaping	Christenfeld, Wagner, Pastva, & Acrish, 1989; Grosenick & Hatmaker, 2000; Holahan & Saegert, 1973; Potthoff, 1995; Shepley et al., 2016; Shepley et al., 2017
Choose furnishings that resist damage and are easily replaced and repaired	Carr, 2011; Davis, Glick, & Rosow, 1979; Shepley et al., 1999; Shepley et al., 2016; Shepley et al., 2017

General	Citation
Patient Rooms	
Provide private patient rooms	Chou, Lu, & Mao, 2002; Cleary et al., 2009; Izumi, 1968; Shepley et al., 1999; Shepley, et al., 2016; Shepley et al., 2017; Turlington, 2004; Tyson, Lambert, & Beattie, 2002; Ulrich et al., 2012; Wolfe, 1975
Provide lower-density patient rooms (large two-person bedrooms)	Chou et al., 2002; Izumi, 1968; Shepley et al., 2016; Shepley et al., 2017; Turlington, 2004; Ulrich et al., 2012; Wilson et al., 1992; Wolfe, 1975
Dayroom	
Provide dayrooms and common areas that encourage social interaction and promote a sense of community	Davis et al., 1979; Devlin, 1992; Gutkowski, Ginath, & Guttmann, 1992; Holahan & Saegert, 1973; Sidman & Moos, 1973; Turlington, 2004
Facilitate the staff observation of the dayroom and spaces used by patients from the nursing station	Carr, 2011; Chou et al., 2002; Christenfeld et al., 1989; Shepley et al., 1999; Turlington, 2004; Ulrich et al., 2012; Whitehead et al., 1984
Locate a mix of seating arrangements that support social interaction between different groups of patients	Baldwin, 1985; Minde, Haynes, & Rogenburg, 1990; Priebe & Broker, 1999; Shepley et al., 2016; Shepley et al., 2017
Provide smoking rooms	Salerno et al., 2012; Shepley et al., 1999; Tyson et al., 2002
Staff Spaces	
Provide open nurse station	Carr et al., 2011; Shepley et al., 2016; Shepley et al., 2017; Southard et al., 2009; Ulrich, Bogren, & Lundin, 2012; Whitehead et al., 1984
Provide areas suitable for private one-on-one interaction between staff and patients	Gutkowski, Ginath, & Guttmann, 1992; McGuire et al., 1977; Perkins, Prosser, Riley, & Whittington, 2011; Shepley et al., 2016; Shepley et al., 2017; Tyson et al., 2002
Include spaces for staff mental health consultation and therapy	Chen, Huang, Hwang, & Chen, 2010; Salerno et al., 2012; Shepley et al., 2016; Shepley et al., 2017
Light and Nature	
Maximize use of daylight; create well-illuminated interior spaces; combine natural and artificial light	Davis et al., 1979; Gutkowski & Guttmann, 1992; Olver, Love, Daniel, Norman & Nicholls, 2009; Shepley et al., 2016; Shepley et al., 2017; Turlington, 2004; Ulrich et al., 2012
Provide indoor and outdoor spaces for therapeutic activities	Bryan, Rudd, & Wertenberger, 2013; Donald, Duff, Lee, Kroschel, & Kulkarni, 2015; Gjerden, 1997; Sorlie, Parniakov, Rezvy, & Ponomarev, 2010
Provide visual or physical access to nature	Potthoff, 1995; Shepley, 1995; Shepley et al., 1999; Shepley et al., 2016; Shepley et al., 2017; Ulrich et al., 2012; Wagenfeld, Roy-Fisher, & Mitchell, 2013
Safety Features	
Enhance staff safety and security	Delaney & Johnson, 2008; Forster, Cavness, & Phelps, 1999; Lynch, Plant, & Ryan, 2005; Martin, 1995; Salerno et al., 2012; Shepley et al., 2016; Shepley et al., 2017
Eliminate features that might support ligature	Carr, 2011; Geddes, 1999; Jeffers, 1991; Shepley et al., 2016; Shepley et al., 2017; Watts et al., 2012

Unlike some bodies of research, there are very few rigorous studies on the topic of behavioral health facilities. If we were to evaluate the literature identified in this chapter, no more than 20 are sufficiently rigorous to merit the drawing of conclusions, and of those, there is little overlap to generate what might be described as strong evidence. Nevertheless, we attempted to identify recurring patterns in the literature, as reflected in Figure 9.2, and to categorize them as emerging evidence. Future researchers should consider addressing one of these topics to elevate the issue to strong evidence.

9.5.2 *Studies requiring additional corroboration*

The list of items that fell into the category of *requiring additional corroboration* were topics that were suggested by at least one researcher or research team and are supported by experience from practice. (See Figure 9.3.) Multiple rigorous studies are needed on each of these conclusions to consider them to be evidence. The reader should also be cautioned that the recommendations need to be placed in the context of the particular study and patient type, and associated articles should be reviewed prior to application to a specific project.

Figure 9.3: *Studies requiring additional corroboration (Based on: Shepley & Pasha et al., 2013)*

General	
Provide locked doors between units	Wilson, Soth, & Robak, 1992
Accentuate functional uses and humanistic values through color and graphics	Whitehead, Polsky, Crookshank, & Fik, 1984
Include open closet arrangements	Watts et al., 2012
Use art that is realistic and displays social engagement	Nanda, Eisen, Zadeh, & Owen, 2010
Provide spaces with clear territorial designations	Shepley, Frohman, & Wilson, 1999
Provide an entrance that is visible from staff locations in the building interior	Shepley, 1995
Provide high-quality air filtration systems	Salerno et al., 2012
Avoid ambiguity	Izumi, 1968
Create egress from each area to an area of refuge	Jeffers, 1991
Provide good temperature control	Devlin, 1992
Provide small wards for patients to support a wide range of choices and large wards for patients to support isolated passive behavior	Salerno et al., 2012
Play music selected by ward therapist	Hunter & Love, 1996
Create a welcoming reception area	Gutkowski & Guttmann, 1992
Define different function units with clear boundaries	Gutkowski & Guttmann, 1992
Separate public and private areas	Gutkowski & Guttmann, 1992
Facilitate closer contact between the hospital and its neighborhood	Donald et al., 2015; Geddes, 1999; Gutkowski et al., 1992
Provide acoustic privacy when needed	Carr, 2011

Dayroom	
Provide direct orientation of seating for more affiliative behavior; provide greater distance between seating to decrease social pressure	Mehrabian & Diamond, 1971
Create smaller activity spaces to create a stronger sense of community	Townley, Kloos, & Wright, 2009
Patient Spaces	
Provide a large closet in adolescent rehab	Potthoff, 1995
Provide a central meeting area or living room for staff and patients and families and patients	Carr, 2011
Provide space for exercise and sports in adolescent rehab	Potthoff, 1995
Reduce restraint space	Perkins, Prosser, Riley, & Whittington, 2011
Provide on-site child care for substance abuse patients	Grosenick & Hatmaker, 2000
Staff Spaces	
Provide a psychiatric physician office that is visible during the daytime	Wilson, Soth, & Robak, 1992
Provide an intern office	Wilson, Soth, & Robak, 1992
Minimize staff walking distances	Carr, 2011
Make nursing station and doctor's office accessible to patients	Gutkowski & Guttmann, 1992
Design staff rooms to lower authoritarianism	Anderson, Good, & Hurtig, 1976
Light and Nature	
Provide direct sunlight in patient rooms	Benedetti , Colombo, Barbini, Campori, & Smeraldi, 2001
Provide access to the main courtyard during meals	Hunter & Love, 1996
Safety	
Implement mental health environment of care to reduce suicide rates	Wilson et al., 1992
Reduce patient density to reduce violence	Kumar & Ng, 2001; Ng, Kumar, Ranclaud, & Robinson, 2001
Limit the number of large shared spaces to reduce violence	Perkins et al., 2011

The third category is design considerations, or best practice as suggested by experts. The items in this category encompass design strategies and are discussed in Chapter 2.

9.6 Research summary

The research we uncovered in this review commonly focuses on traditional psychiatric hospitals as the primary care sites for people with mental illness. Studies on the design of mental health facilities generally fall into one of three categories: (1) the relationship between the physical environment and social behavior, (2) pre- and post-occupancy studies, and (3) the relationship between the physical environment and inappropriate and harmful behavior. Karlin and Zeiss (2006) categorized the domains that can impact patient outcomes in psychiatric hospitals as ambient features, architectural features, and social features. These elements can be part of any of the three topic areas.

9.6.1 Physical environment and social behavior

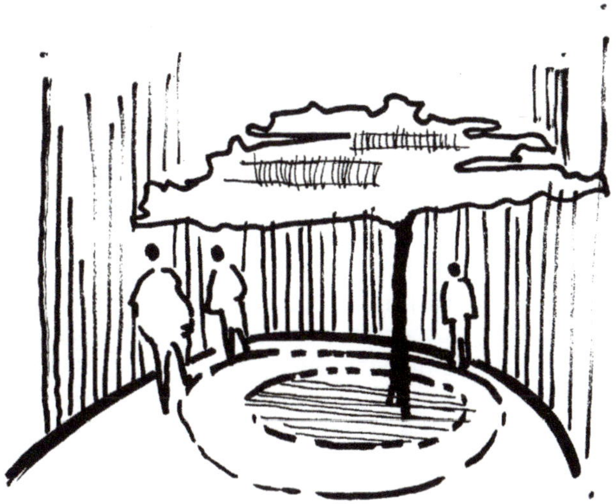

Physical environment and social behavior

The appropriate number of patients per bedroom has been a significant topic of discussion regarding social behavior. In one of the first environment and behavior studies in a psychiatric facility, Ittleson, Proshansky, and Rivlin (1970) examined the impact of bedroom size (based on number of occupants) on adult patient behavior. Comparing patient rooms ranging from singles to 12-bed dormitories, they concluded that the higher the number of occupants, the higher the percentage of isolated passive behaviors, which may run counter to the objectives of a facility. Contrary to the hypothesis, increased density did not increase social interactions.

Additionally, private rooms were found to support a more diverse range of behaviors, while multiple-bed rooms were more likely to provoke a patient's withdrawal. To place this in context, Willer, Staslak, Pinfold, and Rogers (1974) found that patients spend a significant amount of time in their rooms (25.8%) and, while there, engage primarily in passive activities (73.2%). Studies in substance abuse rehabilitation facilities demonstrate that control over privacy can lead to healthy social interactions and peer support that are instrumental in the success of the treatment program (Novonta, Urbanoski, & Rush, 2011). Similarly, Grosenick and Hatmaker (2000) provided evidence that environmental qualities including comfort, perceived attractiveness, noise, privacy, size, and location can contribute to achieving goals of the rehabilitation treatment plan. The treatment goals in the Grosenick and Hatmaker study included reducing drug use, enhancing physical health, feeling good about oneself, interacting well with others, and preparing for independent living.

Wolfe (1975) confirmed the Ittleson, Proshanky, and Rivlin (1970) findings regarding the high frequency of isolated passive behavior for pediatric populations. Wolfe also noticed that children in private rooms used their rooms the most, followed by children in three-bed and four-bed rooms, and lastly by children in two-bed rooms. Wolfe argued that a two-bed room forces a social intimacy that may be intimidating and detrimental to interaction and concluded that (1) activity type rather than mathematical density should dictate room size, (2) private rooms will be used most frequently, (3) the use of the room and interactive behaviors decreases as the number of beds per room increases, and (4) two-person rooms require more than double the space required for a one-person room. Rivlin and Wolfe (1979) note that room size and group size interact to create behavioral responses.

Kho, Sensky, Mortimer, and Corcos (1998) studied incidents in psychiatric acute admission wards that differed in size and design. Three of the units were new wards with single-patient rooms, and the other units were older with shared living spaces. A higher frequency of aggression took place in the older units with shared living space. While these researchers provide support for the hypothesis that private rooms may be appropriate for some patients, other researchers/practitioners argue that shared rooms support patient safety (as the presence of a roommate might prevent a potential suicide) and that private rooms have the negative impact of encouraging withdrawal from therapeutic group interaction.

Apart from the discussion about private and shared rooms, other behavioral outcomes discussed in the literature include the impact of furnishings and color. Mehrabian and Diamond (1971) found that furniture arrangements and the presence of sculpture or art increased social interaction among psychiatric patients. Holahan (1972, 1974, 1979) noted that mixed sociofugal (seating arrangements in which seats face away from one another, as is common in a bus station) and sociopetal seating (seating arrangements in which chairs face toward one another) supported interaction more effectively than sociofugal or free seating (at the discretion of the patient).

Investigating social behavior of schizophrenic patients, Holahan and Saegert (1973) found patients socialized more in a newly remodeled ward with bright colors compared to a ward with old and worn furniture and a dark and dull color scheme. They observed no difference in levels of nonsocial active behavior between the two wards. (See Figure 9.4.)

In a related study, not limited to social interaction, Fairbanks et al. (1977) investigated the way that the physical environment impacted social organization and behavior, whether there were variations in staff and patient use of space, and whether room designation or furniture arrangement impacted behavior. Using behavior observation, they found (1) patients heavily used the dayroom and TV room in addition to the hallway adjacent to the nurses' station or window, (2) patients frequently used areas with furniture, and (3) staff often sequestered themselves in the nurses' station or the adjacent hallway. In a related study, Barton and Mishkin (1984) found that behaviors tended to be directly linked to specific spaces with little overlap and that social interaction most commonly took place around the perimeter of rooms.

Social factors are also critical with regard to counseling environments. Evidence suggests that the physical environment affects client overall comfort, as well as the establishment of a relationship

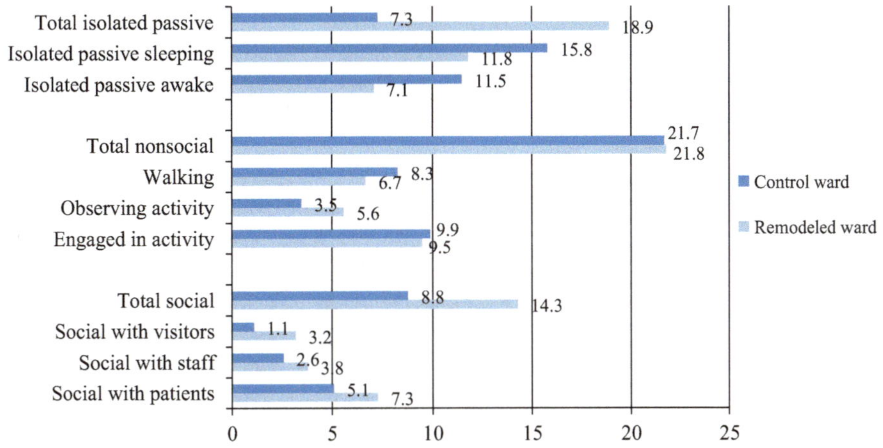

Figure 9.4: *Number of observations of social behaviors pre- and post-occupancy (Data source: Holahan & Saegert, 1973)*

(Backhaus, 2008; Morrow & McElroy, 1981), communication and self-disclosure (Chaikin, Derlega, & Miller, 1976; Miwa & Hanyu, 2006), impressions of therapists' credibility, skills, and expertise (Backhaus, 2008; Devlin et al., 2009, Miwa & Hanyu, 2006), and stress (Kagan & Kigli-Shemesh, 2005; Kweon, Ulrich, Walker, & Tassinary, 2008; Rashid & Zimring, 2008). These factors can also affect the counseling professionals' health and ability to provide quality therapeutic care (Lynes, 2011).

The following five studies are pre- and post-occupancy evaluations but, as they have a strong emphasis on social interaction, we have included them here rather than the subsequent section of this chapter. Social behavior facility evaluation studies range from the redesign of a hallway to the examination of multiple units. Examples are:

- Research conducted at Dykebar Hospital (Edgerton, n.d.) focused on effects of a new corridor design commissioned by an artist. Changes included new paint color, glass replacement, additional trees planted outside the facility, new floor covering, introduction of structure to alter the visual perspective, timber seating elements, and artwork. After the change, the number of patients using the corridor did not increase, but those who did use it were more likely to converse and walk.
- McGuire et al. (1977) observed behavior in four wards and recorded environmental variables. Changes that were noted in modified environments were: (1) removal of glass windows at the nurses' station resulted in more staff visual observations, but did not increase staff-patient interactions and (2) the probability of a conversation between two people increased when only two were in the room.
- Using interview and behavior mapping techniques, Holahan and Saegert (1973) found significantly more socializing and less isolated passive behavior in a newly remodeled unit than in a control unit. Additionally, patient attitudes toward the new space were more positive. In a subsequent study, Holahan (1976, 1979) examined the impact of a unit remodeling that influenced changes in staff roles, communication, distribution of power between staff and patients, ward social systems, and patient behavior using behavioral mapping techniques. The research

included data on interactions between investigators and ward staff, daily ward routines, and critical incidents. After remodeling, patients were significantly more engaged in social behavior, and researchers observed reductions in the hierarchical structure, better communication, and expansion in roles.

- Minde, Haynes, and Rogenburg (1990) examined the impact of a remodeled dayroom (new pictures, plants, furniture, comforters) on a psychogeriatric unit and found increased room usage and more frequent visiting.
- Apart from interaction between patients, researchers are interested in the interaction between staff and patients. Tyson et al. (2002) evaluated staff in old and new psychiatric units using behavior observation and job satisfaction self-ratings. The percentage of time spent in staff-patient interaction increased from 13.9% to 23.0%, and the proportion of positive quality interactions increased from 17.7% to 98.8%.

The following section describes occupancy evaluations that were developed to address a variety of responses in addition to social behavior. Facility evaluation is a time-honored method for gathering data regarding building outcomes.

9.6.2 *Pre- and post-occupancy evaluations*

A major concern of clinicians and researchers in the field of psychiatry is evaluation of therapeutic techniques used or models of care implemented with regard to treatment outcomes. Consequently, pre- and post-occupancy evaluations (Pre-OE and POE) of psychiatric facilities often evaluate change of treatment plans (Okin, 1995) or deinstitutionalization of the environment of care through a shift from psychiatric hospital ward to the community (e.g., Hobbs, Newton, Tennant, Rosen, & Tribe, 2002). Another challenge is that the nature of the physical changes vary enormously and, in many cases, are not described in detail, making interpretation of the design factors that may have led to changes in observed behavior difficult to assess.

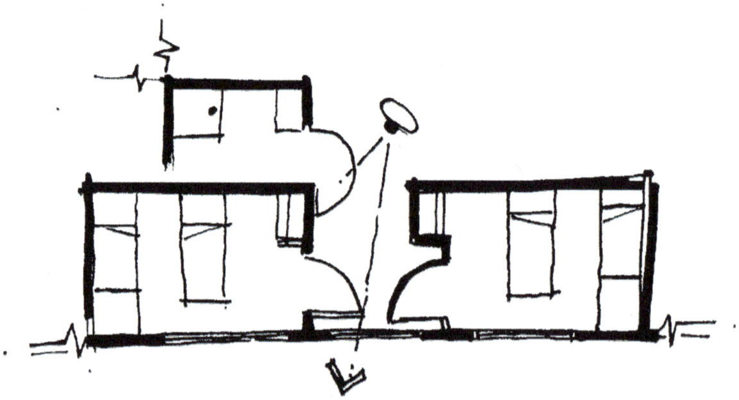

Pre-OE and POE

9.6.2.1 Multiple facility studies

One of the most extensive MBH post-occupancy evaluations was conducted by Rivlin and Wolfe (1979). The researchers gathered data from longitudinal interviews and behavioral observation in eight 24-bed houses, addressing a broad range of physical elements including site, administration, infirmary, school, occupational therapy, recreation, and components of the residential units. Apart from a critique of the effectiveness of these spaces relative to the design intentions, the authors note that, regardless of certain environmental changes, programs are likely to fall back on institutional models of treatment delivery. It is noteworthy that a review of several mental health facilities by Chrysikou (2013) revealed that designs of mental health facilities rarely follow the model of care and organizational policies they will house.

In another broad evaluation study, Devlin (1992) examined the impact of renovations on four wards of a 40-year-old psychiatric facility. Staff were asked to rate the wards pre- and post-renovation. Behavior mapping of patients and staff was conducted on one unit. The survey addressed the day hall, sleeping areas, and bathrooms. Also addressed were ventilation, privacy, furnishings, color, lighting, wayfinding, temperature, socializing areas, plants, safety features, clocks/calendars, and air quality. The behavior mapping protocol recorded subject location, subject status, and patient activity. Categories included sitting, walking, standing, lying down, eating, sleeping, talking, stereotypy (repetitive behavior), playing cards, writing, charting, working, and smoking. Based on the survey, it was concluded that staff rated most environmental variables higher in the new than the old facility. Also noted were reductions in patient stereotypy in the new facility. There was no improvement in general staff morale or ward stimulation.

While most of the literature described in this book focuses on settings in the United States, Canada, and Australia, the issue of lack of quality MBH environments is an international problem. A multisite study involving 164 of 231 psychiatric intensive care units (PICUs) and low-security units (LSUs) in the United Kingdom revealed that 37.5% of the PICUs and 36.5% of the LSUs failed on multiple issues (Pereira, Chaudhry, Pietromartire, Dale, & Halliwell, 2006). Shortcomings included lack of gender-specific facilities, the absence of an enclosed garden, and lack of seclusion facilities. In a pre- and post-evaluation of new psychiatric facilities resulting from the UK National Health Service (NHS) initiative "Enhancing the Healing Environment," increased satisfaction and reduced incidents of aggression were recorded (Payne & May, 2009).

9.6.2.2 Satisfaction

Patient and staff satisfaction is one of the most common outcomes in mental and behavioral health facility design, as represented in the following studies.

- Corey, Wallace, Harris, and Casey (1986) found that even superficial changes such as furniture and finishes had a positive impact on staff and patients. Patient satisfaction encourages patients to participate in care (Vuori, 1991). Additionally, acceptance of treatment by patients with schizophrenia can positively influence results of the patient treatment (Broker, Rohricht, & Priebe, 1995; Priebe & Broker, 1999). However, satisfaction with care can vary depending on the patient diagnosis. For example, lower satisfaction with care is found in patients diagnosed with depression (Koivumaa-Honkanen et al., 1996).
- Improved living conditions, leading to patient satisfaction with the physical or social environment, may reduce rates of patient unauthorized absence. Nijman and colleagues (2011) found a 30%

decrease in absconding among acutely mentally disordered patients when the ward doors were locked during the entire shift. They found a positive correlation between patient unauthorized absence and the following: poor ward environment quality, unqualified staff, conflict behaviors, alcohol and drug use, verbal aggression, and self-harm. However, the authors argue that door locking is far from a final solution.

- Anderson et al. (1976) performed an evaluation of a replacement facility for a county hospital. The new mental health center was examined using 12 open-ended interview questions. Patients indicated their satisfaction regarding the external facility, interior spaces, and general environment. However, the residential units provoked more negative responses. The researchers suggest the negative response to the residential units may have resulted from the change from open to locked connections between units. Related to this, in a study comparing two wards, Müller, Schlosser, Kapp-Steen, Schanz, and Benkert (2002) found that satisfaction with pharmacotherapy was significantly higher in patients in the open ward compared to the patients in the closed ward for similar patient populations.
- Potthoff conducted two studies involving adolescents in residential drug treatment facilities during which satisfaction was evaluated (Potthoff, 1991, 1995). These studies are discussed in detail in Chapter 5.
- Gutkowski, Ginath, and Guttmann (1992) found that the addition of formal entrances in a mental health center resulted in better accessibility, greater sense of freedom, and improved unit identity. In their research paper, they reported that the therapeutic atmosphere of a day hospital was reinforced by modifying the lighting, opening a stairway, and defining separate living and dining spaces. Regarding the day hospital, the designers also added bright colors and enhanced lighting and a separate entrance from the rehabilitation ward, which resulted in an improved experience (Gutkowski et al., 1992).
- Townley, Kloos, and Wright (2009) conducted interviews, solicited drawings, and used a global positioning system (GPS) to determine the relationship between activity zones and satisfaction, sense of community, and attitudes toward recovery in patients living in supportive housing in community versus traditional residential facilities. Individuals whose activity territories were larger (up to 37.40 square miles [96.9 square kilometers]) had higher life satisfaction, more positive attitudes toward recovery, and decreased sense of community compared with those with more limited activity ranges (as small as 0.06 square miles (0.16 square kilometers).
- During a mental health facility relocation, Cleary, Hunt, and Walter (2009) interviewed patients to measure their satisfaction with comfort, safety, cleanliness, privacy, food, information about the facility, and perceptions of care. Likewise, Long, Langford, Clay, Craig, and Hollin (2011) used the WAS and found patients to feel the environment was more home-like, but this change did not result in negative behavioral outcomes. Gjerden (1997) studied psychiatric patients' satisfaction with their stay by mailing a standardized questionnaire to patients discharged from the unit. The questionnaire included categories in which discharged patients would rate their satisfaction with ward staff, physical environment, information and influence, and treatment.

In summary, studies of mental health facilities should be mindful of models of care, as well as organizational and cultural factors.

9.6.2.3 Staff behavior

As with studies involving the social behavior of patients, occupancy evaluation researchers have been interested in staff behavior. Dorr, Honea, and Ponzer (1980) found a positive correlation between psychiatric nurse job satisfaction and higher scores on Moos' Ward Atmosphere Scale (WAS) (Moos, 1989; Moos & Houts, 1968). Tyson et al. (2002) evaluated staff in old and new psychiatric units by examining burnout rates and analyzing job satisfaction surveys. The results indicated that staff in the new ward experienced less emotional exhaustion and an increased sense of personal accomplishment. However, staff burnout rose due to increased engagement with patients, and there was no change in job satisfaction. Tuvesson, Eklund, and Wann-Hansson (2011) used the WAS and found that involvement and psychosocial work environment were indicators of perceived stress.

Setting-Response Inventory (SRI) is another tool developed by researchers and used to obtain staff input regarding various settings in psychiatric wards. Using a 7-point scale, Moos and Daniels (1967) asked staff members to describe eight different ward settings and concluded that different staff members function best depending on their expertise, seniority, and personality.

Other organizational or social factors may also influence staff job satisfaction and quality of life. Chen, Huang, Hwang, and Chen (2010) studied the correlation between health-related quality of life and workplace physical violence (WPV) among the nurses in a psychiatric hospital in Taipei. They found a negative correlation between number of WPVs and years of employment; a 40% reduction was observed in number of WPVs reported among the staff that was employed over five years. Their findings also demonstrated a positive correlation between staff feelings of worry at work and number of WPVs reported.

9.6.3 Harmful behavior and stress

Most environmental psychologists agree that the physical environment can reinforce and encourage appropriate behavior (Gabb, Speicher, & Lodl 1992). An environment can positively impact the behavior of patients and create a more supportive, stabilized environment for schizophrenic patients (Gabb et al., 1992). Conversely, avoidance of potentially harmful behaviors is a common objective in behavioral facilities.

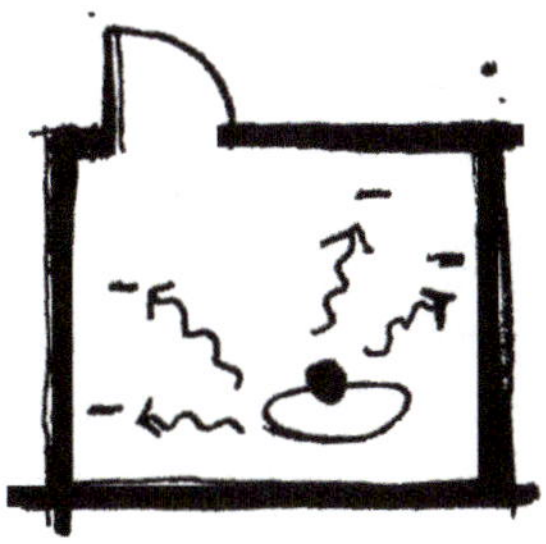

Harmful behavior and stress

9.6.3.1 Suicide

Safety is a critical objective in the design of facilities, and more work is required to create a secure environment (Brickell & McLean, 2011). Direct supervision at all times is difficult, and remote monitoring is controversial (Desai, 2010). The most harmful behaviors, of course, are attempted suicide or suicide. The Centers for Disease Control and Prevention (2013) reported that in 2013 there were 41,149 suicides in the United States. In 2003, the American Psychiatric Association (2003) estimated that each year, 1,500 suicides take place in U.S. inpatient mental health units. Bowers et al. (2012) recommend staff visual access to patients at all times, especially individuals at risk of suicide, self-harm, or aggressive behavior. Physical objects and design features that can be exploited by aggressive or suicidal patients should be eliminated or safeguarded.

For example, Li et al. (2008) and Stewart, Ross, Watson, James, and Bowers (2012), among several other researchers, suggest that building fixtures such as handles, doors, fittings, pipes, curtains, shower heads, grab bars, plumbing, HVAC, and lighting be eliminated to reduce risk of self-harm. Dobrohotoff and Llewellyn-Jones (2011) recommend high ceilings to hinder access to ceiling fixtures that can be used as anchor points for hanging. They also recommend collapsible curtain rails to reduce risk of hanging.

Gournay and Bowers (2000) recommend controlled access to rooftop and window openings where jumping may be possible. Watts et al. (2012) used the Mental Health Environment of Care Checklist (MHEOCC) to ensure compliance of all Veterans Health Administration (VHA) hospitals with safety measures. They found a significant reduction in number of completed suicides in VHA hospitals after implementation of MHEOCC.

Other factors, such as time past admission, can influence suicide rates as well. Hunt et al. (2013) reported that almost half of suicides take place within the first three days of admission. Their research suggests improvements to the ward environment to increase staff supervision and decrease patient distress, especially during admission and the first days of hospitalization. In general, guidelines recommend easy accessibility and proximity of security stations to inpatient units to allow quick response times (Yeager et al., 2005).

9.6.3.2 Stress

Less focus has been given to the impact of the environment on stress in outpatient settings. One group of researchers, however, recently studied the relationship between art displays and patient anxiety in an acute care psychiatric unit. Nanda, Eisen, Zadeh, and Owen (2010) found a significant positive correlation between presence of realistic art displays and anxiety reduction.

Stahler, Frazer, and Rappaport (1984) made observations of patient behavior in a remodeled ward and a predecessor ward. Immediately after relocation, patient-staff interaction increased in the remodeled ward, but patients expressed increased stress as well as lower sociability and self-maintenance. Five weeks later, however, it was found that negative behavior had decreased below the levels experienced in the old unit, and no changes took place in the un-remodeled ward. Interviews indicated that the remodeling improved morale among patients and staff.

9.6.3.3 Pathological behavior

Higgs (1970) noted a decrease in pathological behavior and behavioral inappropriateness in schizophrenic patients after they had moved to a modernized unit. Similarly, Whitehead, Polsky,

Crookshank, and Fik (1984) conducted behavioral observations to compare new and old facilities and found that the renovated environments were characterized by a reduction in pathological behaviors.

Christenfeld et al. (1989) had partially conflicting results in their study on the impact of physical changes in the interior design of a ward on staff and severely regressed psychotic inpatients. The researchers compared renovated wards to similar traditional wards. Staff mood level improved, and unscheduled absences were reduced by 50%. However, the researchers did not report improvement in ward atmosphere or patient functioning. The patients reported improvement in self-image, but not in irritability, depression, or isolation. On the other hand, patients were significantly more satisfied with the dayroom, and patient violence decreased by almost 50%. Teglbjaerg (2011) conducted a qualitative study on the impact of art therapy on pathological behavior of schizophrenic patients. Those findings suggested that engagement in the artistic process, either through creation of a new artwork or reflection on an existing one, can help schizophrenic patients gain a strong sense of self, boost their self-esteem, and improve their social competencies. Studies in this area may suggest incorporation of artwork into the design of mental health facilities.

9.6.3.4 Aggression and violence

Fear of patient aggressive or self-destructive behavior is one of the major concerns of the staff in psychiatric wards (Salerno et al., 2012). Salerno et al. (2012) reported a correlation between involuntary admission and incidents of aggressive behavior among psychotic patients. Other studies include:

- McGuire et al. (1977) found inappropriate behavior was highest when patients were alone and decreased in the presence of other patients. However, aggressive patient behaviors are more likely to take place in areas of high patient concentration (Kumar & Ng, 2001; Ng, Kumar, Ranclaud, & Robinson, 2001; Palmstierna, Huitfeldt, & Wistedt, 1991). In line with this observation, dining rooms have been noted as time/locations with high incidents of aggressive behavior (Fottrell, 1980; Hunter & Love, 1996; Kennedy, Harrison, Hillis, & Bluglass, 1995). Middelboe, Schjødt, Byrsting, and Gjerris (2001) used the WAS, clinical assessments, and a satisfaction questionnaire and found that, among similar patient groups, patients in locked wards displayed more anger and aggression.
- Feeney, Kavanagh, Kelly, and Mooney (2007) used hospital computerized admissions data and found that, after moving to a purpose-built acute psychiatric care unit, fewer patients left the new facility against medical recommendation; they also found a reduction in overall aggression. Other results have been more mixed. Daffern, Mayer, and Martin (2004) found that the number of aggressive acts remained the same when relocating to a new unit, but the nature of the aggressive acts changed. In a study on the impact of the manipulation of seating into conversational clusters, Baldwin (1985) noted less reliance on physical removal of patients and a higher number of patient incentive points.
- Vaaler, Morken, and Linaker (2005) recorded patient symptoms and satisfaction, and violent episodes using Brøset Violence Checklist or the Global Assessment of Function, as well as length of stay. They reported that their study on noninstitutional versus traditional design of an acute ward failed to support the relationship between incidents of dangerous behavior and interior design and finishes. Their data, however, showed a higher level of well-being in females experiencing the noninstitutional atmosphere.

- For patients with extreme assaultive behavior, seclusion rooms have been used in the past (Renvoize, 1991). However, seclusion rooms have been questioned for numerous clinical, ethical, and practical reasons (e.g., Tooke & Brown, 1992). As an alternative to seclusion rooms, extra care areas, living space closely supervised by staff, have been suggested (Dix, 2001), but not fully studied.
- Available research suggests a link between inactivity and aggressive behavior (Lloyd, 1995). While providing opportunities for recreation and therapeutic activities, safety and security measures should be considered. Janner and Delaney (2012) sought feedback from 100 psychiatric units that implemented the Star Wards program, which is designed to promote staff and patient engagement through "practical, accessible, and inspirational resource ideas" (Janner & Delaney, 2012). They found that boredom and poor staff-patient engagement can contribute to prevalence of aggressive and violent behavior.
- Alternatively, implementation of the Star Wards program promoted staff morale as well as the ward atmosphere. The seven major categories incorporated into the Star Wards program include recreation and conversation, physical health and activity, visitors' accommodation, care planning, talking therapies, ward community, and patient participation in care process and evaluation (Janner & Delaney, 2012). More specifically, the physical environment can be influential in supporting recreational activities and accommodating visitors. However, the available body of research has not focused on attributes of the physical environment that support such programs.
- In a recent study, Ulrich, Bogren, and Lundin (2012) compared outcomes in two hospitals and showed that a bundle of design guidelines can decrease patient aggression. These items include private rooms, less crowding, movable furniture, better acoustics, nature window views, nature art, higher daylight exposure, homelike design, and proximity and visibility of common spaces to the staff station.

9.6.3.5 Issues regarding smoking

The negative effects of cigarette smoking and secondhand smoke on human health have prompted many healthcare facilities, among other institutions, to ban smoking on their premises (World Health Organization, 1997). However, smoking bans may lead to challenges in psychiatric wards, more specifically because of a higher prevalence of disruptive behavior as well as higher rates of smoking among psychiatric inpatients (Lasser et al., 2000).

On the other hand, without an indoor smoking policy, staff job satisfaction and staff and patients' health are at risk (Salerno et al., 2012), especially due to the high percentage of smokers. Crockford, Kerfoot, and Currie (2009) studied psychiatric patient behavior changes before and after opening a smoking room in a psychiatric unit with a smoking ban. The smoking room was embedded in a psychiatric unit and shared by two adjacent units, ventilated to the outside air, and only available to psychiatric inpatients for a maximum of one cigarette per hour. The researchers used staff surveys and chart reviews of 180 inpatients to gather data regarding incidents of disruptive behavior and concluded that implementation of a smoking room did not have a significant impact on reducing incidents of disruptive behavior.

Regardless, staff was in support of allowing the use of the smoking room to avoid spending time discussing smoking privileges with patients. The findings of this study are in alignment with the review conducted by el-Guebaly, Cathcart, Currie, Brown, and Gloster (2002). Evidence is also available that assumes a direct link between assaultive behavior and smoking bans. Setting limits, such as denying off-site privileges or restrictions on cigarettes, were found to provoke aggression (e.g., Chou, Lu, & Mao, 2002).

9.7 Trends

The lack of research on MBH environments is a critical issue in providing evidence-based facilities. Future research must respond to trends, increase awareness of potential confounding variables, and fit within a research strategy.

The first step in setting a research agenda is to establish theoretical structures around which studies can be built, some of which are discussed in Chapter 2. Golembiewski (2010) offers Antonovsky's salutogenic theory as a model. As mentioned previously, salutogenic theory proposes that health is supported by coherence, and coherence is supported when the environment is comprehensive, manageable, and meaningful (Golembiewski, 2010). This theory partners well with other theories, such as the attention restoration theory proposed by the Kaplans (Kaplan & Kaplan, 1989), Appleton's prospect and refuge theory (Appleton, 1996), Powell Lawton's environmental competence press theory (Lawton & Nahemow, 1973), and the long-documented need for individuals to be able to exercise choice and control, particularly when their health status is challenged. Other theories, such as Ulrich's theory of supportive environments (Ulrich, 1997), are also relevant. Future researchers should consider contextualizing their studies in the framework of one or more of these theories, with an emphasis on the particular needs of patients and their families and staff in behavioral health settings.

In this context, specific topics might build upon the predecessor studies identified in Figure 9.2. Focusing on these topics will allow for the formulation of strong evidence that can be used to back up proposed guidelines. When addressing these subjects, future studies should: (1) be designed with more precision regarding identification of patient demographics and type of illness; (2) acknowledge differences between staff and patient perceptions; (3) use appropriate, pre-tested tools and methods; (4) corroborate or disprove existing design guidelines; and (5) provide better control of confounding variables.

Unfortunately, most of the existing studies are confounded by extraneous variables, such as changes to care protocols, and transitions in staff and patient populations. One of the primary difficulties in interpreting these studies is limiting the number of independent variables and discerning which component of the physical environment (e.g., color, views of nature) is impacting the behavior. The lack of clarity regarding the relevant components of the physical environment limits the generalizability of the studies to other MBH settings. Much more detailed descriptions of the physical environment are necessary so we can make intelligent interpretations of what factors might be associated with what outcomes.

Other topics for research might include focusing on the innovations associated with alternative care strategies, looking at research that enhances patient safety, and addressing those areas that are rarely examined such as patient outreach, continued care, and outpatient and community-based mental healthcare. A variety of other critical issues, which have been addressed in other health facility guidelines (and supported by research studies in those settings), have not been studied in MBH facilities. Prominent among these is the impact of noise levels and daylight and access to nature. More studies, such as those conducted by Kanakri (2012) in facilities for persons with autism, are needed. Other critical factors that need to be considered and described in detail include organizational culture, management style, pharmacological patterns, and technology. In other words, much more attention should be paid to the system characteristics, not just the design of facilities.

References

American Psychiatric Association. (2003). Practice guideline for the assessment and treatment of patients with suicidal behaviors. *American Journal of Psychiatry*, *160*(11, suppl.), 1–60.

Anderson, S., Good, L., & Hurtig, W. (1976). Designing a mental health center to replace a county hospital. *Hospital and Community Psychiatry*, *27*(11), 807–813.

Appleton, J. (1996). *The experience of landscape*. New York: Wiley.

Backhaus, K. L. (2008). *Client and therapist perspectives on the importance of the physical environment of the therapy room: A mixed methods study* (Doctoral dissertation). Texas Women's University, Denton, TX.

Baldwin, S. (1985). Effects of furniture arrangement on the atmosphere of wards in a maximum-security hospital. *Hospital and Community Psychiatry*, *36*(5), 525–528.

Barton, M., & Mishkin, D. (1984). Behavior patterns related to spatially differentiate areas of a psychiatric ward dayroom. In M. Spivack (Ed.), *Institutional settings: An environmental design approach* (pp. 117–128). New York: Human Sciences Press.

Benedetti, F., Colombo, C., Barbini, B., Campori, E., & Smeraldi, E. (2001). Morning sunlight reduces length of hospitalization in bipolar depression. *Journal of Affective Disorders*, *62*(3), 221–223.

Bowers, L., Hammond, N., James, K., Quirk, A., Robson, D., & Stewart, D. (2012). Characteristics of acute wards associated with the presence of a psychiatric intensive care unit, and transfers of patients to it. *Journal of Psychiatric Intensive Care*, *8*(2), 66–77.

Brickell, T. A., & McLean, C. (2011). Emerging issues and challenges for improving patient safety in mental health: A qualitative analysis of expert perspectives. *Journal of Patient Safety*, *7*(1), 39–44.

Broker, M., Rohricht, F., & Priebe, S. (1995). Initial assessment of hospital treatment by patients with paranoid schizophrenia: A predictor of outcome. *Psychiatry Research*, *58*, 77–81.

Brunt, D., & Rask, M. (2008). Patient and staff perception of the ward atmosphere in a Swedish maximum-security forensic psychiatry hospital. *The Journal of Forensic Psychiatry & Psychology*, *16*(2), 263–276.

Bryan, C.J., Rudd, M.D., & Wertenberger, E. (2013). Reasons for suicide attempts in a clinical sample of active duty soldiers. *Journal of Affective Disorders*, *144*(2023), 148–152.

Carr, R. (2011). Psychiatric facility. *Whole Building Design Guide*. Retrieved from www.wbdg.org/design/psychiatric.php

Center for Health Design. (2015). *A safety risk assessment for healthcare facility environments*. Concord, CA: Center for Health Design.

Centers for Disease Control and Prevention (CDC). (2013, 2011). Web-Based Injury Statistics Query and Reporting System (WISQARS). National Center for Injury Prevention and Control, CDC. Retrieved from www.cdc.gov/injury/wisqars/index.html

Chaikin, A. L., Derlega, V. J., & Miller, S. J. (1976). Effects of room environment on self-disclosure in a counseling analogue. *Journal of Counseling Psychology*, *23*(5), 479.

Chen, W., Huang, C., Hwang, J., & Chen, C. (2010). The relationship of health-related quality of life to workplace physical violence against nurses by psychiatric patients. *Quality of Life Research Journal*, *19*, 1155–1161.

Chou, K., Lu, R., & Mao, W. (2002). Factors relevant to patient assaultive behavior and assault in acute inpatient psychiatric units in Taiwan. *Archives of Psychiatric Nursing*, *16*, 187–195.

Christenfeld, R., Wagner, J., Pastva, G., & Acrish, W. P. (1989). How physical settings affect chronic mental patients. *Psychiatric Quarterly*, *60*, 253–264.

Chrysikou, E. (2013). Accessibility for mental healthcare. *Facilities*, *31*(9/10), 418–426.

Cleary, M., Hunt, G., & Walter, G. (2009). A comparison of patient and staff satisfaction with services after relocating to a new purpose-built mental health facility. *Environments and Facilities*, *17*(3), 212–217.

Connellan, K., Gaardboe, M., Riggs, D., Due, C., Reinschmidt, A., & Mustillo, L. (2013). Stressed spaces: Mental health and architecture. *HERD: Health Environments Research & Design Journal*, *6*(4), 127–168.

Corey, L., Wallace, M., Harris, S., & Casey, B. (1986). Psychiatric ward: A before and after look at how refurbishing affects staff and patient perceptions. *Journal of Psychosocial Nursing*, *24*(10), 10–16.

Crockford, D., Kerfoot, K., & Currie, S. (2009). The impact of opening a smoking room on psychiatric inpatient behavior following implementation of a hospital-wide smoking ban. *Journal of the American Psychiatric Nurses Association*, *15*, 393.

Daffern, M., Mayer, M. M., & Martin, T. (2004). Environment contributors to aggression in two forensic hospitals. *International Journal of Forensic Mental Health*, *3*(1), 105–114.

Davis, C., Glick, I., & Rosow, I. (1979). The architectural design of the psychotherapeutic milieu. *Hospital Community Psychiatry*, *30*, 453–460.

Delaney, K. R., & Johnson, M. E. (2008). Psychiatric nursing: Why safety must be the key deliverable. *Archives of Psychiatric Nursing*, *22*(6), 386–388.

Department of Health Estates and Facilities (2008). *A Staff and Patient Environment Calibration Toolkit* (ASPECT). London, UK: Department of Health, NHS.

Desai, S. (2010.) Violence and surveillance: Some unintended consequences of CCTV monitoring within mental health hospital wards. *Surveillance & Society*, *8*(1), 85–92.

Devlin, A. (1992). Psychiatric ward renovation. *Environment and Behavior*, *24*(1), 66–84.

Devlin, A., & Arneill, A. B. (2003). Health care environments and patient outcomes: A review of the literature. *Environment & Behaviour*, *35*(5), 665–694.

Devlin, A., Donovan, S., Nicolov, A., Nold, O., Packard, A., & Zandan, G. (2009). "Impressive?" Credentials, family photographs, and the perception of therapist qualities. *Journal of Environmental Psychology*, *29*(4), 503–512.

Dijkstra, K., Piesterse, M., & Pruyn, A. (2006). Physical environmental stimuli that turn healthcare facilities into healing environments through psychologically mediated effects: Systematic review. *Journal of Advanced Nursing*, *56*(2),166–181.

Dix, R. (2001). *Psychiatric environments*: *Physical environment*. London, UK: Greenwich Medical Media.

Dobrohotoff, J. T., & Llewellyn-Jones, R. H. (2011). Psychogeriatric inpatient unit design: A literature review. *International Psychogeriatrics*, *23*(2), 174–189.

Donald, F., Duff, C., Lee, S., Kroschel, J., & Kulkarni, J. (2015). Consumer perspectives on the therapeutic value of a psychiatric environment. *Journal of Mental Health*, *24*(2), 63–67.

Dorr, D., Honea, S., & Ponzer, R. (1980). Ward atmosphere and psychiatric nurses' job satisfaction. *American Journal of Community Psychology*, *8*(4), 455–461.

Edgerton, E. (n.d). *An evaluation of a redesigned corridor at Dykebar Psychiatric Hospital.* Retrieved from www.findingspace.org/healthcare3.html

Eklund, M., & Hansson, L. (2001). Ward atmosphere, client satisfaction, and client motivation in a psychiatric work rehabilitation unit. *Community Mental Health Journal, 37*(2), 169–177.

el-Guebaly, N., Cathcart, J., Currie, S., Brown, D., & Gloster, S. (2002). Public health and therapeutic aspects of smoking bans in mental health and addiction settings. *Psychiatric Services, 53*, 1617–1622.

Evans, G. (2003). The built environment and mental health. *Journal of Urban Health: Bulletin of the New York Academy of Medicine, 80*(4), 536–555.

Fairbanks, L., McGuire, M., Cole, S., Shordone, R., Silers, F., & Richards, M. (1977). The ethological study of four psychiatric wards: Patient, staff and system behaviors. *Journal of Psychiatric Research, 13*, 193–209.

Feeney, L., Kavanagh, A., Kelly, B., & Mooney, M. (2007). Moving to a purpose built acute psychiatric unit on a general hospital site – does the new environment produce change for the better? *Irish Journal of Medicine, 100*(3), 391–393.

Forster, P. L., Cavness, C., & Phelps, M. A. (1999). Staff training decreases use of seclusion and restraint in an acute psychiatric hospital. *Archives of Psychiatric Nursing, 13*(5), 269–271.

Fottrell, E. (1980). A study of violent behavior amongst patients in psychiatric hospitals. *British Journal of Psychiatry, 136*, 216–221.

Gabb, B., Speicher, K., & Lodl, K. (1992). Environmental design for individuals with schizophrenia: An assessment tool. *Journal of Applied Rehabilitation Counseling, 23*, 35–40.

Geddes, J. R. (1999). Suicide and homicide in mentally ill patients. *British Medical Journal, 318*, 1225–1226.

Gjerden, P. (1997). A survey of patient satisfaction as a means of evaluating quality of care in an open psychiatric ward. *Nord Journal of Psychiatry, 51*, 235–242.

Golembiewski, J. (2010). Start making sense: Applying a salutogenic model to architectural design for psychiatric care. *Facilities, 28*(3/4), 100–117.

Gournay, K., & Bowers, L. (2000). Suicide and self-harm in in-patient psychiatric units: A study of nursing issues in 31 cases. *Journal of Advanced Nursing, 32*(1), 124–131.

Griffin, W., Mauritzen, J., & Kasmar, J. (1969). The psychological aspects of the architectural environment: A review. *American Journal of Psychiatry, 125*(8), 1057–1062.

Grosenick, J., & Hatmaker, C. (2000). Perceptions of the importance of physical setting in substance abuse treatment. *Journal of Substance Abuse Treatment, 18*, 29–39.

Gutkowski, S., Ginath, Y., & Guttmann, F. (1992). Improving psychiatric environments through minimal architectural changes. *Hospital Community Psychiatry, 43*, 920–923.

Gutkowski, S., & Guttmann, F. (1992). Program and process: Designing the physical space of a day hospital. *Israel Journal of Psychiatry and Related Sciences, 29*(3), 167–173.

Higgs, W. (1970). Effects of gross environmental change on behavior of schizophrenics: A cautionary note. *Journal of Abnormal Psychiatry, 26*, 421–422.

Hobbs, C., Newton, L., Tennant, C., Rosen, A., & Tribe, K. (2002). Deinstitutionalization for long-term mental illness: A 6-year evaluation. *Australian and New Zealand Journal of Psychiatry, 36*, 60–66.

Holahan, C. (1972). Seating patterns and patient behavior in an experimental dayroom. *Journal of Abnormal Psychology, 80*, 115–124.

Holahan, C. (1974). Experimental investigations of environment-behavior relationships in psychiatric facilities. *Man Environment Systems, 4*, 109–113.

Holahan, C. (1976). Environmental change in a psychiatric setting: A social systems analysis. *Human Relations, 29*(2), 153–166.

Holahan, C. (1979). Environmental psychology in psychiatric settings. In D. Canter & S. Canter (Eds.), *Designing for therapeutic environments* (pp. 213–232). Sussex, UK: John Wiley & Sons.

Holahan, C., & Saegert, S. (1973). Behavioral and attitudinal effects of large-scale variation in the physical environment of psychiatric wards. *Journal of Abnormal Psychology*, *82*, 454–462.

Hunt, I. M., Bickley, H., Windfuhr, K., Shaw, J., Appleby, L., & Kapur, N. (2013). Suicide in recently admitted psychiatric in-patients: A case-control study. *Journal of Affective Disorders*, *144*(1–2), 123–128.

Hunter, M., & Love, C. (1996). Total quality management and the reduction of inpatient violence and costs in a forensic psychiatric hospital. *Psychiatric Services*, *47*, 751–754.

Ittleson, W., Proshansky, H., & Rivlin, L. (1970). Bedroom size and social interaction of the psychiatric ward. *Environment and Behavior*, *2*, 255–270.

Izumi, K. (1968). Architectural considerations in the design of places and facilities for the care and treatment of the mentally ill. *Journal of Schizophrenia*, *2*(1), 42–52.

Janner, M., & Delaney, K. R. (2012). Safety issues on British mental health wards. *Journal of the American Psychiatric Nurses Association*, *8*(2), 104–111.

Jeffers, T. (1991). Safety considerations in the psychiatric setting. *The Psychiatric Hospital*, *22*(3), 119–122.

Kagan, I., & Kigli-Shemesh, R. (2005). Relocating into a new building and its effect on uncertainty and anxiety among psychiatric patients. *Journal of Psychiatric and Mental Health Nursing*, *12*, 603–606.

Kanakri, S. (2012). The impact of acoustical environmental design on children for autism. *EDRA 43 SEATTLE: Emergent Placemaking: Proceedings of the 43rd Annual Conference of the Environmental Design Research Association*, *43*, 54–59.

Kaplan, R., & Kaplan, S. (1989). *The experience of nature: A psychological perspective*. New York: Cambridge University Press.

Karlin, B. E., & Zeiss, R. A. (2006). Environmental and therapeutic issues in psychiatric hospital design: Toward best practices. *Psychiatric Services*, *57*(10), 1376–1378.

Kasmar, J., Griffin, W., & Mauritzen, J. (1968). Effect of environmental surroundings on outpatients' mood and perception of psychiatrics. *Journal of Consulting and Clinical Psychology*, *32*(2), 223–226.

Kennedy, J., Harrison, J., Hillis, T., & Bluglass, R. (1995). Analysis of violent incidents in a regional secure unit. *Medical Science Law*, *35*, 255–260.

Kho, K., Sensky, T., Mortimer, A., & Corcos, C. (1998). Prospective study into factors associated with aggressive incidents in psychiatric acute admission wards. *British Journal of Psychiatry*, *172*, 38–43.

Koivumaa-Honkanen, H. T., Viinamäki, H., Honkanen, R., Tanskanen, A., Antikainen, R., Niskanen, L., Jääskeläinen, J., & Lehtonen, J. (1996). Correlates of life satisfaction among psychiatric patients. *Acta Psychiatrica Scandinavica*, *94*, 372–378.

Kumar, S., & Ng, B. (2001). Crowding and violence on psychiatric wards: Explanatory models. *Canadian Journal of Psychiatry*, *46*(5), 433–437.

Kweon, B. S., Ulrich, R. S., Walker, V. D., & Tassinary, L. G. (2008). Anger and stress: The role of landscape posters in an office setting. *Environment and Behavior*, *40*(3), 355–381.

Lasser, K., Boyd, W., Woolhandler, S., Himmelstein, D., McCormick, D., & Bor, D. (2000). Smoking and mental illness: A population-based prevalence study. *Journal of the American Medical Association*, *284*, 2606–2610.

Lawton, P., & Nahemow, L. (1973). Ecology and the aging process. In C. Eisdorfer & M. Lawton (Eds.), *The psychology of adult development and aging* (pp. 619–674). Washington, DC: American Psychological Association.

Li, J., Ran, M. S., Hao, Y., Zhao, Z., Guo, Y., Su, J., & Lu, H. (2008). Inpatient suicide in a Chinese psychiatric hospital. *Suicide and Life Threatening Behavior, 38*(4), 449–455.

Lloyd, C. (1995). *Forensic psychiatry for health professionals, therapy in practice*. London, UK: Chapman & Hall.

Long, C. G., Langford, V., Clay, R., Craig, L., & Hollin, C. (2011). Architectural change and the effects on the perceptions of the ward environment in a medium secure unit for women. *British Journal of Forensic Practice, 13*, 205–212.

Lynch, M. F., Plant, R. W., & Ryan, R. M. (2005). Psychological needs and threat to safety: Implications for staff and patients in a psychiatric hospital for youth. *Professional Psychology: Research and Practice, 36*(4), 415–425.

Lynes, D. (2011). *The effects of the physical environment on a counselor's well-being and ability to provide optimal care* (Doctoral dissertation). Capella University, Minneapolis, MN.

Main, S., McBride, A., & Austin, K. (1991). Patient and staff perceptions of a psychiatric ward environment. *Issues in Mental Health Nursing, 12*, 149–157.

Marcheschi, E. (2012). *The interaction between the physical and social environment in supported housing for people with severe mental illness* (Doctoral dissertation). Lund University, Sweden.

McGonagle, I., & Allan, S. (2002). A comparison of behavior in two differing psychiatric long-stay rehabilitation environments. *Journal of Psychiatric and Mental Health Nursing, 9*(4), 493–499.

McGuire, M., Fairbanks, L., Cole, R., Shordone, R., Silvers, M., Richards, M., & Akers, J. (1977). The etiological study of four psychiatric wards: Behavior changes associated with new staff and new patients. *Journal of Psychiatric Research, 13*, 211–244.

Martin, J. H. (1995). Improving staff safety through an aggression management program. *Archives of Psychiatric Nursing, 9*(4), 211–215.

Mehrabian, A., & Diamond, S. (1971). Effects of furniture arrangement, props, and personality on social interaction. *Journal of Personality and Social Psychiatry, 20*(1), 18–30.

Middelboe, T., Schjødt, T., Byrsting, K., & Gjerris, A. (2001). Ward atmosphere in acute psychiatric in patient care: Patients' perceptions, ideals and satisfaction. *Acta Psychiatrica Scandinavica, 103*(3), 212–219.

Minde, R., Haynes, E., & Rogenburg, M. (1990). The ward milieu and its effect on the behavior of psychogeriatric patients. *Canadian Journal of Psychiatry, 35*, 133–138.

Miwa, Y., & Hanyu, K. (2006). The effects of interior design on communication and impressions of a counselor in a counseling room. *Environment and Behavior, 38*(4), 484–502.

Moos, R. (1989). *The Ward Atmosphere Scale manual*. Palo Alto, CA: Consulting Psychologists Press.

Moos, R., & Daniels, D. (1967). Differential effects of ward settings on psychiatric staff. *Archives of General Psychiatry, 17*(1), 75–82.

Moos, R., & Houts, P. (1968). Assessment of the social atmospheres of psychiatric wards. *Journal of Abnormal Psychiatry, 73*, 595–604.

Morrow, P. C., & McElroy, J. C. (1981). Interior office design and visitor response: A constructive replication. *Journal of Applied Psychology, 66*(5), 646–650.

Müller, M., Schlosser, R., Kapp-Steen, G., Schanz, B., & Benkert, O. (2002). Patients' satisfaction with psychiatric treatment: Comparison between open and closed ward. *Psychiatric Quarterly, 73*(2), 93–107.

Nanda, U., Eisen, S., Zadeh, R. S., & Owen, D. (2010). Effect of visual art on patient anxiety and agitation in a mental health facility and implications for the business case. *Journal of Psychiatric and Mental Health Nursing, 185*, 386–393.

New York City Departments of Design and Construction, Health and Mental Hygiene, Transportation, City Planning, and Office of Management and Budget. (2010). *Active design guidelines:*

Promoting physical activity and health in design. New York: NYC Departments of Design and Construction, Health and Mental Hygiene, Transportation, City Planning, and Office of Management and Budget.

Ng, B., Kumar, S., Ranclaud, M., & Robinson, E. (2001). Ward crowding and incidents of violence on an acute psychiatric inpatient unit. *Psychiatric Services*, *46*(5), 433–437.

NHS Estates. (2013). *AEDET evolution design evaluation toolkit*. Retrieved from www.wales.nhs.uk/sites3/documents/254/AEDET_Evolution_documentation_v100605.pdf

Nijman, H., Bower, L., Haglund, K., Muir, E., Simpson, A., & Vender Merwe, M. (2011). Door locking and exit security measures on acute psychiatric admission wards. *Journal of Psychiatric and Mental Health Nursing*, *18*, 614–621.

Novonta, G., Urbanoski, K., & Rush, B. (2011). Client-centered design of residential addiction and mental healthcare facilities: Staff perceptions of their work environment. *Qualitative Health Research*, *21*(11), 1527–1538.

Okin, R. L. (1995). Testing the limits of deinstitutionalization. *Psychiatric Services*, *46*, 569–574.

Olver, J., Love, M., Daniel, J., Norman, T., & Nicholls, D. (2009). The impact of a changed environment on arousal levels of patients in a secure extended rehabilitation facility. *Australasian Psychiatry*, *17*, 207–211.

Palmstierna, T., Huitfeldt, B., & Wistedt, B. (1991). The relationship between crowding and aggressive behavior in the psychiatric intensive care unit. *Hospital and Community Psychiatry*, *42*, 1237–1240.

Payne, H., & May, D. (2009). Evaluation of a refurbishment scheme incorporating the King's Fund 'Enhancing the healing environment' design principles. *Journal of Facilities Management*, *7*, 74–89.

Pereira, S. M., Chaudhry, K., Pietromartire, S., Dale, J., & Halliwell, J. (2006). Design in psychiatric intensive care units: Problems and issues. *Journal of Psychiatric Intensive Care*, *1*(2), 70–76.

Perkins, E., Prosser, H., Riley, D., & Whittington, R. (2011). Physical restraint in a therapeutic setting: A necessary evil? *International Journal of Law and Psychiatry*, *35*, 43–49.

Potthoff, J. (1991). Young adult male satisfaction with drug and alcohol rehabilitation facilities: Interior design implications. *Journal of Alcohol and Drug Education*, *37*(1), 38–45.

Potthoff, J. (1995). Adolescent satisfaction with drug/alcohol treatment facilities: Design implications. *Journal of Alcohol and Drug Education*, *41*, 62–73.

Priebe, S., & Broker, M. (1999). Prediction of hospitalizations by schizophrenia patients' assessment of treatment: An expanded study. *Journal of Psychiatric Research*, *33*, 113–119.

Rashid, M., & Zimring, C. (2008). A review of the empirical literature on the relationships between indoor environment and stress in health care and office settings problems and prospects of sharing evidence. *Environment and Behavior*, *40*(2), 151–190.

Renvoize, E. (1991). The association of medical officers of asylums and hospitals for the insane, the Medico-Psychological Association, and their president. In G. Berrios & H. Freeman (Eds.), *150 years of British psychiatry, 1841–1991* (pp. 29–78). London, UK: Gaskell.

Rice, C., Berger, D., Klett, S., Sewall, L., & Lemkau, P. (1963). The Ward Evaluation Scale. *Journal of Clinical Psychology*, *16*(2), 251–258.

Richter, D., & Hoffmann, H. (2014). Architecture and design of mental health institutions: Systematic review on the consequences of the physical environment on adult psychiatric patients. [Architecktur und design psychiatrischer einrichtungen: Eine systematische literaturubersicht zu den effekten der ramlichen umgebung auf patienten in der erwachsenenpsychiatrie]. *Psychiat Prax*, *41*(3), 128–134.

Rivlin, L., & Wolfe, M. (1979). Understanding and evaluating therapeutic environments for children. In D. Canter & S. Canter (Eds.), *Designing for therapeutic environments* (pp. 29–61). Sussex, UK: John Wiley & Sons.

Salerno, S., Forcella, L., Di Fabio, U., Figa Talamance, I., & Boscolo, P. (2012). Ergonomics in the psychiatric ward towards workers or patients? *Work*, *41*, 1832–1835.

Schjødt, T., Middelboe, T., Mortensen, E. L., & Gjerris, A. (2003). Ward atmosphere in acute psychiatric inpatient care: Differences and similarities between patient and staff perceptions. *Nordic Journal of Psychiatry*, *57*, 215–220.

Shepley, M. (1995). The location of behavioral incidents in a children's psychiatric facility. *Children's Environments*, *12*(3), 352–361.

Shepley, M. (2011). Health facility evaluation for design professionals. Myersville, MD: Asclepion Publishing.

Shepley, M., Frohman, B., & Wilson, P. (1999). Designing for persons with AIDS: A post-occupancy study at the Bailey-Boushay House. *Journal of Architectural & Planning Research*, *16*(1), 17–32.

Shepley, M., Pasha, S., Ferguson, P., Huffcut, J.C., Kiyokawa, G., Martere, J., . . . & Malone, E. (2013). *Design research and mental and behavioral health facilities*. Concord, CA: The Center for Health Design.

Shepley, M., Watson, A., Pitts, F., Garrity, A., Spelman, E., Kelkar, J., & Fronsman, A. (2016). Mental & behavioral health facilities: Critical considerations for facility design. *General Hospital Psychiatry*, *42*, 15–21.

Shepley, M., Watson, A., Pitts, F., Garrity, A., Spelman, E., Fronsman, A., Kelkar, J. (2017). Mental and behavioral health settings: Importance & effectiveness of environmental qualities & features as perceived by staff. *Journal of Environmental Psychology*, *50*, 37–50.

Sidman, J., & Moos, R. (1973). On the relation between psychiatric ward atmosphere and helping behavior. *Journal of Clinical Psychology*, *29*(1), 74–78.

Sorlie, T., Parniakov, A., Rezvy, G., & Ponomarev, O. (2010). Psychometric evaluation of the Ward Atmosphere Scale in a Russian psychiatric hospital. *Nordic Journal of Psychiatry*, *64*(6), 377–383.

Southard, K., Jarrell, A., Shattell, M. M., McCoy, T. P., Bartlett, R., & Judge, C. A. (2002). Enclosed versus open nursing stations in adult acute care psychiatric settings: does the design affect the therapeutic milieu? *Journal of Psychosocial Nursing Mental Health Services*, *50*, 28–34.

Stahler, G., Frazer, D., & Rappaport, H. (1984). The evaluation of an environmental remodeling program on a psychiatric geriatric ward. *The Journal of Social Psychology*, *123*, 101–113.

Stewart, D., Ross, J., Watson, C., James, K., & Bowers, L. (2012). Patient characteristics and behaviors associated with self harm and attempted suicide in acute psychiatric wards. *Journal of Clinical Nursing*, *21*(7–8), 1004–1013.

Tapak, D. M. (2012). *Don't speak about us without us: Design considerations and recommendations for inpatient mental health environments for children and adolescents* (Unpublished master's thesis). University of Manitoba, Winnipeg, Canada.

Teglbjaerg, H. (2011). Art therapy may reduce psychopathology in schizophrenia by strengthening the patients' sense of self: A qualitative extended case report. *Psychopathology*, *44*, 314–318.

Timko, C. (1996). Physical characteristics of residential psychiatric and substance abuse programs: Organization determinants and patient outcomes. *American Journal of Community Psychology*, *24*(1), 173–192.

Tooke, K., & Brown, J. (1992). Perception of seclusion: Comparing patient and staff reactions. *Journal of Psychogical Nursing*, *30*, 23–26.

Townley, G., Kloos, B., & Wright, P. A. (2009). Understanding the experience of place: Expanding methods to conceptualize and measure community integration of persons with serious mental illness. *Health and Place*, *15*(2), 520–531.

Turlington, R. (2004). Creating a Planetree inpatient psychiatric unit. *Health Facilities Management Magazine*, *17*(6), 12–13.

Tuvesson, H., Eklund, M., & Wann-Hansson, C. (2011). Perceived stress among nursing staff in psychiatric inpatient care: The influence of perceived atmosphere and the psychosocial work environment. *Issues in Mental Health Nursing*, *32*(7), 441–448.

Tyson, G., Lambert, G., & Beattie, L. (2002). The impact of ward design on the behavior, occupational satisfaction and well-being of psychiatric nurses. *International Journal of Mental Health Nursing*, *11*, 94–102.

Ulrich, R. (1997). A theory of supportive design for healthcare facilities. *Journal of Healthcare Design*, *9*, 3–7.

Ulrich, R., Bogren, L., & Lundin, S. (2012). Towards a design for reducing aggression in psychiatric facilities. In *Arch 12: Architecture/Research/Care/Health*. Gothenberg: Chalmers. Retrieved from http://vbn.aau.dk/files/71203129/FINAL_pdf_UlrichBogren_Lundin_Toward_a_design_theory_for_reducing_aggression_Oct_2_.pdf

Vaaler, A., Morken, G., & Linaker, O. (2005). Effects of different interior decorations in the seclusion area of a psychiatric acute ward. *Nordic Journal of Psychiatry*, *59*(1), 19–24.

Vuori, H. (1991). Patient satisfaction – does it matter? *Quality Assurance in Health Care*, *3*, 183–189.

Wagenfeld, A., Roy-Fisher, C., & Mitchell, C. (2013). Collaborative design: Outdoor environments for veterans with PTSD. *Facilities*, *31*(9/10), 391–406.

Watts, B. V., Young-Xu, Y., Mills, P., DeRosier, P., Kemp, J., Shiner, B., & Duncan, W. (2012). Examination of the effectiveness of the Mental Health Environment of Care Checklist in reducing suicide on inpatient mental health units. *Archives of General Psychiatry*, *69*(6), 588–592.

Whitehead, C., Polsky, R., Crookshank, C., & Fik, E. (1984). Objective and subjective evaluation of psychiatric ward design. *American Journal of Psychiatry*, *82*, 454–462.

Willer, B., Staslak, E., Pinfold, P., & Rogers, M. (1974). Activity patterns and the use of space by patients and staff on the psychiatric ward. *Canadian Psychiatric Association Journal*, *14*, 561.

Wilson, M., Soth, N., & Robak, R. (1992). Managing disturbed behavior by architectural changes: Making spaces fit the program. *Residential Treatment for Children and Youth*, *10*(2), 63–74.

Wolfe, M. (1975). Room size, group size, and density behavior patterns in a children's psychiatric facility. *Environment and Behavior*, *7*, 199–224.

World Health Organization. (1997). *Tobacco or health: A global status report*. Geneva, Switzerland: WHO.

Yeager, K. R., Saveanu, R., Roberts, A. R., Reissland, G., Mertz, D., Cirpili, A., & Makovich, R. (2005). Measured response to identified suicide risk and violence: What you need to know about psychiatric patient safety. *Brief Treatment and Crisis Intervention*, *5*(2), 121–141.

Part Four: Guidelines and future directions

Guidelines

10

10.1 Introduction

Guidelines and standards for behavioral health design help to inform the planning, programming, and design process. They may be generated by the building and design industry (e.g., Facility Guidelines Institute), or federal healthcare systems (e.g., Military Health Services System), or national standards (e.g., Australian and Canadian healthcare standards), and are intended to provide minimum standards for behavioral health design. However, guidelines and standards are not typically substantiated by research. One purpose for future research should be the substantiation and expansion of design guidelines and standards to enhance the value of the environments that are produced. Value is perceived by stakeholders as design features that, in addition to meeting code requirements, result in improved clinical outcomes, patient/staff safety, or cost savings.

Standards and guidelines have different definitions. Standards typically refer to governmental mandated requirements, while guidelines are recommendations. In some cases guidelines may be adopted by agencies to serve as standards. However, in reviewing the literature these terms are often used interchangeably.

10.2 Organizations providing standards and guidelines

The majority of the behavioral health standards and guidelines described in this chapter were identified by the behavioral research subcommittee that led to the publication of *Design Research and Behavioral Health Facilities* (Shepley & Pasha et al. 2013). The BH guideline and standards assessment team reviewed documents from seven organizations: Australasian Health Infrastructure Alliance & New South Wales Health, Canadian Standards Association (CSA), Department of Defense (DoD), Facility Guidelines Institute (FGI), National Association of Psychiatric Health Systems (NAPHS), New York State Office of Mental Health, and Department of Veterans Affairs (DVA). To expand the international content of the book, we have added the Royal College of Psychiatrists (RCP). A brief history of each of these organizations and their associated standards and guidelines documents follows.

10.2.1 Australasian Health Infrastructure Alliance & New South Wales Health

The Australasian Health Infrastructure Alliance (AHIA), previously known as the Health Capital Asset Managers' Consortium of Australia and New Zealand, was founded in 2004 and incorporates representatives from all health jurisdictions in Australia and New Zealand (Carthey, 2013). The purpose of the organization is to support the activities of organizations that plan and manage health infrastructure.

The AHIA contracted the Centre for Health Assets Australasia (CHAA) at the University of New South Wales to create health design guidelines (*Australasian Health Facility Guidelines* [AusHFG]) in order to inform the programming and design of health facilities (Carthey, 2013). The new guidelines were based on those created by the Victoria Department of Health and Human Services in 2001–2002, published as the *New South Wales Health Facility Guidelines* (NSWHFG) (Carthey, 2013). The AusHFG were distributed in December 2006 and officially replaced the NSWHFG in 2007. Victoria uses the *Design Guidelines for Day Procedure Centres* (Carthey, 2013).

In 2010, a survey was conducted to explore the effectiveness of the new guidelines in three of the nine potential regions. The electronic survey gathered demographic information as well as benefits and suggestions for improvement. Evaluations were generally positive, but confusion was demonstrated regarding the purpose and limitations of the guidelines (Carthey, 2013).

10.2.2 Canadian Standards Association

CSA is an organization dedicated to the development of standards, testing, and certification. The Canadian Standards Association had its roots in the Canadian Engineering Standards Association in 1919. In the 1940s, it became the certification agency for electrical equipment and later changed its name to the Canadian Standards Association and established a certification mark. In the 1970s, this standard became the base for the ISO9000 quality management (Canadian Standards Association, 2011).

In September 2011, CSA Z8000, the first edition of *Canadian Health Care Facilities*, was published. The document was developed by the Subcommittee on the Design and Construction of Health Care Facilities under the combined auspices of the Strategic Steering Committee on Health Care Technology and the Technical Committee on Health Care Facility Engineering and Physical Plant (CSA, 2016).

10.2.3 Military Health Services System (MHSS): Department of Defense

At the close of World War II, the Department of War and the Department of the Navy were combined into the Department of Defense. In 1956, Congress passed the Military Medical Act that was amended in 1966 and resulted in the Civilian Health and Medical Program of the Uniformed Services (CHAMPUS) (Jones, 2001).

Among the DoD/VA/Federal Healthcare Services are the Military Health Services System, Department of Veterans Affairs, Federal Healthcare Services, Navy Deployment Health Centers, and National Guard/Reserve (DHCC, 2016). The mission of the Military Health Services System (MHSS) is to manage the health of service personnel so that they can carry out their missions and be supported with healthcare during time of war (Best, 2005). The MHSS includes the Department of Defense medical services that are provided to dependents and to retirees. CHAMPUS (Civilian Health and Medical Program of the Uniformed Services), which was founded in 1966, reimburses beneficiaries for a percentage of the cost of care from civilian providers. To coordinate the medical services, the DoD set up TRICARE, a system that offers beneficiaries access to provider options (Best, 2005).

The DoD Medical Space Planning Criteria are broken into the categories of purpose, scope, definitions, policies, program elements, and criteria that address 38 topics ranging from dental clinics to food service to physical therapy. Two categories are pertinent to behavioral health: Behavioral Health Clinic, and Behavioral Health/Partial Hospitalization/Substance Abuse/Alcohol Rehabilitation.

10.2.4 Facility Guidelines Institute (FGI) and the American Institute of Architects

General standards were part of the *Federal Register* in 1947 in association with the Hill-Burton program (AIA, 1996). The Hill-Burton Hospital Survey and Construction Act was passed by Congress in 1946 and was intended to support the construction of new healthcare facilities via financial support earmarked to improve hospital facilities (Lave & Lave, 1974). The document was renamed the *Minimum Requirements of Construction and Equipment for Hospital and Medical Facilities* in 1973 to reinforce the notion that the recommendations were minimum rather than ideal (AIA, 1996). In 1984, Health and Human Services removed the regulations for construction, renovation, and equipment previously dictated by Titles VI and XVI of the Public Health Service Act (AIA, 1996). The associated loan program expired and the federal government did not find it necessary to retain the guidelines in regulatory format. The title was changed to reflect the non-regulatory designation. Shortly thereafter, the Health Guidelines Revision Committee (HGRC) was formed and eventually published the 1992–1993 edition (AIA, 1996). In 1997, the title was amended to be *Guidelines for Design and Construction of Hospital and Health Care Facilities*, and in 2006, the title evolved into *Guidelines for Design and Construction of Health Care Facilities*.

Design Considerations for Mental Health Facilities was published as a separate document by the American Institute of Architects (AIA) Committee on Architecture for Health in 1993, but was largely reorganized and incorporated into the subsequent *Guidelines for Design and Construction of Hospital and Health Care Facilities*, which was published by the Academy of Architecture for Health (AAH) with assistance from the U.S. Department of Health and Human Services.

The organization currently known as the Academy of Architecture for Health was founded approximately 50 years ago under the auspices of the AIA (Peck, 2008). Originally called the Committee of Architecture for Health, its primary contribution has been reviewing guidelines, presenting at conferences, and sponsoring student design charrettes (Peck, 2008).

The FGI was founded in 1998 and exists to this day (FGI, 2014). The mission of the organization is to "establish and promote consensus-based guidelines and publications, advised by research, to advance quality health care." These guidelines are pursued throughout the world, particularly in countries that lack their own guidelines.

10.2.5 National Association of Psychiatric Health Systems

The National Association of Psychiatric Health Systems (NAPHS) was founded in 1933. The mission of the association is to support treatment and prevention programs for children and adults with mental and substance abuse disorders. NAPHS merged with the Association of Behavioral Group Practices in 1999. Membership in the organization includes health systems, inpatient and outpatient facilities, and children through older adults (NAPHS, 2016).

The guidelines were first published in 2003 (Hunt & Sine, 2014). They focus on architectural accessories, interior finishes, and furniture as they relate to adult patient and staff safety. These guidelines have been described as serving to augment regulatory requirements (Hunt & Sine, 2014).

10.2.6 New York State Office of Mental Health

The New York State (NYS) Office of Mental Health (OMH) serves approximately 700,000 individuals annually (OMH, 2016). The office is charged with operating NYS psychiatric centers and regulating 4,500 outpatient, residential, family, and community programs; regulations are those adopted by the New York Commissioner of Mental Health (OMH, 2016).

The current document, *Patient Safety Standards, Materials and Systems Guidelines* (PSSMSG), is the 15th edition. These guidelines were coauthored by the firm architecture+ in Troy, NY. The intention was to provide guidance concerning patient safety features in inpatient settings in NYS, and the document addresses existing NYS-operated facilities, psychiatric units (Article 28), and hospitals (Article 31) and is part of a multiple component approach that includes patient and facility risk assessment, staff training, appropriate products, and installation (OMH, 2006). PSSMSG identifies three levels of risk: high, medium, and low. High-risk areas include patient bedrooms, bathrooms, seclusion rooms, comfort rooms, and spaces with ceilings lower than 9 feet. Living rooms, dining rooms, group rooms, and corridors fall into the category of medium risk. Medication rooms, offices, and clean and soiled utility rooms are considered to be low risk.

10.2.7 Royal College of Psychiatrists

The Royal College of Psychiatrists was founded in 1841 as the Association of Medical Officers of Asylums and Hospitals for the Insane (Bewley, 2008). Subsequent names were the Medico-Psychological Association (1865) and the Royal Medico-Psychological Association (1926). In 1972, it assumed its current title (Bewley, 2008). The organization provides information through publications and other venues to the public and is the primary organization for psychiatrists in the United Kingdom.

The Royal College of Psychiatrists authors *Accreditation for Inpatient Mental Health Services* (AIMS) standards. The standards cover general topics, admissions, safety, environment and facilities, and activities and therapies. Standards are described in three levels: those that are essential, those that are expected, and those "that an excellent ward would be expected to meet" (Royal College of Psychiatrists, 2016). Separate AIMS documents are provided for each sub-typology. They are:

- wards for working-age adults,
- assessment wards for working-age adults,
- wards for older people,
- psychiatric intensive care units,
- inpatient learning disability services,
- inpatient rehabilitation units, and
- adult inpatient eating disorder services.

The content of these documents addresses recommended unit size and scale, bathroom location, privacy, accessibility, security, and lines of sight, among other things (von Sommaruga Howard, 2004).

10.2.8 Veterans Affairs

In 1918, the U.S. Congress directed the Bureau of War Risk Insurance and Public Health Service to operate hospitals specifically for World War I veterans. Currently, the Veterans Health Administration (VHA) is a national healthcare delivery system and the largest of the three administrations that constitutes the Department of Veterans Affairs (VA) (U.S. Department of Veterans Affairs, 2015). The VA supports 152 hospitals, 800 outpatient clinics, 126 nursing homes, and 35 domiciliaries (U.S. Department of Veterans Affairs, 2015). The VHA employs approximately 53,000 licensed healthcare practitioners and serves more than 8,300,000 veterans annually (U.S. Department of Veterans Affairs, 2015). For a detailed history of the U.S. Department of Veterans Affairs, see Chapter 6.

To develop their document, the U.S. Department of Veterans Affairs (VA) used in-house teams from both the Veterans Health Administration and the VA's Construction and Facility Management organization. The DoD hired HDR Architecture as a consultant to update the design criteria and engaged The Design Partnership in San Francisco, California, to serve as peer reviewers. The version described here consolidates previous VA standards including six VHA Space Planning Criteria Chapters (patient care units, substance abuse, clinics, day treatment, psychology service, and domiciliaries) as well as a variety of preexisting specifications (OCFM, 2010). Among the most commonly treated health conditions are depression disorder, substance abuse disorder, post-traumatic stress disorder, anxiety disorders, and serious mental illness (bipolar, schizophrenia, psychotic disorders) (OCFM, 2010). Specialized demographic subgroups are the aged, women, vets with physical disabilities or traumatic brain injury, bariatric patients, and airborne infection isolation patients (OCFM, 2010).

A brief summary of each of these guidelines and standards is provided in Figure 10.1. The information provided includes the organization that produced the document, the document name, date of the current edition, intended audience, general topics covered, and intent. The intended audience and overall intent is typically quoted verbatim from the source, the references for which can be found at the end of the chapter.

Figure 10.1: *Summary of guidelines and standards (Based on: Shepley et al., 2013)*

BH Guideline Title/ Author	*Pub Date*	*Intended Audience*	*BH Clinical Areas Addressed*	*Overall Intent of Guidelines/ Standards*
Australasian Health Infrastructure Alliance & New South Wales Health				
Australasian Health Facility Guidelines/ Australasian Health Infrastructure Alliance & New South Wales Health	2010	"This document provides design information for Health Facilities in Australia and New Zealand. . . . Generally designs that depart from these Guidelines will not be approved by the responsible Health Authority unless clear patient, service and cost benefits can be demonstrated and justified."	Addresses "public hospitals; licensed facilities contracted to provide services to public patients; day procedure units; ambulatory care facilities; rehabilitation centers; oral health units; palliative care centers; multipurpose healthcare facilities; birthing centers." Does not address facilities for the aged; medical practitioner consulting; pharmacies.	"The primary objective of the Guidelines is to achieve a desired performance result or service. . . . Where specific measurements, capacities or other standards are described, equivalent alternative solutions may be deemed acceptable if it is demonstrated that the intent of the standards has been met and the specific service can be safely and appropriately delivered. . . . The main aims of these Guidelines are to: provide general guidance to designers seeking information on the special needs of typical Health Care Facilities; promote the design of Health Care Facilities with due regard for the safety, privacy and dignity of patients, staff and visitors; maintain public confidence in the standard of Health Care Facilities; achieve affordable solutions for the planning and design of Health Care Facilities; eliminate design features that result in unacceptable practices; eliminate duplication between various existing Guidelines; minimize recurrent costs and encourage operational efficiencies."
Canadian Standards Association				
CSA Z8000–11 Canadian Health Care Facilities/ Canadian Standards Association	2011	This Standard "is intended to be used by all facilities providing health care services regardless of type, size, location, or range of services.	Addresses "inpatient and outpatient mental health and addictions units for adult patients, and the planning	"This Standard was developed to provide a consistent methodology and practical requirements for health care facilities (HCFs)

BH Guideline Title/ Author	*Pub Date*	*Intended Audience*	*BH Clinical Areas Addressed*	*Overall Intent of Guidelines/ Standards*
		This Standard was developed for use by architects, engineers, planning and project managers, contractors and builders, commissioning teams, facility managers, maintenance managers, infection prevention and control personnel, and other health care professionals."	of these units for pediatric and adolescent patients. It addresses psychiatric intensive care units (PICUs), a tertiary-level service that admits acute mental health and addictions patients requiring containment, security and intensive clinical management, and observation. It also addresses forensic patient care units, which have specialized security requirements."	across the country, to achieve the following benefits: (a) establish a common standard that Canadian authorities can adopt and enforce within their jurisdictions; (b) share best practice between provinces and regions, and between larger and smaller facilities; (c) promote consistency in the physical layout of Canadian facilities, thereby increasing operational efficiency and helping to reduce the risk of error by newly hired or visiting staff from other facilities; (d) enhance facility operational efficiency, optimize quality of service delivery, and maintain high levels of worker and patient health and safety; and (e) provide a common terminology and design approach, to improve communication between the organizations and individuals involved in HCF design and construction, to reduce construction errors, and to facilitate the movement of knowledge and skilled tradespeople between regions."
Department of Defense				
Space Planning Criteria 318: Behavioral Health Clinic/U.S. Department of Defense	2015	Addresses all behavioral health Military Treatment Facilities.	"Criteria for outpatient behavioral health clinics within the Military Health Services System including freestanding community-based facilities, as well as ambulatory clinics in or directly adjacent to hospital-based services.	To provide "space planning criteria guidance in support of planning, programming and budgeting for DoD Military Health System (MHS) facilities."

BH Guideline Title/ Author	*Pub Date*	*Intended Audience*	*BH Clinical Areas Addressed*	*Overall Intent of Guidelines/ Standards*
			Specifically covered in this chapter are Behavioral Health, Child and Adolescent Services, the Family Advocacy Program, and the Substance Abuse Alcohol Rehabilitation Program."	
Space Planning Criteria 410: Nursing Units (Substance Abuse/Alcohol Rehabilitation)/ Department of Defense	2015	Inpatient behavioral health and substance abuse/alcohol rehabilitation units for all Military Treatment Facilities in the Military Health System.	Inpatient and rehabilitation. No specified Inpatient Behavioral Health criteria. Instead the Nursing Unit criteria include Substance Abuse and Alcohol Rehab guidelines are part of overall Nursing Unit guidelines. Medical/ Psychiatric rooms are not included as they are part of a Medical-Surgical unit.	"To provide space planning criteria guidance in support of planning, programming and budgeting for DoD Military Health System (MHS) facilities."
Facility Guidelines Institute				
*Guidelines for Design and Construction of Hospital and Outpatient Facilities/*Facility Guidelines Institute	2014	Intended for public and private use including "reference in laws, codes, rules and regulations as well as in private self-regulation."	Standards for design and construction of long-term care psychiatric nursing units in general hospitals, psychiatric hospitals, outpatient facilities, and psychiatric centers.	To provide minimum space requirements that are recommended or mandatory for specific program functional requirements as they relate to an inpatient unit, an entire BH hospital, or clinic settings.
National Association of Psychiatric Health Systems				
Design Guide for the Built Environment of Behavioral Health Facilities/ Hunt & Sine and National Association of Psychiatric Health Systems	2014	"Designers, operators, and clinicians who are entrusted with both the care of behavioral health patients and with the environment of care in which those patients are cared for and treated."	Addresses "the built environment of the general adult inpatient behavioral healthcare unit." Does not address "child and adolescent patients, patients with medical care needs, geriatric patients, and	"This document is not a replacement for regulatory requirements, but rather augments them to detail practical means of protecting patients and staff."

BH Guideline Title/ Author	Pub Date	Intended Audience	BH Clinical Areas Addressed	Overall Intent of Guidelines/ Standards
			some patients with diagnoses such as substance abuse and eating disorders."	
NYS Office of Mental Health				
Patient Safety Standards, Materials and Systems Guidelines/ New York State Office of Mental Health & architecture+	2016	"With respect to NYS-OMH operated facilities, these Guidelines apply solely to new construction and major renovation projects. Existing facilities should use these Guidelines as a reference document whenever they make improvements."	"Patient safety features in the inpatient psychiatric environments throughout New York State. It grows out of the standards of new construction for the New York State Office of Mental Health's inpatient hospitals in order to provide guidance for: existing NYS-OMH state-operated inpatient facilities; psychiatric units in NYS-OMH licensed Article 28 and 31 hospitals." Not addressed: outpatient psychiatric facilities.	"The purpose of these guidelines is to provide a selection of materials, fixtures, and hardware that the NYS-OMH has reviewed and supports for use within inpatient psychiatric units to further the agency's goal of reducing the risk of harm to individuals in inpatient settings. Utilization of any of these products is not mandatory."
Royal College of Psychiatrists				
Accreditation for Inpatient Health Services Standards/ Royal College of Psychiatrists	2010 or 2014 based on sub-section	"Standards incorporate national requirements and recommendations; aligned with: Dept of Health Policy Implementation Guides; Confidential Inquiry into Suicide and Homicide; NICE guidance; recommendations by NHS Estates and Royal College of Psychiatrists about ward design; National Patient Safety Agency's Safer Wards	Addresses wards for working-age adults, psychiatric intensive care units, inpatient learning disability services, inpatient rehabilitation units, and adult inpatient eating disorder services.	"The standards reflect the issues which make a difference to the experience of the person using the service. . . . For this reason, the standards follow the patient pathway through care and how the service interfaces with other services. As far as possible, standards are written from the service user perspective, with an emphasis on a purposeful admission."

BH Guideline Title/ Author	*Pub Date*	*Intended Audience*	*BH Clinical Areas Addressed*	*Overall Intent of Guidelines/ Standards*
		for Acute Psychiatry Initiative; and National Audit of Violence."		
Veterans Administration				
Mental Health Facilities Design Guide/ Department of Veterans Affairs Office of Construction & Facilities Management	2010	VA facility planners and designers	Inpatient/outpatient/ rehab; "includes aspects of the external facility, which serves as a. . . first introduction to the facility and impacts initial impressions and expectations. This also includes external grounds and visual and physical access to nature." Other topics are "size, layout, and configuration of space. The interior design level includes furniture, flooring, wall color, texture, trim, use of artwork, and other aesthetic features."	"The goal of the Design Guide is to facilitate the design process and to ensure excellent quality, effectiveness, efficiency, and consistency of VA facilities while controlling construction and operating costs. This document is intended to be used as a guide and to supplement VA Space Planning Criteria, technical criteria, and other related VHA policies for mental health services in VA Medical Centers and Clinics."
Mental Health Environment of Care Checklist/ VHA National Center for Patient Safety, Department of Veterans Affairs	2015	VA clinicians, facility planners, and designers having inpatient psychiatric units treating currently suicidal patients (including both locked and unlocked mental health units).	"Any mental health unit where actively suicidal patients might be treated." Not for "Residential Rehab Programs, Domiciliaries, Dementia Care Units, Nursing Home Care Units, or Medical Units."	"To prospectively identify and eliminate environmental risks for inpatient suicide. . . to heighten the awareness of clinical staff regarding environmental hazards on locked psychiatric units. . . to focus specific attention on psychiatric unit safety, above and beyond the routine inspections."

10.3 Challenges to development of guidelines and standards

Three significant challenges face the development of guidelines and standards: the lack of research to support recommendations, difficulty enforcing recommendations (in the case of nongovernmental organizations), and the conflicts within content.

Although most organizations actively seek research to support their recommendations, there are simply insufficient data to provide adequate evidence to fully endorse most design decisions. Lacking these data, authors of guidelines and standards rely on input from designers and clinicians regarding best practice. Guidelines, when not mandated by government agencies, lack enforcement. This is particularly true when the recommended amenities will increase the cost of a project, which is commonly the case. More studies need to be undertaken on return on investment. In some cases guidelines may be adopted by code agencies that have been approved in particular geographic areas. A frequent challenge when pursuing the directives of standards and guidelines is resolving conflicts. For example, the National Fire Protection Association (NFPA) Life Safety Code may have conflicts with mandates for Joint Commission accreditation (Shepley et al., 2013). In some cases recommendations are contradictory, and in other cases they exceed one another.

10.4 Differences between guidelines and standards

The guidelines and standards are summarized in Figure 10.2 for the purposes of comparison. Some of the guidelines include safety, security, interior design, concept development (such as a healing environment), interior finishes, discussion of industry standards, and space planning standards. The NY State Office of Mental Health guidelines focus on materials, hardware, and furnishings to achieve patient safety. Both the VA and DoD guidelines serve as mechanisms to inform the design process, as well as planning and financial programming. Additionally, they emphasize equipment planning and placement.

The Australasian HFG are similar, but they also address less tangible aspects of the design process such as innovation and the role of culture in design. The FGI applies general hospital requirements as well as specialty requirements for inpatient and outpatient settings. The CSA guidelines address inpatient and outpatient facilities including psychiatric intensive care and forensic care. The National Association of Psychiatric Health Systems focuses on adult inpatient care. These guidelines do not address pediatric patients, patients with medical care needs, geriatric patients, and some patients with double diagnoses such as substance abuse and eating disorders. The Royal College of Psychiatrists AIMS guidelines also focus on adults, but include disability, rehabilitation, and eating disorders. Sorting out the contributions of each is complicated. Figure 10.2 represents an effort to compare the emphases of each of the guidelines and standards.

10.5 Guideline research agenda

In order to take full advantage of research in the development of standards and guidelines, some organizations use a multistep process when new research becomes available; potentially relevant studies are described in document appendices and incorporated when they gain credence and have been vetted by the professional public.

There are three main steps to consider when establishing research priorities in support of guidelines and standards:

1. Clearly define the variables of interest (e.g., safety), as well as their application and measurement tools (how to quantify).

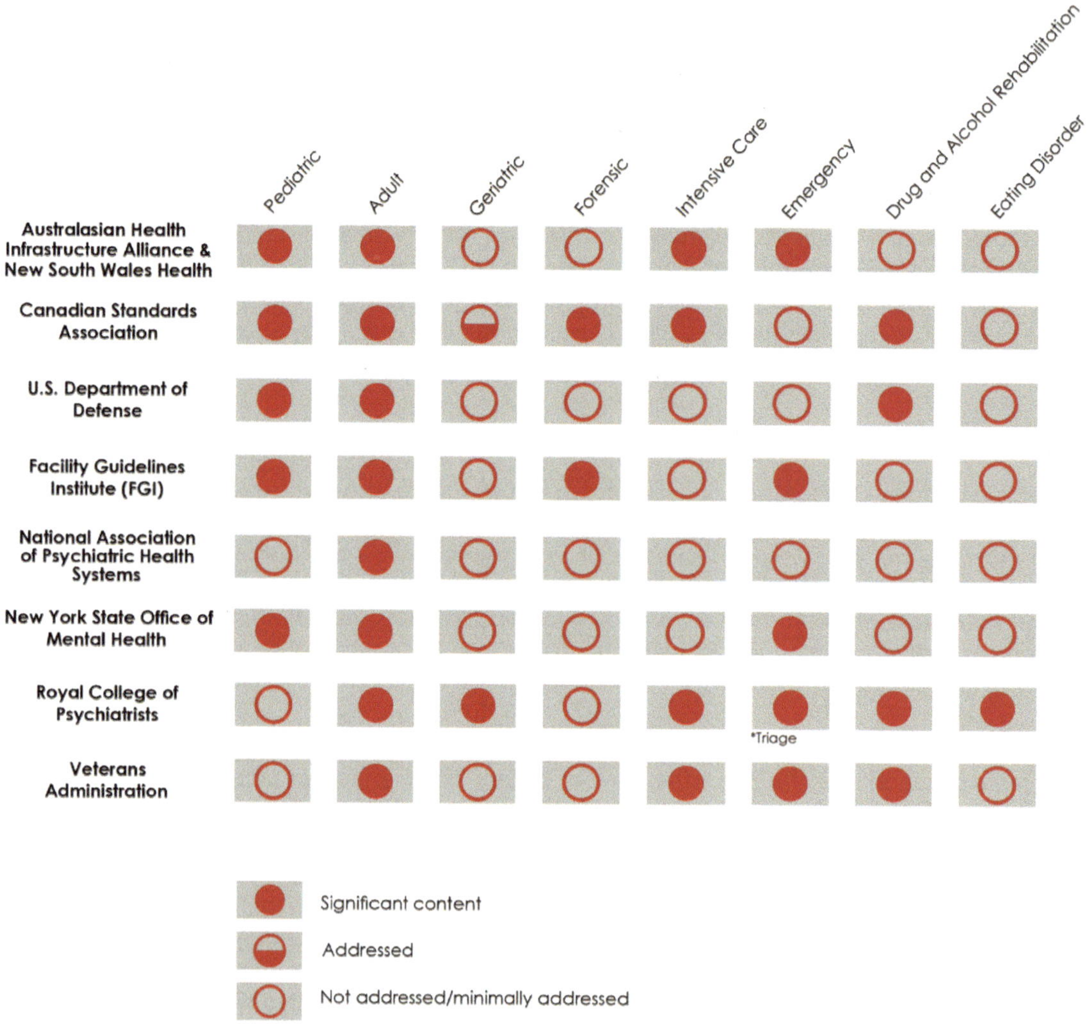

Figure 10.2: *Comparison of guidelines and standards relative to population served*

2. Identify the subsets of populations and differences in their needs based on vulnerability and demographics such as age, length of stay, or gender. The guidelines might need to be categorized or grouped to clarify which treatment objective the design might impact.
3. Identify salient, controversial topics. The two most currently hotly debated topics in residential settings are open versus closed nurse stations and private versus shared patient rooms. In emergency room design, proximity to nonpsychiatric emergency rooms is an issue that is difficult to resolve. In psychiatric outpatient settings, furniture arrangements in offices relative to the safety of counselors has been raised as a multidimensional issue (Shepley et al., 2013).

As mentioned in the introduction to this chapter, the relationship between guidelines/standards and research is critical to the creation of appropriate environments. Researchers who are aware of the content of these documents should be encouraged to conduct studies that substantiate them.

References

American Institute of Architects (AIA). (1996). *Guidelines for design and construction of hospital and health care facilities*. Washington, DC: American Institute of Architects.

Best, R. A. (2005). *Military medical care services: Questions and answers*. Washington, DC: Congressional Research Service, The Library of Congress.

Bewley, T. (2008). *Madness to mental illness: A history of the royal college of psychiatrists*. London, UK: The Royal College of Psychiatrists.

Canadian Standards Association (CSA). (2011). *Canadian health care facilities*. Toronto, Ontario: Canadian Standards Association.

Canadian Standards Association (CSA). (2016). *CSA Group; History*. Retrieved from www.csagroup.org/about/history/

Carthey, J. (2013). *Australasian Health Facility Guidelines (AusHFG) User survey – South Australia*. Sydney: Centre for Health Assets Australasia.

Deployment Health Clinical Center (DHCC). (2016). *Healthcare and support services*. Retrieved from www.pdhealth.mil/hss/healthcare_services.asp

Facility Guidelines Institute (FGI). (2014). *Guidelines for design and construction of hospitals and outpatient facilities* (2014 ed.). Chicago, IL: American Society for Healthcare Engineering.

Hunt, J. M., & Sine, D. M. (2014). *Design guide for the built environment of behavioral health facilities*. Washington, DC: National Association of Psychiatric Health Systems.

Jones, D. E. C. (2001). *Unification of the military health system: A half-century of unresolved debate*. Carlisle Barracks, PA: U.S. Army War College.

Lave, J. R., & Lave, L. B. (1974). *The hospital construction act: An evaluation of the Hill-Burton program, 1948–1973* (Vol. 16). Washington, DC: American Enterprise Institute Press.

National Association of Psychiatric Health Systems (NAPHS). (2016). *History*. Retrieved from www.naphs.org/about/history

New York State Office of Mental Health (OMH). (2016). *About OMH*. Retrieved from www.omh.ny.gov/omhweb/about/

Office of Construction & Facilities Management, Department of Veterans Affairs (OCFM). (2010). *Mental health facilities design guide*. Washington, DC: U.S. Department of Veterans Affairs.

Peck, R. L. (2008). Welcome to the academy of architecture for health. *Healthcare Design*, *8*(4), 20.

Royal College of Psychiatrists. (2016). *AIMS Accreditation for Inpatient Mental Health Services*. Retrieved from www.rcpsych.ac.uk/workinpsychiatry/qualityimprovement/ccqiprojects/adultinpatientservices/aims.aspx

Shepley, M. M., Pasha, S., Ferguson, P., Huffcut, J. C., Kiyokawa, G., Martere, J., . . . Malone, E. (2013). *Design research and behavioral health facilities*. Concord, CA: The Center for Health Design.

U.S. Department of Veterans Affairs. (2015). *Department of Veterans Affairs (VA)*. Retrieved from www.va.gov/

von Sommaruga Howard, T. (2004). The physical environment and use of space. In P. Campling, S. Davies, & G. Farquharson (Eds.), *From toxic institutions to therapeutic environments: Residential settings in mental health services* (pp. 69–78). Glasgow, UK: The Royal College of Psychiatrists.

Conclusion 11

11.1 Where we've been

Ponder the following quotation:

> *If the goal of the medical-care delivery systems is the improvement of health, a great deal of money has been spent with no discernible effect. Prices and expenditures have risen, but the indices of health, such as life expectancy or mortality rates, have shown no improvement.*
>
> *One reason for the ineffectiveness of increased healthcare expenditures is the inefficient allocation of these resources. Too much is spent on expensive inpatient care and too little on ambulatory care. More should be done to improve the basic health level of the population – for example, by improving public health, health education and people's health habits, and by cleaning the environment.*

Written in 1994? Or perhaps in 2010 when the Affordable Care Act became effective? This surprisingly contemporary statement is a quotation from Lave and Lave's (1974) booklet on the Hospital Construction Act (1948–1973) (p. 1). The fact that we are still facing the same issues more than 40 years later is troubling.

Certainly, there have been improvements during that time frame. We have evidence that healthcare environments are becoming more humane. The wellness movement is alive and well, and it manifests itself in the proliferation of fitness facilities and greater awareness of nutritional needs (Kickbusch & Payne, 2003). However, we seem unable globally, and specifically in the United States, to successfully provide healthcare services for all. Some success has been experienced in other countries, but the lack of attention to providing behavioral and mental health treatment is a serious concern.

Apart from the importance of relieving the suffering of those with behavioral and mental health diagnoses, the lack of psychiatric services has broad implications on society, health systems, and public health. Worldwide, about 22.2% of all disability-adjusted life years (DALYs) are due to mental and behavioral disorders (Murray, Vos, Lozano, Naghavi, & Flaxman 2013). Once this group of disorders co-occurs with other diseases, it causes poorer health outcomes (Pike, Susser, Galea, & Pincus 2013). To provide holistic care to individuals, integrated care may target health behaviors that can contribute to chronic medical illnesses, ineffective patterns of healthcare utilization, as well as mental health and substance abuse conditions (Peek and the National Integration Academy Council, 2013).

11.2 Where we're headed

11.2.1 Transitions in mental and behavioral health practice

In this context, transitions in the medicine of behavioral health continue. According to Bewley (2008), practice trends include: (1) the increasing importance of the biological nature of psychiatric research, (2) the expanding influence of users, (3) the increase in the number of clinical guidelines, and (4) those transitions in culture and dynamics that change social behavior.

Regarding the first trend, chemical means of addressing behavioral and mental health have grown in sophistication over the years, and the role of our genetic makeup in MBH disorders has become more apparent. Pharmacological solutions continue to advance. However, progress is dependent upon commitment by researchers and clinicians, policy makers, and society (Millan, Goodwin, Meyer-Lindenerg, & Ogren, 2015). Supported in part by the logarithmical development of technology, evolution in the biological nature of psychiatric research and treatment can only be expected to mature. Smoller (2014) notes three main implications of psychiatric genetics: the identification of DNA markets that will support the selection of treatment options, awareness regarding treatment boundaries due to subgroup identification, and pharmacogenetic profiles that lead to clearer understanding of responses.

Developments in technology will also have an impact. In the case of overcrowded emergency departments and long psychiatric boarding times, a bundle of interventions is suggested by the Emergency Medicine Practice Group at the American College of Emergency Physicians (2014). The interventions span from inclusion of telecare to incorporation of treatment protocols. Additionally, the impact of technology may influence design practice by decreasing the number of involuntary inpatient facilities and increasing the number of ambulatory behavioral health facility settings. Programs such as those provided at Fountain House, where individuals transition more informally to societal integration, may become more commonplace.

Bewley's statement regarding the increased participation of clients and patients in the process of treatment is an interesting one and parallels trends in the design process that embrace the contributions and advice of all building occupants. On a broader scale, perhaps enhanced global awareness of psychiatric issues and destigmatization of mental illness will encourage those suffering with behavioral health issues to come forward and engage on these topics. Bewley, in his history of the Royal College of Physicians, reflects on this notion in his conclusion:

> There will no doubt be continuing efforts to combat the fear and misunderstanding that colour people's notions of mental illness. I would like to be able to hope that there will be an increasing recognition, by the general public, politician and the media, of the high prevalence and disabling consequences of mental illness.
>
> (Bewley, 2008, p. 153)

Regarding the third topic – the growth in guidelines – this will likely be impacted by changes in technology and changes in public awareness and participation. Increased research on psychiatric healthcare environments will also be of influence; the more information we have, the more substance we can bring to recommended standards.

Concerning broad cultural behaviors, based on the events of the last 50 years, Bewley predicts that there will be an increase in the number of criminals, disturbed adolescents, and others who "offend against the social canons." We could easily add those who have a predilection toward violence to this list, due to the apparent growth in terrorism and gun violence.

11.2.2 Trends in behavioral health environments

A new system of care delivery will have new design implications. Proximity and collocation of mental health clinics and primary health centers will require research and innovation (SAMHSA National Council, 2013). Design should be able to support the flexibility required for integration.

In general, the body of research on MBH facilities is limited and lacks rigor, making it premature to establish evidence-based guidelines. However, the process of writing this book has enabled us to draw some preliminary conclusions.

- Our research and project review suggest a trend in mental and behavioral health facilities from the creation of visually plain environments (so as not to overstimulate patients) to richer, more complex spaces and increased access to the outdoors (Cochran, 1978). According to Levin (2007), the primary trends in contemporary psychiatric facility design address environments that support recovery, induce shorter stays, and allow patients to participate in their treatment. Environments that support recovery are more likely to involve access to natural light and the outdoors and artwork involving nature.
- Means of increasing patient safety while reducing the use of medications, seclusion, and restraints are another area of research advocated by medical practitioners (Borckardt et al., 2007). Our survey of the design programs associated with new facilities supported this evolving emphasis. Use of alternative interventions is also being discussed in the literature. Gaskin, Elsom, and Happell (2007) reviewed literature on interventions that can reduce use of seclusion. They found that staff utilize a combination of various tactics and resources ranging from emergency response strategies to pharmacological interventions to decrease need for seclusion. Perkins, Prosser, Riley, and Whittington (2012) argued that using physical restraints is a coercive and traumatic procedure with escalatory effects and should be decreased through improvements in practice and use of alternatives.
- Increased sense of control was also identified as a factor contributing to the healing of a variety of mental illnesses. Providing environmental flexibility (acoustics, lighting, and furniture options) may be helpful in supporting this goal. Spaces that support participation in treatment are those that provide environments that are sufficiently flexible in configuration as to allow for a variety of activities. Other trends include the increased need to provide environments that address program spaces for drug and alcohol addiction (Carr, 2011) and the more common use of single-patient rooms.
- Open nurse stations are being used increasingly, but responses are mixed. For example, Shattell et al. (2015) examined the responses of patients and nurses before and after the removal of a Plexiglas enclosure. Nurses had mixed assessments of the enclosure and were concerned about the resultant lack of confidentiality and ability to concentrate but agreed that it created a barrier to communication. Patients were unanimously in support of the removal of the barrier, indicating that the absence resulted in an increased sense of freedom, better interaction with nurses, and greater safety.
- The movement toward private rooms has also been described in detail in this book. While intuitively an appropriate direction, there are no data available that substantiate the safety of

these private room environments. Shepley et al. (2016) found support for private rooms in their interviews of expert academics, practitioners, and healthcare administrators, but the impact of private rooms versus shared rooms on safety has yet to be established.

- One topic that is not limited to design and planning of mental health facilities per se is improvements in the design of communities, as adjunct support to mental health services. Nelson and Prilleltensky (2010) discuss ameliorative versus transformative change, which, respectively, focus on improving existing infrastructure in contrast to revisiting the system's values and operations. Nelson (2010) identified supported housing and care for persons with mental health diagnoses as an example of transformative change. Designers may investigate best practices for housing and similar interventions, thus allowing this population to live in the community successfully.

In the international context, the burden of mental illnesses on economic development, public health status, and quality of life among various geographic regions was discussed. We examined limitations in services and the trauma imposed on each community and its subsequent impact on the mental health of its members. Although much of the book's content deals with information on the situation in North America, we addressed global research and design when the data were available. Again, in surveying the solutions and best practices put forward globally, we identified guidelines, tools, supportive programs, and built facilities, which are mainly rooted in the developed world.

In this book we have gathered basic information regarding mental and behavioral health history, design theories, building typologies, research, and guidelines. At times we have gone out on a limb by attempting to integrate limited information into a format that might be useful to designers and design terms. We have surveyed international healthcare challenges, blended the recommendations of various designers and clinicians into a cohesive summary, consolidated research into design guidelines, and compared the content of multiple standards. Integration of knowledge, as we have endeavored to do here, is consistently harder than parroting information, and we welcome the input of our readership.

References

Bewley, T. (2008). *Madness to mental illness: A history of the royal college of psychiatrists*. London, UK: The Royal College of Psychiatrists.

Borckardt, J. J., Grubaugh, A. L., Pelic, C. G., Danielson, C. K., Hardesty, S. J., & Frueh, B. C. (2007). Enhancing patient safety in psychiatric settings. *Journal of Psychiatric Practice®*, *13*(6), 355–361.

Carr, R. (2011). Psychiatric facility. *Whole Building Design Guide*. Retrieved March 21, 2012, from www.wbdg.org/design/psychiatric.php

Cochran, B. (1978). Design and planning of psychiatric facilities. *Hospital and Community Psychiatry*, *29*(8), 533–537.

Emergency Medicine Practice Group. (2014). *Care of the psychiatric patients in the emergency department–A review of the literature*. American College of Emergency Physicians. Retrieved from www.acep.org/uploadedFiles/ACEP/Clinical_and_Practice_Management/Resources/Mental_Health_and_Substance_Abuse/Psychiatric%20Patient%20Care%20in%20the%20ED%20 2014.pdf

Gaskin, C., Elsom, S., & Happell, B. (2007). Interventions for reducing the use of seclusion in psychiatric facilities. *British Journal of Psychiatry*, *191*, 283–303.

Kickbusch, I., & Payne, L. (2003). Twenty-first century health promotion: The public health revolution meets the wellness revolution. *Health Promotion International*, *18*(4), 275–278.

Lave, J. R., & Lave, L. B. (1974). *The hospital construction act: An evaluation of the Hill-Burton program, 1948–1973* (Vol. 16). Washington, DC: American Enterprise Institute Press.

Levin, A. (2007). Psychiatric hospital design reflects treatment trends. *Psychiatric News*, *42*(2), 9.

Millan, M., Goodwin, G., Meyer-Lindenerg, A. & Ogren, S. (2015). Learning from the past and looking to the future: Emerging perspectives for improving the treatment of psychiatric disorders. *European Neuropsychopharmacology*, *25*(5), 599–656.

Murray, C. J., Vos, T., Lozano, R., Naghavi, M., & Flaxman, A. D., (2013). Disability adjusted life years (DALYs) for 291 diseases and injuries in 21 regions, 1990–2010: A systematic analysis for the global burden of disease study 2010. *Lancet*, *380*, 2197–2223.

Nelson, G., (2010). Housing for people with serious mental illness: Approaches, evidence, and transformative change. *Journal of Sociology & Social Welfare*, *37*, 123–146.

Nelson, G., & Prilleltensky, I. (2010). *Community psychology: In pursuit of liberation and wellbeing*. New York: Palgrave Macmillan.

Peek, C. J., & The National Integration Academy Council (2013). *Lexicon for behavioral health and primary care integration: Concepts and definitions developed by expert consensus* (AHRQ Publication No.13-IP001-EF). Rockville, MD: Agency for Healthcare Research and Quality.

Perkins, E., Prosser, H., Riley, D., & Whittington, R. (2012). Physical restraint in a therapeutic setting: A necessary evil? *International Journal of Law and Psychiatry*, *35*, 43–49.

Pike, K., Susser, E., Galea, S., & Pincus, H. (2013). Towards a healthier 2020: Advancing mental health as a global health priority. *Public Health Reviews*, *35*(1), 1–25.

SAMHSA National Council for Community Behavioral Healthcare. (2013). *A standard framework for levels of integrated healthcare*. SAMHSA-HRSA Center for Integrated Health Solutions. Retrieved from www.integration.samhsa.gov/integrated-care-models/A_Standard_Framework_for_Levels_of_Integrated_Healthcare.pdf

Shattell, M., Bartlett, R., Beres, K., Southard, K., Bell, C., Judge, C. A., & Duke, P. (2015). How patients and nurses experience an open versus an enclosed nursing station on an inpatient psychiatric unit. *Journal of the American Psychiatric Nurses Association*, *21*(6), 398–405.

Shepley, M., Watson, A., Pitts, F., Garrity, A., Spelman, E., Kelkar, J., & Fronsman, A. (2016). Mental and behavioral health facilities: Critical issues. *General Hospital Psychiatry*, *42*, 15–22.

Smoller, J. (2014). Psychiatric genetics and the future of personalized treatment. *Depression and Anxiety*, *31*, 893–898.

Glossary

Ambulatory care Outpatient care, or care provided without admission to a hospital or other inpatient facility (www.medpac.gov/-research-areas-/ambulatory-care-settings).

Anthroposophy A philosophy emphasizing the attainment of well-being through exploratory means such as physical or nonverbal artistic therapies (Hamre et al., 2006).

Clubhouse An alternative support system for those with mental illnesses, fostering a sense of community and autonomy by encouraging members to additionally contribute to the offering of social services, instead of passively receiving services (Doyle et al., 2013).

Day treatment/Day hospital A healthcare facility offering services to patients who are able to return home overnight, but still require daily therapeutic services (http://medical-dictionary.thefreedictionary.com/day+hospital).

Evidence-based design (EBD) A process carefully utilizing current research-grounded evidence to make informed design decisions (Hamilton & Watkins, 2009, p. 9).

Generative design Design of social spaces supported by the physical environment that encourage the improvement of health and well-being (Ruga, 2008).

Institute for Patient-Centered Design A patient-centered care organization focusing specifically on the physical environment's impact on healing (Institute for Patient-Centered Design, Inc., n.d.).

Partially supervised group housing A model of residential mental healthcare nested between supervised group housing and supported housing; residents are not under custodial care, but do not live as independently as those in supportive housing (NAMI, 2016).

Patient-centered care The primary objective of the U.S. healthcare system currently, focusing specifically on patient needs in hopes of improving clinical outcomes, satisfaction, and cost-effectiveness (Cliff, 2012).

Planetree A patient-centered care organization providing an innovative healthcare model that includes the incorporation of accessible and homelike environments (Planetree, 2014).

Residential mental health facility A variety of mental health facility aimed at fostering independent living and community involvement, either within the immediate community or the larger community containing the facility (Burt, 2006; Fitzpatrick, 2007).

Salutogenic design A holistic design approach based upon the concept of salutogenesis, emphasizing the role of facilitating social interaction and providing opportunities for control and spaces for relaxation as components of a coherent environment aiding the healing process (Heerwagen et al., 1995).

Setting-Response Inventory (SRI) A metric of gauging staff opinions on settings within the psychiatric ward environment (Moos & Daniels, 1967).

Sociofugal grouping An environmental arrangement offering privacy from others (http://psychologydictionary.org/sociofugal/).

Sociopetal grouping An environmental arrangement offering opportunities for interaction with others (http://psychologydictionary.org/sociopetal/).

Supervised group housing A custodial model of residential mental health offering in-house staff members who are available to assist residents with treatment and daily tasks (NAMI, 2016).

Supportive housing A model of residential mental healthcare wherein residents live nearly independently, but have access to resources if needed (NAMI, 2016).

Transformational design A design concept implemented within the clubhouse environment aimed at making activities accessible to members through means such as structured schedules and opportunities to exercise choice (Doyle et al., 2013).

Ward Atmosphere Scale A metric evaluating both client and staff perceptions of the psychiatric ward atmosphere (www.mindgarden.com/156-ward-atmosphere-scale).

References

Burt, M. (2006). *Characteristics of transitional housing for homeless families*. Urban Institute, Washington, DC. Retrieved from www.urban.org/sites/default/files/alfresco/publication-pdfs/411369-Characteristics-of-Transitional-Housing-for-Homeless-Families.PDF

Cliff, B. (2012). The evolution of patient-centered care. *Journal of Healthcare Management, 57*(2), 86.

Doyle, A., Lanoil, J., & Dudek, K. (2013). *Fountain House: Creating community in mental health practice*. New York: Columbia University Press.

Fitzpatrick, H. (2007). *Supportive housing for mental health recovery: A bio-psycho-social approach* (Unpublished masters thesis). University of Waterloo, Ontario.

Hamilton, D.K., & Watkins, D.H. (2009). *Evidence-based design for multiple building types*. Hoboken, NJ: John Wiley & Sons.

Hamre, H.J., Witt, C.M., Glockmann, A., Ziegler, R., Willich, S.N., & Kiene, H. (2006). Anthroposophic therapy for chronic depression: A four-year prospective cohort study. *BMC Psychiatry, 6*(1), 1.

Heerwagen, J.H., Heubach, J.G., Montgomery, J., & Weimer, W.C. (1995). Environmental design, work, and well being: Managing occupational stress through changes in the workplace environment. *AAOHN Journal: Official Journal of the American Association of Occupational Health Nurses, 43*(9), 458–468.

Institute for Patient-Centered Design (n.d.). *About*. Retrieved June 23, 2016, from www.institutepcd.org/about

Moos, R., & Daniels, D. (1967). Differential effects of ward settings on psychiatric staff. *Archives of General Psychiatry, 17*(1), 75–82.

National Alliance for Mental Health (NAMI). (2016). *Dual diagnosis*. Retrieved from www.nami.org/Learn-More/Mental-Health-Conditions/Related-Conditions/Dual-Diagnosis#sthash.97jKwhDT.dpuf

Planetree. (2014). *Planetree designated sites*. Retrieved from http://planetree.org/planetree-designated-sites/

Ruga, W. (2008). Your general practice environment can improve your community's health. *British Journal of General Practice, 58*(552), 460–462.

Index

Note: Page numbers in *italics* indicate figures.